New Insights into Veterinary Science

New Insights into Veterinary Science

Editor: Melisa Bradshaw

FOSTER ACADEMICS

www.fosteracademics.com

www.fosteracademics.com

FOSTER ACADEMICS

Cataloging-in-Publication Data

New insights into veterinary science / edited by Melisa Bradshaw.
p. cm.
Includes bibliographical references and index.
ISBN 978-1-63242-868-4
1. Veterinary medicine. 2. Animals--Diseases. 3. Animal health. I. Bradshaw, Melisa.
SF745 .N49 2020
636.089--dc23

Foster Academics,
118-35 Queens Blvd., Suite 400,
Forest Hills, NY 11375, USA

ISBN 978-1-63242-868-4 (Hardback)

Contents

Preface

Veterinary science is concerned with the study of animal diseases and disorders, as well as the diagnosis, treatment, management and prevention of these. It is practiced for both wild and domesticated animal species suffering from a wide range of conditions. Surgery is an important domain of veterinary science. It falls within the broad categories of soft tissue surgery, orthopedics and neurosurgery. Some of the surgical procedures performed on animals are complex wound management, spaying, minor mass excisions, fracture fixation, skin grafts, joint replacement, balloon valvuloplasty, cystotomy, Caesarean section, etc. The stethoscope, thermometer, laryngoscope, glucometer, centrifuge and autoclave are some of the general tools used in veterinary medicine. ECG, ultrasound, biochemistry analyzer, X-rays, pulse oximeter and refractometer are some of the diagnostic technologies. The objective of this book is to give a general view of the different areas of veterinary medicine. It studies, analyzes and upholds the pillars of animal ethics and animal welfare and their utmost significance. For someone with an interest and eye for detail, this book covers the most significant topics in veterinary science and medicine.

Various studies have approached the subject by analyzing it with a single perspective, but the present book provides diverse methodologies and techniques to address this field. This book contains theories and applications needed for understanding the subject from different perspectives. The aim is to keep the readers informed about the progresses in the field; therefore, the contributions were carefully examined to compile novel researches by specialists from across the globe.

Indeed, the job of the editor is the most crucial and challenging in compiling all chapters into a single book. In the end, I would extend my sincere thanks to the chapter authors for their profound work. I am also thankful for the support provided by my family and colleagues during the compilation of this book.

Editor

1

Risk factors for canine cognitive dysfunction syndrome in Slovakia

Stanislav Katina[1†], Jana Farbakova[2†], Aladar Madari[2†], Michal Novak[3] and Norbert Zilka[3,4*]

Abstract

Background: Increasing prevalence of cognitive impairment in an aging canine population poses a serious health problem. Identifying risk factors, which may influence the onset of cognitive decline, is becoming increasingly important. Here we investigated whether age, sex, weight, nutrition, dogs' housing and reproductive state were associated with increased risk of canine cognitive dysfunction syndrome (CCDS) in Slovakia.

Results: Age was associated with cognitive decline and nutrition emerged as a significant predictor variable. Dogs fed controlled diets had 2.8 times lower odds of developing CCDS when compared with dogs fed uncontrolled diets. Sex, weight, reproductive state and dogs' housing were not significantly associated with cognitive decline. Further, the prevalence of CCDS was similar in both small and medium/large sized dogs aged 8–11 years, but differed in dogs at an age of 11–13 years.

Conclusion: Age was found to be the most prominent risk factors of CCDS. Nutrition may influence the cognitive state of dogs. This finding suggests that nutritional interventions may modify canine cognitive functions.

Keywords: Canine cognitive dysfunction syndrome, Cognitive decline, Risk factors, Prevalence, Epidemiology, Nutrition

Background

Canine cognitive dysfunction syndrome (CCDS) is a complex of behavioural symptoms in aged dogs characterised by deficits in learning, memory, perception, awareness and by impairment of social interactions and sleeping patterns [1]. Improvements in nutrition, elimination of most infectious diseases, better hygiene and adoption of antibiotics and vaccines have increased the life expectancy of dogs. The immediate consequence of the extended life span is an increased number of aged dogs. It has been estimated that there are more than 45 million dogs around 7-years-old in USA and Europe [2]. Because ageing is the main risk factor of CCDS, aged dogs likely represent a large population with a great risk of developing CCDS [3]. Indeed, Neilson et al. [4] showed that the prevalence of CCDS was 28 % in 11–12 years old dogs and 68 % in 15–16 years old dogs. Similarly, Azkona et al. [5] demonstrated that 22.5 % of dogs older than 9 years displayed cognitive impairment.

As a result of the increasing number of cognitively impaired dogs, increasing emphasis is being placed on management and therapy of an age-related canine cognitive impairment [3]. Thus identifying modifiable risk factors and developing preventive strategies for CCDS represent important goals. Currently, there are only limited data available about the risk factors of CCDS, as only a few studies dealing with the risk factors of CCDS have been conducted over the last decade. A study carried out in Spain suggested an association between sex, size, reproductive state and cognitive function of aged dogs [5]. That study showed that females and neutered dogs were significantly more affected than males and intact dogs. Moreover, small breeds had greater odds of showing age-related cognitive impairment than medium or large sized dogs, although weight was not a statistically significant predictor variable. The major drawback of the

*Correspondence: norbert.zilka@savba.sk
†Stanislav Katina, Jana Farbakova and Aladar Madari contributed equally to this work
[4] Institute of Neuroimmunology, No., Dvorakovo Nabrezie 45, Bratislava, Slovak Republic

study lied in structured phone interviews that did not take into account the subjective evaluation of pet owners. Similarly, Hart et al. [6] demonstrated that sexually intact male dogs were significantly less likely than neutered dogs to progress from mild impairment to severe impairment. Another study, conducted in Denmark, showed that neither sex nor weight correlated with cognitive decline [7]. Contradictory results are likely caused by different methodologies used for detection of canine cognitive decline.

The aim of the present study was to test several variables, age, sex, reproductive status, bodyweight, dogs' housing and nutrition in order to identify possible risk factors for CCDS.

Methods

Animals

Study animals were identified among all dogs visiting the Small Animal Veterinary Clinic of the University of Veterinary Medicine and Pharmacy in Kosice, Slovak Republic for regular vaccination, parasite treatments and various health complaints. The age of study dogs ranged from 8 to 18 years (mean = 11 years), there were 116 males and 99 females of different breeds, body weights ranged from 2.3 to 55 kg (mean = 19.6 kg) and reproduction state was neutered males (n = 88), neutered females (n = 79); intact males (n = 25), and intact females (n = 23).

Haematology and biochemistry

An integral part of the diagnosis was haematological and biochemical blood tests. The following haematological variables were analysed by IDEXX ProCyte Dx® Hematology Analyzer: HCT, RBC, HGB, MCV, MCH, MCHC, red cell distribution width (RDW), reticulocytes (absolute number and percentage), WBC, neutrophils, lymphocytes, monocytes, eosinophils, and basophils (number and percentage), platelets [number, MPV, platelet distribution width (PDW) and PCT], band neutrophils (when presence suspected) and nRBCs (nucleated red blood cells, when presence suspected). Biochemical blood parameters were analysed by Cobas C 111 analyzer (Roche). These variables included ALT, AST, ALP, pAMS, LIP, Crea, UREA, Glu, Chol, TP, Alb, Ca, P, Mg, NH3, K, Na, Cl. All dogs included in this study were assessed by neurological examination, orthopaedic, radiology, ultrasound and ECG examination, as well as by blood and urine analyses. Eighty-five dogs were excluded from the study because of other medical causes interfering with cognitive decline such as blindness, deafness, diabetes mellitus, cushing syndrome, urinary tract infection, incontinence of urine or faeces, cardiological patients, head trauma and other disease conditions.

Cognitive evaluation

Behavioural investigation included observation of geriatric dogs by a veterinary clinician and collection of information provided by pet owners. The investigator was pro-active in asking about behavioural abnormalities to identify even subtle signs that often go unrecognized by pet owners. Data collected by using questionnaire was important for calculation of the final score. The questionnaire also included basic information about dog characteristics and lifestyle variables such as sex, age, weight, reproductive state, dog's housing and type of diet. The composite scale–CAnine DEmentia Scale (CADES) used in this study was adapted and modified from the questionnaires proposed by Osella, et al. [8] and Salvin et al. [9]. It contained 17 items distributed into four domains (spatial orientation, social interactions, sleep-awake cycles and house soiling) related to changes in dog's behaviour. The value of each item corresponded to the frequency of abnormal behaviour. We used a 5-point scale for easy evaluation of behaviour: 0—abnormal behaviour of the dog had never observed; 2—abnormal behaviour of the dog was detected at least once within the last 6 months; 3—abnormal behaviour appeared at least once per month; 4—abnormal behaviour was seen several times per month; 5—abnormal behaviour was observed several times a week. The score from each domain was added up to obtain a final quantitative score that reliably reflected the qualitative evaluation of cognitive decline. We validated CADES as a screening tool for CCDS [10]. Dogs were divided into two subgroups: dogs with no or very mild cognitive impairment (MiCI) and dogs with an advanced cognitive decline. The first group consists of cognitively normal dogs (NA; CADES score 0–7) and dogs with MiCI (CADES score 8–23). The second group consists of dogs with moderate cognitive impairment (MoCI; CADES score 23–44) and dogs with severe cognitive impairment (CADES score higher than 44).

Prevalence calculation

The prevalence of CCDS in three age groups was calculated. All tested dogs were divided into age groups based on estimated life expectancies [11]: short-lived, 6–11 years; medium-lived, 11–13 years and long-lived, >13 years, as proposed by Salvin et al. [9]. The prevalence was calculated by dividing the number of dogs in each tested group (NA, MiCI, MoCI, CD) by the number of individuals examined in each age category.

Data analysis

Statistical analyses were performed with R software [12]. Univariable logistic regression analysis (two-sample Z-test of log odds) [13] was used to assess relationships between cognitive impairment as dependent variable (moderate and severe CCDS vs normal ageing and mild cognitive impairment) and risk factors such as sex (males vs females), reproductive state (neutered vs entire dogs), food (uncontrolled-scrabs, commercial dry or wet food low quality or mix of different kind of food vs controlled diet—commercial dry or wet food for specific breed, age or life stages—obese, neutered, intact, working dogs), dog's housing (outside—dogs spending much of their time outside the house vs inside—dogs spending much of their time inside the house or flat) and weight (under 15 kg vs over 15 kg, under 15 kg means smaller or equal than 15 kg in the paper) as independent variables. All age and weight related intervals used in the text are open from left and closed from right, e.g. 11–13 years means greater than 11 and smaller or equal than 13 (except for the first in the range, which is closed from both sides, e.g. 8–11 years means greater or equal than 8 and smaller or equal than 11). The risk was considered to be positive with respect to cognitive impairment when the estimate of odds ratio (OR) was greater than one, and negative when OR was less than one. Additionally, Wald 95 % empirical confidence intervals for OR were calculated. To test correlation between age (in years) and composite CADES score, one-sample Fisher Z-test of zero correlation was used. Additionally, Wald 95 % empirical confidence intervals for Pearson product-moment correlation coefficient were calculated. All of the null hypotheses were tested against two-sided alternatives on significance level $\alpha = 0.05$. Finally we also used saturated additive multivariable logistic regression model with interaction (of sex and reproductive state) of the form-cognitive impairment ~ sex + reproductive state + diet + housing + weight + (sex: reproductive state), where the log odds were tested similarly as in univariate analyses equivalent to univariable logistic regression model.

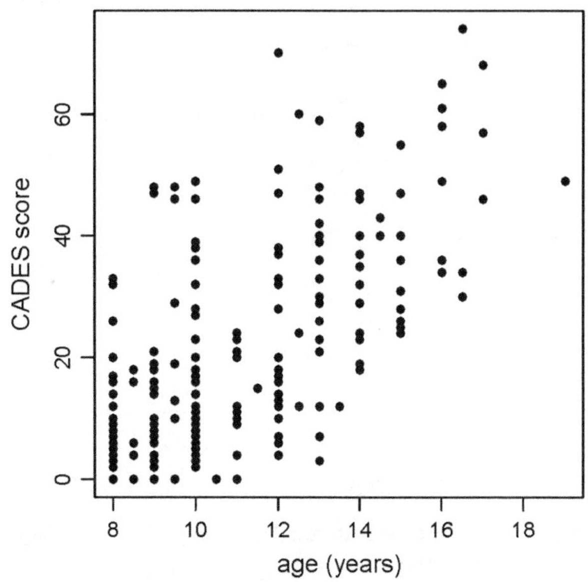

Fig. 1 The positive correlation of CADES score and age of dogs

Results

Correlation of age and CCDS

First, we focused on relationship between advancing age and CADES score reflecting degree of cognitive impairment. There was positive correlation between both advancing age and CADES score (estimate of Pearson product-moment correlation coefficient $r = 0.662$, $t = 12.895$, $df = 213$, $P < 0.0001$, 95 % CI: (0.580, 0.731); Fig. 1).

Association between nutrition and CCDS

For the study of putative risk factors, the dog population with a slightly uneven sex ratio [54 % males, 46 % females] was classified as follows: weights—small size breeds (less than or equal to 15 kg; 112 dogs) or medium/large size breeds (over 15 kg; 103 dogs), nutrition-controlled diets (113 dogs) or uncontrolled diets (102 dogs), dogs' housing-outside (78 dogs) or inside (137 dogs) and reproductive status—neutered (167 dogs) or entire dogs (48 dogs); see Table 1.

Univariable analyses demonstrated that there was a significant association between nutrition and CCDS ($P < 0.001$). Dogs fed with controlled diet displayed 2.8 times lower odds of CDS when compared to dogs fed uncontrolled diets (OR = 2.8). Sex ($P = 0.11$), weight ($P = 0.14$), reproductive status ($P = 0.32$) and dogs' housing ($P = 0.42$) were not significant at the univariable level (Table 2; Fig. 2). Multivariable analyses showed similar results. Sex, reproductive state, housing, weight, and interaction of sex and reproductive state were all ruled out from saturated model and the only statistically important variable is diet (OR = 2.8, $P < 0.001$).

The prevalence of CCDS increased with age

We found that the prevalence of fully developed CCDS (MoCI + CD) was 13 % (7 dogs, below 15 kg) and 16 % (12 dogs, over 15 kg) in the age period 8–11 years, 41 % (11 dogs, below 15 kg) and 65 % (13 dogs, over 15 kg) in the age period 11–13 years and 87 % (26 dogs, below 15 kg) and 100 % (9 dogs, over 15 kg) in the age over 13 years. Further, 52 % (28 dogs, below 15 kg) and 42 % (31 dogs, over 15 kg) of 8–11 years old dogs and 37 % (10 dogs, below 15 kg) and 35 % (7 dogs, below 15 kg) of 11–13 years old dogs were classified as mildly affected (MiCI). Prevalence of CCDS was similar in both small and medium/large sized dogs in the age period 8–11 years (13 vs 16 %), and differed in older dogs, 11–13 years old (41 vs 65 %); see Table 3; Fig. 3. In dogs older than 13 years, we did not find any cognitively intact dog.

Discussion

The cognitive decline of aged dogs represents serious medical and social problem. Increasing number of dogs older than 7 years is leading to a higher prevalence of CCDS worldwide [2]. The aging profile of dogs varies

Table 1 Distribution of dogs throughout selected categories and stages of canine dementia

Categories	Total number of dogs	Weight		Nutrition		Sex		Dogs' housing		Reproductive status	
		Over 15 kg	Below 15 kg	Uncontrolled diet	Controlled diet	Females	Males	Inside	Outside	Neutered	Entire
Normal ageing	56	31	25	21	35	30	26	34	22	43	13
Mild cognitive impairment	80	38	42	31	49	37	43	52	28	64	16
Moderate cognitive impairment	49	23	26	30	19	19	30	32	17	38	11
Severe cognitive impairment	30	11	19	20	10	13	17	19	11	22	8

Table 2 The results of statistical analyses of the risk factors—weight, nutrition, sex, dogs' housing and reproductive state for canine dementia

Variable (group 1 vs group 2)	n_1	N_1	n_2	N_2	OR	sd (OR)	LB	UB	*Z*-statistics	*P* value
Weight OR (under 15 kg vs over 15 kg)	45	112	34	103	1.36	0.21	0.78	2.38	1.0879	0.1383
Nutrition OR (uncontrolled vs controlled diet)	50	102	29	113	2.79	0.82	1.57	4.94	3.5006	*0.0002*
Sex OR (males vs females)	47	116	32	99	1.43	0.20	0.81	2.50	1.2401	0.1075
Dogs' housing OR (outside vs inside)	51	137	28	78	1.06	0.28	0.59	1.89	0.1943	0.4230
Reproductive state OR (neutered vs entire dogs)	60	167	19	48	0.86	0.39	0.44	1.65	−0.4627	0.3218

n_1 the number of moderate and severe cognitive impaired dogs in group 1 (weight below 15 kg, nutrition-uncontrolled diet, males, housing inside, neutered), n_2 the number of moderate and severe cognitive impaired dogs in group 2 (weight above 15 kg, nutrition-controlled diet, females, housing outside, entire), N_1, N_2 total number of dogs in group 1 and group 2, *OR* odds ratio, *sd (OR)* standard deviation of odds ratio, *LB* lower bound, *UB* upper bound of Wald 95 % empirical confidence interval (CI) for OR, *Z-statistics* two-sample *Z*-test about log OR (*P* values related to statistically significant results are highlighted in italics; the bounds of CI are back transformed bounds of CI for log OR)

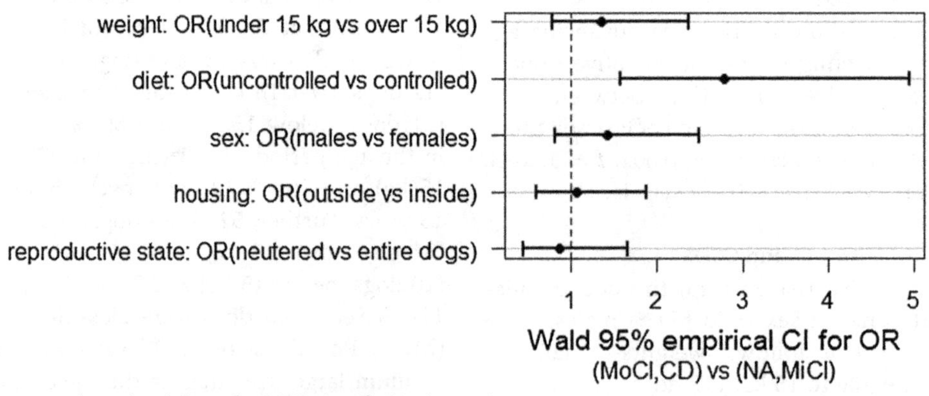

Fig. 2 Nutrition represents the only risk factor for CCDS identified in the study

between breeds, generally smaller dogs can live up to 10–14 years, while medium and large sized breeds live up to 8 years [14]. Today, dogs are generally living longer than previously thanks to increasing knowledge about nutritional needs and advances in veterinary medicine. Increasing life span does not equal increasing life quality as shown by higher prevalence of age-related disorders or healthy problems such as arthritis and joint problems, prostate enlargement, urinary incontinence, constipation, hearing and vision loss.

Several studies have shown that the prevalence of CCDS raises with increased age [4, 5, 8, 9]. However,

Table 3 The prevalence of CCDS

Current paper			
	8–11 years	11–13 years	Over 13 years
Small breed (%)	13	41	87
Medium/large breed (%)	16	55	100
Salvin et al. [9]			
8–10 years	10–12 years	12–14 years	Over 14 years
3.4 %	5 %	23.3 %	41 %
Azkona et al. [5]			
	9–11 years	12–14 years	15–17 years
Small breed (%)	22.7	32.7	50.0
Medium/large breed (%)	10.3	26.9	40

telephone interviews used in some studies cannot exclude various medical causes of CCDS and thus the prevalence of CCDS can be overestimated. To strengthen the design of the study, we combined structured interviews with pet owners with direct clinical evaluation. Previously, Salvin et al. [9] showed that the prevalence of CCDS increased with age. Similarly, Azkona et al. [5] demonstrated increased prevalence of CCDS in both small breeds and medium/large breeds. In contrast, we observed greater prevalence of CCDS in medium/large sized breeds compared with small sized breeds in the age group of 11–13 years, while no difference was observed in the age group of 8–11 years. Our findings are in accordance with a previous study that focused on the relationship between body size and life span [14]. The researchers clearly demonstrated that while there was no clear correlation between body size and the onset of senescence, there was a strong positive relationship between size and aging rate. Finally, they concluded that dogs of large breeds died younger than small breed dogs, mainly because they aged more quickly. We plan to increase the total number of dogs to identify whether some of the breeds are more vulnerable to CCDS than the others.

The increasing incidence of CCDS highlights the importance of identification of putative aetiological risk factors. Unfortunately, knowledge regarding risk factors of CCDS is still quite limited and some data are rather contradictory, e.g., one study found that sex and size of breeds had no association with CCDS [7], while another study indicated that small sized dogs and females had a greater risk of developing signs of CCDS [5]. Another proposed risk factor was the reproductive state. Azkona et al. [5] demonstrated a higher risk of CCDS in neutered female and male dogs in comparison to intact dogs. Similarly, Hart [6] showed that sexually intact male dogs were significantly less likely than neutered dogs to progress from mild impairment to severe impairment. Surprisingly, our data did not support the contribution of sex, reproductive status and weight to the disease progression. We also did not find any correlation between dogs' housing and cognitive decline. In case of dogs' housing and reproduction state, we are aware of the fact, that the number of dogs in each group (neutered vs entire, outside vs inside) is not equal. In our study, we recruited much more neutered dogs than intact dogs and the majority of dogs lived inside of houses or flats. This uneven distribution may have influenced the outcome of the study.

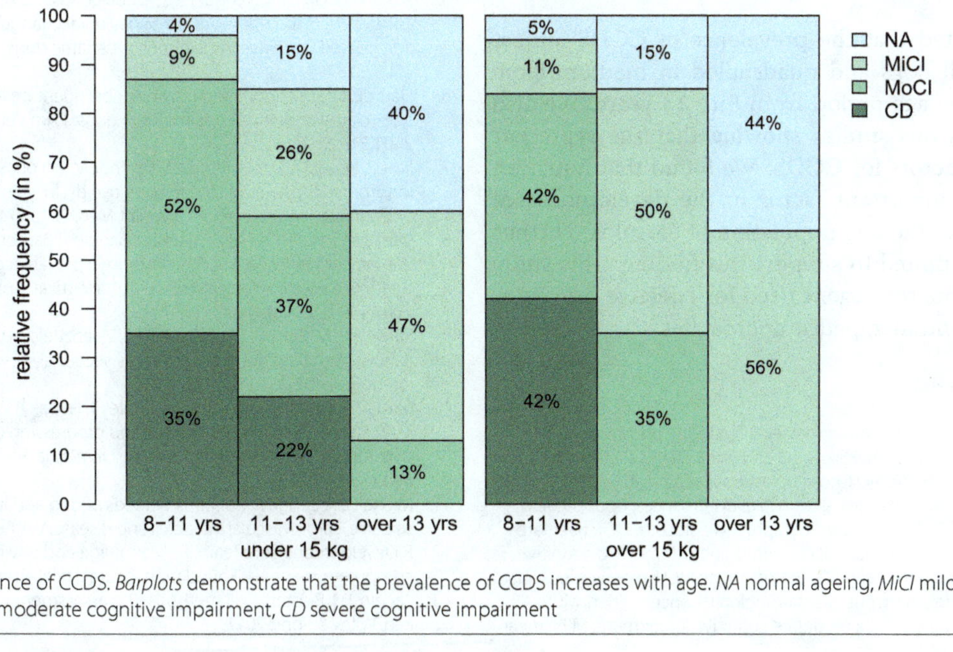

Fig. 3 The prevalence of CCDS. *Barplots* demonstrate that the prevalence of CCDS increases with age. *NA* normal ageing, *MiCI* mild cognitive impairment, *MoCI* moderate cognitive impairment, *CD* severe cognitive impairment

On the other hand, we found for the first time that nutrition may represent an important factor for development of CCDS. We defined two groups of diets as proposed by Hand et al. [15]: controlled diet and uncontrolled food. In this study, controlled diet is characterized as high-quality commercial food purchased for the size of the breed or age or healthy status demands (Hill's, Royal Canine, Specific etc.). Uncontrolled diet represents kitchen waste, unspecified feed mixture or low-quality commercial food, which is not purchased for the size of the breed or age or healthy status demands. Our study revealed that uncontrolled diets may increase a dog's risk of developing CCDS. Based on our results we suggest that controlled diets could be more protective against cognitive damage than homemade or mixed diets. Our findings may explain why nutritional manipulation through the use of special diets and dietary supplements may be beneficial for treatment and prevention of CCDS [16]. We suggest that CCDS is an aging-related multifactorial disorder that may be modified by a properly balanced diet.

We are aware of strengths and weaknesses of our study. While this study included only a small number of subjects and conducted in one clinic in Slovakia, and therefore, may represent regional and/or cultural group, the results are consistent with several independent nutritional studies showed that controlled diet can significantly improve, or slow the decline of learning and memory in aged dogs [17, 18]. Moreover, it has been demonstrated that antioxidants and mitochondrial cofactors, and long-term supplementation with medium-chain triglycerides improve cognitive function in aged dogs [19].

Conclusions

We demonstrated that the prevalence of CCDS almost tripled in small dogs and quadrupled in medium/large dogs, within the age period from 8 to 13 years. We also confirmed previous studies showing that age represent the main risk factors for CCDS. We found that nutrition may represent important factor in the development of CCDS at least in the dog population of Slovakia. Further studies are warranted to support this finding. This study further highlights the urgent need for effective preventative strategies and therapeutic approaches.

Abbreviations

Alb: albumin; ALT: alanine aminotransferase; ALP: alkaline phosphatase; AST: aspartate aminotransferase; CADES: canine dementia scale; CCDS: canine cognitive dysfunction syndrome; Chol: cholesterol; Crea: creatine; DISHA: disorientation, interaction changes, sleep/wake disturbances, house soiling and activity changes; ECG: electrocardiography; Glu: glucose; HCT: haematocrit; LIP: lipase; RBC: red blood cells; HGB: haemoglobin; MiCI: mild cognitive impairment; MCI: human mild cognitive impairment; MCH: mean corpuscular hemoglobin; MCHC: mean corpuscular hemoglobin concentration; MCV: mean corpuscular volume; MoCI: moderate cognitive impairment; MPV: mean platelet volume; NA: normal ageing; nRBCs: nucleated red blood cells; OD: odds ratio; PCT: plateletcrit; pAMS: amylase; PDW: platelet distribution width; RDW: red cell distribution width; TP: total protein.

Authors' contributions

SK performed the statistical analyses and performed the final correction of the manuscript. AM and JF performed the behavioural examination of dogs. NZ and MN analysed and interpreted data. All authors participated in the writing of the manuscript. All authors read and approved the final manuscript.

Author details

[1] Department of Mathematics and Statistics, Masaryk University, Kotlarska 2, Brno, Czech Republic. [2] University of Veterinary Medicine and Pharmacy, Komenskeho 73, Kosice, Slovak Republic. [3] Institute of Neuroimmunology, Slovak Academy of Sciences, Dubravska cesta 9, Bratislava, Slovak Republic. [4] Institute of Neuroimmunology, No., Dvorakovo Nabrezie 45, Bratislava, Slovak Republic.

Acknowledgements

This work is dedicated to Prof. Marian Kozak, the father of the cognitive research in Slovak veterinary medicine. This work was supported by research Grants APVV 0206-11 and EU structural fund 26240220046.

Competing interests

The authors declare that they have no competing interests.

References

1. Landsberg GM, Nichol J, Araujo JA. Cognitive dysfunction syndrome: a disease of canine and feline brain aging. Vet Clin North Am Small Anim Pract. 2012;42:749–68.
2. Bosch MN, Pugliese M, Gimeno-Bayón J, Rodríguez MJ, Mahy N. Dogs with cognitive dysfunction syndrome: a natural model of Alzheimer's disease. Curr Alzheimer Res. 2012;9:298–314.
3. Sanabria CO, Olea F, Rojas M. Cognitive dysfunction syndrome in senior dogs. In: Kishore U, editor. Neurodegenerative diseases, 2013. p. 615–628.
4. Neilson JC, Hart BL, Cliff KD, Ruehl WW. Prevalence of behavioral changes associated with age-related cognitive impairment in dogs. J Am Vet Med Assoc. 2001;218:1787–91.
5. Azkona G, García-Belenguer S, Chacón G, Rosado B, León M, Palacio J. Prevalence and risk factors of behavioural changes associated with age-related cognitive impairment in geriatric dogs. J Small Anim Pract. 2009;50:87–91.
6. Hart BL. Effect of gonadectomy on subsequent development of age-related cognitive impairment in dogs. J Am Vet Med Assoc. 2001;219:51–6.
7. Fast R, Schütt T, Toft N, Møller A, Berendt M. An observational study with long-term follow-up of canine cognitive dysfunction: clinical characteristics, survival, and risk factors. J Vet Int Med. 2013;27:822–9.
8. Osella MC, Re G, Odore R, Girardi C, Badino P, Barbero R, Bergamasco L. Canine cognitive dysfunction syndrome: prevalence, clinical signs and treatment with a neuroprotective nutraceutical. Appl Anim Beh Sci. 2007;105:297–310.
9. Salvin HE, McGreevy PD, Sachdev PS, Valenzuela MJ. Under diagnosis of canine cognitive dysfunction: a cross-sectional survey of older companion dogs. Vet J. 2010;184:277–81.
10. Madari A, Farbakova J, Katina S, Smolek T, Novak P, Weissova T, Novak M, Zilka N. Assessment of severity and progression of canine cognitive dysfunction syndrome using CAnine DEmentia Scale (CADES). Appl Anim Behav Sci. 2015;171:138–45.
11. Michell AR. Longevity of British breeds of dog and its relationships with sex, size, cardiovascular variables and disease. Vet Rec. 1999;145:625–9.
12. R Development Core Team. R: A language and environment for statistical computing. Vienna: R Foundation for Statistical, Computing; 2014.
13. Lachin JM. Biostatistical methods. The assessment of relative risks. Hoboken: Wiley & Sons; 2011.

2

Magnetic resonance imaging and computed tomography as tools for the investigation of sperm whale (*Physeter macrocephalus*) teeth and eye

Aage Kristian Olsen Alstrup[1*], Ole Lajord Munk[1], Trine Hammer Jensen[2], Lasse Fast Jensen[3], Abdi Hedayat[4] and Brian Hansen[5]

Abstract

Background: Scanning techniques such as magnetic resonance imaging (MRI) and computed tomography (CT) are useful tools in veterinary and human medicine. Here we demonstrate the usefulness of these techniques in the study of the anatomy of wild marine mammals as part of a necropsy. MRI and CT scans of sperm whale teeth ($n = 4$) were performed. The methods were compared and further compared to current standard methods for evaluation of tooth layering. For MRI a zero echo time sequence was used, as previously done for imaging of intact human teeth. For CT two different clinical scanners were used.

Results: The three scanners did not provide sufficient information to allow age estimation, but both MRI and CT provided anatomical information about the tooth cortex and medulla without the need for sectioning the teeth. MRI scanning was also employed for visualizing the vascularization of an intact eye from one of the stranded sperm whale.

Conclusions: Clearly, MRI was useful for investigation of the retinal vasculation, but optimum results would require well-preserved tissue. It was not possible to estimate age based on CT scans of tooth growth lines. Further research is needed to clarify the usability of MRI and CT as tools for marine mammal research when samples need to remain intact or when a spatial (three dimensional) arrangement of features needs to be determined.

Keywords: Imaging techniques, Computer tomography, Magnetic resonance, Sperm whales, Eyes, Teeth

Background

Traditionally, anatomical and pathological knowledge in cetacean research is obtained by dissection of stranded individuals followed by e.g. bacteriological, virological, morphological or histological examinations [1–3]. However, modern scanning techniques have much to offer in this research field—at least as a supplement to dissection: first, modern scanners offer the possibility of non-invasive imaging of organs providing access to data about organ structure in situ, e.g. vasculature of soft tissue organs such as the eye, heart or kidney. Second, many museums find preservation of the intact organ desirable, which can be compromised by traditional examination techniques, in particular necropsy. In toothed whales, for instance, age is estimated by counting growth layers in the teeth after cutting them into halves, which makes the teeth less suited for later display. Non-invasive analyses are also preferable when dealing with samples originating from rare or extinct species. Third, modern imaging techniques and computer aided data visualization offer a better three-dimensional understanding of the organ morphology than simple dissection, which is a benefit e.g. for bone examination in whales [4]. Today, three-dimensional imaging techniques can provide anatomical information more quickly and in a non-invasive way, as

*Correspondence: aagols@rm.dk
[1] Department of Nuclear Medicine and PET Center, Institute of Clinical Medicine, Aarhus University Hospital, Nørrebrogade 44, 10C, 8000 Aarhus, Denmark
Full list of author information is available at the end of the article

described for terrestrial vertebrates by Lauridsen et al. [5].

Both magnetic resonance imaging (MRI) and computed tomography (CT) provide detailed images with millimeter spatial resolution for routine scans and cellular level resolution is attainable when imaging samples [6–9]. In MRI a constant external magnetic field sets up a magnetization in the subject or sample being imaged. This magnetization may be manipulated with radiofrequency pulses to induce a signal in a detector coil. During the scan the magnetization is encoded in frequency and phase by additional time-dependent magnetic fields (called gradients). This encoding makes it possible to reconstruct an image from the signal received in the coil. MRI offers very good soft tissue contrast, but MRI in bony structures is often not feasible due to the very rapid signal decay in these crystalline structures. In comparison, medical CT scanners consist of a rotating X-ray source, which is rigidly linked to an X-ray detector located on the other side of the target [10]. The target is exposed to a fan-shaped X-ray beam, while being translated through the scanner. The CT detectors measure the X-ray transmission through the target at all angles, which allows reconstruction of a three-dimensional density image. The resulting CT image is linearly rescaled into CT numbers in Hounsfield units.

CT is a fast and useful technique for visualizing the normal and pathological anatomy of organs, which has been particularly well-suited for imaging of mineral or crystalline structures such as bones and teeth. For clinical use, contrast-enhanced CT protocols with intravenously or orally administrated iodine-based contrast agents are routinely used to improve tissue differentiation and delineation of anatomic structures, and for ex vivo imaging, iodine staining of soft tissue specimens has recently been shown to improve visualization using diffusible iodine-based contrast-enhanced computed tomography (diceCT) [11]. Both MRI and CT are routinely used in human and veterinary medicine, and they are also useful tools in preclinical and clinical research [12–14].

Recent technological developments have improved both resolution and versatility of MRI and CT scanning techniques. For instance, using ultra-short echo time (UTE) sequences [15, 16] and more recently, zero echo time (ZTE) sequences [17–19] allow MRI to be used on bony structures as well. Thus, Weiger et al. [20] showed that the ZTE technique provides a good delineation of mineralized dentine and enamel layers in human teeth. Likewise, recent developments in CT scanning and reconstruction techniques have increased the resolution significantly.

In cetaceans, scanning techniques have proved useful in anatomical examinations and have been applied in studying e.g. head anatomy of Cuvier's beaked whale (*Ziphius cavirostris)* [21–23] and sperm whale (*Physeter macrocephalus*) [24], brain anatomy of the white whale (*Delphinapterus leucas*) [25] and dwarf sperm whale (*Kogia simus*) [26] and in discovering a sensory organ related to lunge feeding in rorqual whales (*Balaenopteridae*), a technique used to engulf large quantities of concentrated prey [27]. However, scanning techniques are not applied on a routine basis in cetacean research due to the difficulties of getting access to fresh tissue or organ samples as well as logistical challenges and the sheer size of many cetacean species.

In this study the usage of modern MRI and CT scanning techniques in anatomical examinations of sperm whales was evaluated for two challenging samples: thick dense teeth with fine inner structures and an eye with detailed soft-tissue structures. Specifically, we investigate whether MRI and CT scanning of sperm whale teeth are suitable methods for age estimation by identifying tooth growth lines [28] and resolving details of anatomy, including measurement of dentin and enamel thickness. In addition, the anatomical details of retina vasculation in situ and sclera structure in the sperm whale eye were studied by MR imaging and compared to similar scans acquired in an isolated pig eye. This demonstrated possibilities and limitations of using modern clinical and preclinical imaging techniques in cetacean research, for which samples are often not in an ideal state due to various stages of decomposition.

Methods

Teeth (Fig. 1) were sampled from a whale bone collection belonging to the Natural History Museum of Denmark, Copenhagen, Denmark. The teeth (n = 4) were from stranded male sperm whales stranded in 1996 (MCE1654; Rømø, Denmark), 1997 (MCE1652; Rømø, Denmark) and 2014 (MCE1644 and MCE1645; Henne Strand, Denmark). Due to the limited gantry size only teeth from MCE1652 (tooth A) and MCE1654 (tooth B) were MRI

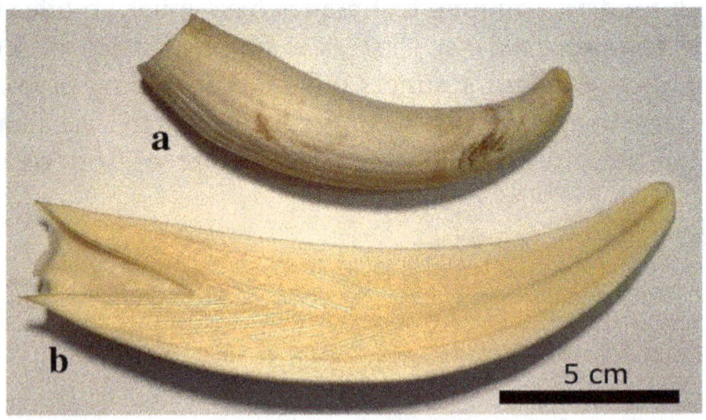

Fig. 1 The two whale teeth (tooth **a** MCE1652 and tooth **b** MCE1654) used for evaluation of the use of ZTE MRI in whale age estimation

scanned, while all four teeth were CT scanned. In 2014, the eye was taken from a stranded whale (MCE1645) a few hours after death at Henne Strand, Denmark. The whale was still alive when it stranded, and the eye was immediately preserved in 4% buffered formaldehyde post mortem. After 2 weeks, the eye was transferred to a 99% ethanol solution until scanning was performed. Similarly, a pig eye was sampled from a female 40 kg domestic pig (*Sus scrofa domesticus*) after euthanasia as part of a different research experiment (approved by The Danish Animal Experiments Inspectorate). The pig eye was processed in the same way as the whale eye.

CT of the whale teeth was performed on two clinical CT scanners: Siemens Biograph 64 Truepoint PET/CT and Siemens Somatom Definition Flash. These or similar modern scanners are widely available. Images of the teeth were comparable for the two scanner systems (Figs. 2 and 3), but the scan settings and reconstruction parameters were important for the quality of the images and visualization of the inner structures of the teeth. We aimed at using parameters for high-resolution imaging. Details of the scan and reconstruction parameters are provided below. The eyes were not CT scanned because good soft tissue CT imaging requires the use of contrast agent, which is only possible for in vivo studies. Thus, MRI is more suitable for this purpose.

MRI of teeth and eyes was performed on a Bruker Biospec 9.4T animal system. Scan details are provided below. Anatomical scans of the eye were performed along three orthogonal directions to ensure a detailed mapping of the anatomical features. For mapping the vasculature of the eye, including the retina we used a fast gradient echo scan which to our experience is very sensitive to the vasculature in this type of sample where blood was not washed out prior to preservation. After scanning, vascular segments in each image plane were segmented out by hand and processed in Matlab (The Mathworks, Natick, MA, USA). In this manner, mapping of the eye vasculature was possible.

MRI method details

Eye vasculature was imaged using an 86 mm quadrature coil and a gradient echo (FLASH) sequence: resolution 180 μm × 180 μm × 500 μm, echo time: 7.2 ms, repetition time: 2.3 s, 20 averages, scan time: 5 h.

The eye anatomy was imaged using a 3D MDEFT sequence. Resolution in the pig eye scans was 120 μm × 120 μm × 250 μm, echo time: 3.5 ms, repetition time: 4.2 s. In the whale eye the resolution was 466 μm × 466 μm × 700 μm.

Teeth were imaged using a 40 mm quadrature coil and a ZTE sequence. For tooth A the scan parameters were: repetition time: 1.92 ms, flip angle: 5°, Bandwidth: 300 kHz, isotropic resolution of 234 μm, 1000 averages were acquired resulting in a total scan time of approximately 21 h. Tooth B was scanned with scan parameters: repetition time 8 ms, flip angle: 10°, Bandwidth: 313 kHz, isotropic resolution of 234 μm, 250 averages were acquired resulting in a total scan time of approximately 22 h. The ZTE sequence does not allow selective excitation and therefore everything within the coil's field of view contributes to the signal. The edges of the coil field of view are seen in Figs. 4 and 5 as a region where the image fades out. In each image, image contrast has been adjusted to improve visibility of the described features. In all cases contrast was adjusted evenly over the whole image. Remaining image background has been masked for presentation.

CT method details

Tooth images were imaged on two CT systems using the following scan- and reconstruction parameters.

Siemens Biograph 64: Protocol name: ExtrUHR, 120 kV, 248 eff. mAs, rotation time: 1.0 s, Pitch factor: 0.9, convolution kernel: U70u, slice thickness: 1.0 mm.

Siemens Somatom Definition Flash: Protocol name: Inner Ear UHR: 120 kV, 195 eff. mAs, rotation time: 1.0 s, Pitch factor: 0.8, convolution kernel I: 50 s, slice thickness: 2.0 mm.

Results

CT scans of whale teeth are shown in Fig. 2 (tooth A and tooth B) and Fig. 3 (tooth B). The CT images from two different clinical CT scanners are shown—the slices are similar, but not exactly from the same plane. The differences between the images are mainly due to different scan settings and reconstruction parameters rather than

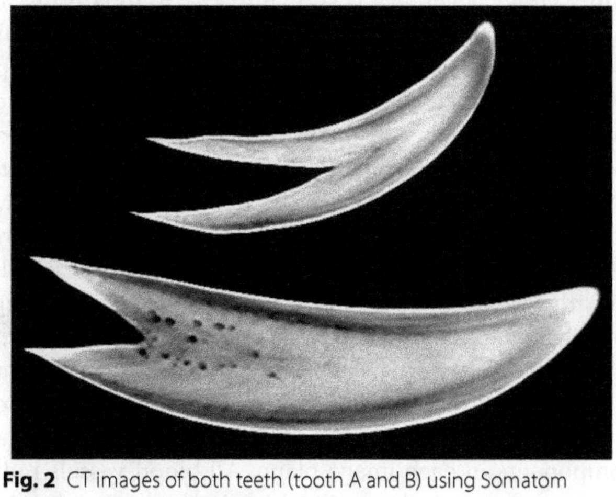

Fig. 2 CT images of both teeth (tooth A and B) using Somatom Definition Flash and the scan- and reconstruction parameters in the CT method details. Coarse inner structures such as *small inner holes* and different densities of enamel and marrow are clearly visualized. Parts of the V-shaped structures can be seen

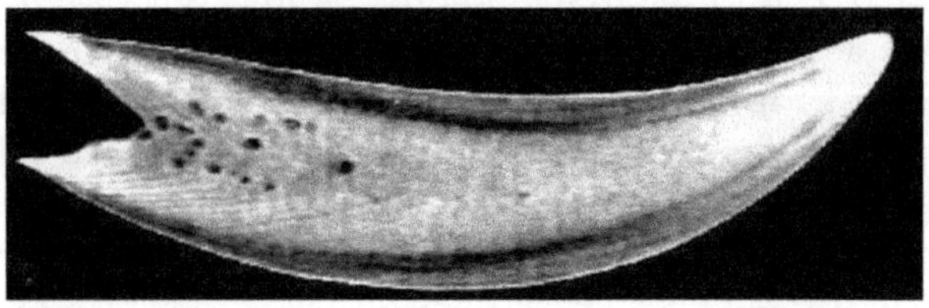

Fig. 3 CT image of tooth B using Biograph 64 and the scan- and reconstruction parameters in the CT method details. The slice is similar (but not exactly the same) as in Fig. 2. This image has smaller slice thickness and the filter was not as smooth as in Fig. 2. Thus, this image has more noise but higher spatial resolution, which improves visualization of the fine V-shaped pattern. Still only parts of the V-shaped structures can be visualized and the total number of layers cannot be determined from these images

the CT scanner hardware. The data shown in Fig. 3 was acquired at higher resolution and is consequently more noisy than the data shown in Fig. 2. Higher resolution improves visualization of the fine V-shaped pattern in the tooth, whereas larger structures such as inner holes and different densities of enamel and marrow are clearly visualized at both resolutions. However, only parts of the V-shaped structures can be visualized and the total number of layers cannot be determined from these images. CT scans of the two other teeth gave similar results (data not shown).

The axial ZTE MRI image of tooth A in Fig. 4 (upper left corner) shows concentric ring-like structures. When shown with a sagittal slice orientation (Fig. 4, upper right corner and lower row) V-shaped patterns are seen. Examples of the ZTE scans of tooth B are shown in Fig. 5. Here the contrast delineates the border between cortex and medulla.

Anatomical MRI scans of the pig eye and the significantly larger whale eye is shown in Fig. 6. In contrast to the pig eye, the deterioration was evident in the whale eye. Furthermore, the whale bulbus is seen to be encapsulated by a very large sclera (and remnants of retractor muscles, which were gently tried off-dissected prior to scanning). Neither of these features were prominent in the pig eye. While the pig eye scan very clearly shows optic nerve, lens, lens suspension, iris and cornea, the whale eye scan only shows optic nerve, lens and iris. In fact, the whale eye lacks major internal structures, e.g. the whale lens lack the suspension (ciliary muscles) seen in the pig eye. The whale eye vasculature of the retina was mapped as shown in Fig. 7, which shows an example of a raw image and a montage showing isolated vascular components in each image plane. All blood vessels radiate from the central retina, which is in agreement with position of a central artery and vein, both of which enter the eye together with the optic nerve in the highly vascularized *rete ophthalmica*.

Discussion

Although adult sperm whales cannot be scanned in commercial scanners, we found that single organ MRI and CT scannings can be suitable tools to gain knowledge of their anatomy. The MRI ZTE sequences and the two different CT scanners showed markedly different performance in elucidating detailed tooth structure. Layering was successfully resolved with MRI in tooth A but was insufficient for age estimation. The concentric appearance of the layers in the axial plane and their V-shaped arrangement in the sagittal plane indicate that the resolved structures are layers in the tooth's cone-shaped growth zones. In the images of tooth B (sagittal plane), the V-shape of these layers is readily seen along with the distinct border between tooth enamel and marrow (see Fig. 1). In the ZTE scans of tooth B (Fig. 5) this border between enamel and tooth marrow was clearly separated which might be useful for non-destructive studies of variation in enamel thickness in archived samples. This is an underexplored field of marine mammals, though enamel thickness is considered to be crucial for tooth strength in humans and therefore under investigation in dental medicine [29]. Layering, however, could not be resolved in tooth B possibly due to the sample drying out during storage in the museum. In the human teeth study [20] the teeth were stored in water to prevent drying prior to ZTE scans. Future studies might benefit from storing the samples in water for an extended period prior to ZTE imaging. In the case of fresh samples storing the teeth in saline immediately after extraction until imaging might be advantageous. On the CT scans, the border between enamel and marrow was easily seen. The V-shaped layering was resolved but not with sufficient detail to allow age estimation. Higher resolution helps to resolve the layering, but at very high resolutions the noise increasingly becomes a problem. New iterative image reconstruction algorithms are likely to produce images with less noise, but these algorithms were not available for the scanners applied in the present study. In this study, we have not tried high quality scanners, such as micro-CT, since we as well as many other research groups do not have access to such equipment. Therefore, we can not rule out if such scanners would have given images with better contrast and resolution.

The anatomical scans allow qualitative comparison between the whale eye and the terrestic porcine eye. All identified structures (and their size and shapes) were similar to what has already been reported for sperm whale eyes by Bjergager et al. [30] and in agreement with the general cetacean eye described by Mass and Supin [31]. In the pig eye, the scans clearly show the optic nerve, lens, lens suspension, iris and cornea. The whale eye was seen to lack internal structures beyond a lens.

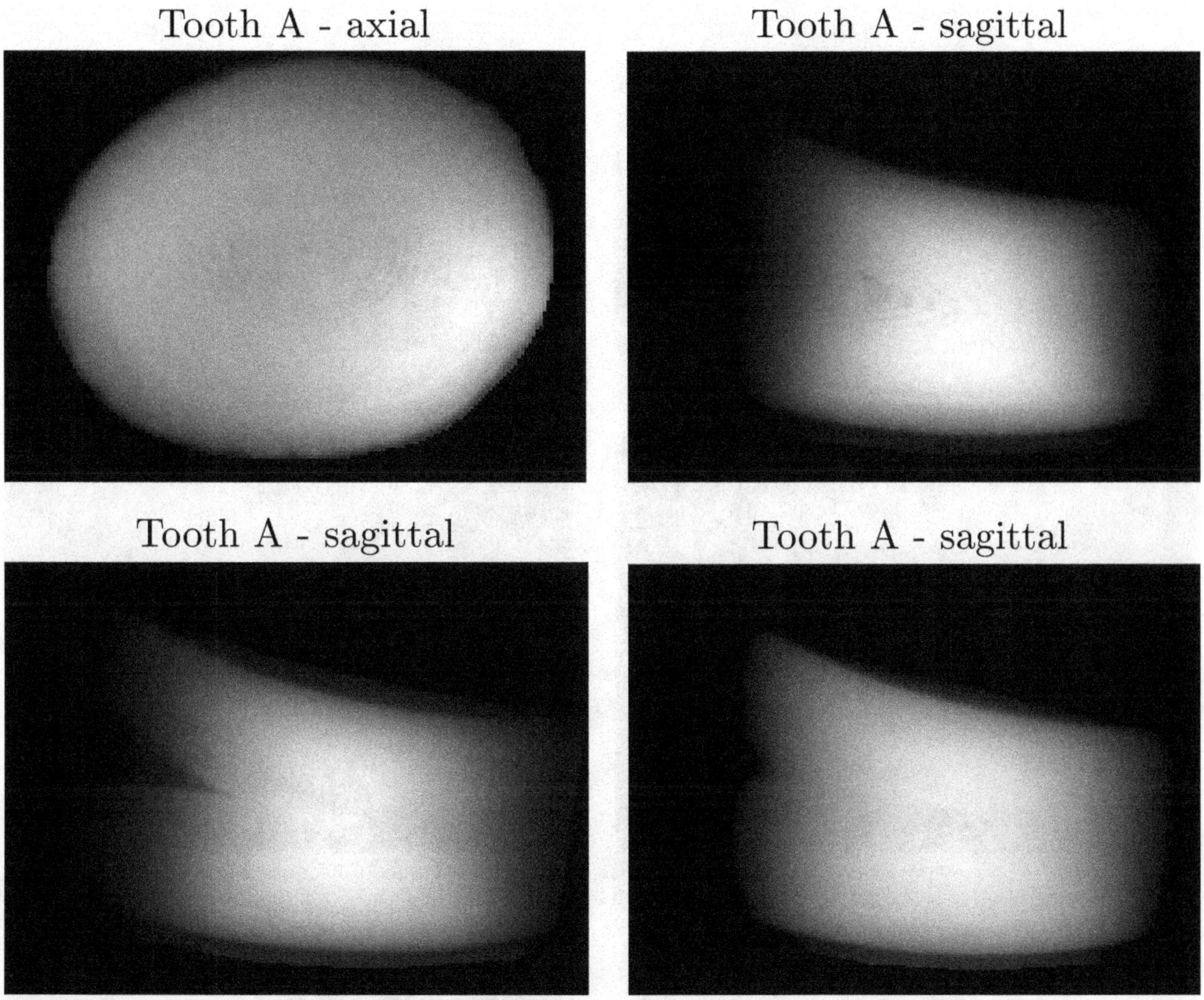

Fig. 4 Examples of ZTE images in tooth *A* (see Fig. 1) along various axis (axial and sagittal). Axial at *top left*. Three sagittal *slice planes* are shown. Note that layering is visible in all examples, but it is not possible to determinate the exact numbers

The optic nerve is clearly visible, as previously described [30]. The findings of this somewhat superficial comparison of the two eyes are in agreement with what is known about the whale eye anatomy and its use as primarily a light detector without the need for focusing ability [31]. The whale eye is thought to be retractable to withstand the high pressures in the deep sea [30]. The anatomical scans of the whale eye show considerable deterioration of the sample even though the sample was extracted and preserved shortly after the time of death. Even though the pig and whale eyes were treated similarly, degradation was much more pronounced in the latter. This is probably because the large size of the eye, and the whale's thick sclera, which are both factors that would slow down the diffusion of formalin into the eye and therefore allow more time for sample degradation. It is also possible that the whale died a few hours earlier than the estimated time of death described herein. Consequently, the sample state made it impossible to visualize e.g. the structure of the sclera in this specimen by MRI. However, even in this state the eye vascular network can be visualized as shown in the 2D visualization in Fig. 7. In the present study, we chose to represent the vasculature as a montage of 2D segmentations, but a three dimensional (3D) reconstruction of the vascularization is entirely possible with the acquired data. In more well preserved samples 3D renderings of the nerves, vasculature and connective tissue would be possible with nerve fiber pathways traced by diffusion tensor tractography [32]. In this manner, the MRI would provide a digital

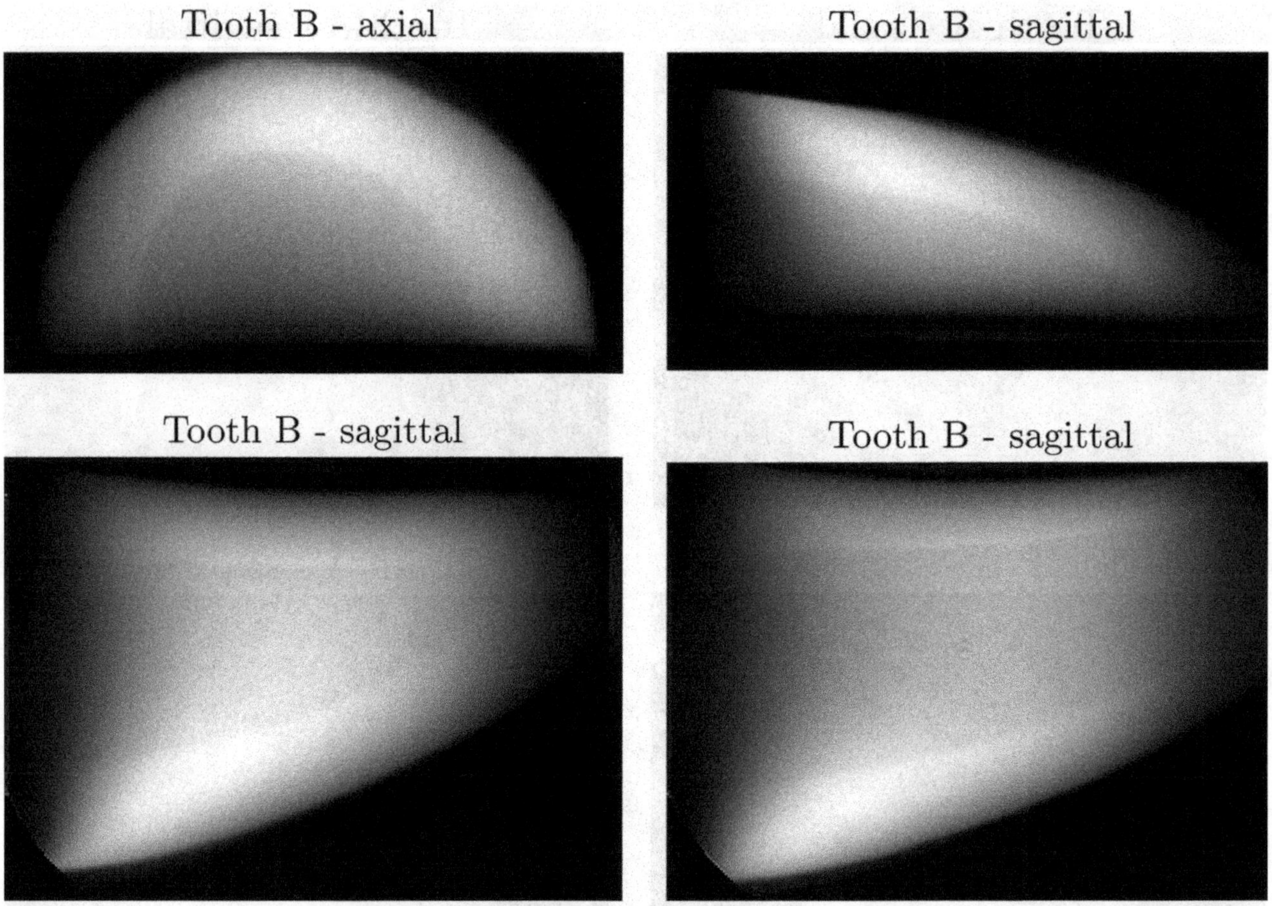

Fig. 5 Examples of ZTE images in tooth *B* (see Fig. 1) along various axis (axial and sagittal). Axial at *top left*. Three sagittal *slice planes* are shown. Here, the layered structure is visible as well as the border between marrow and enamel

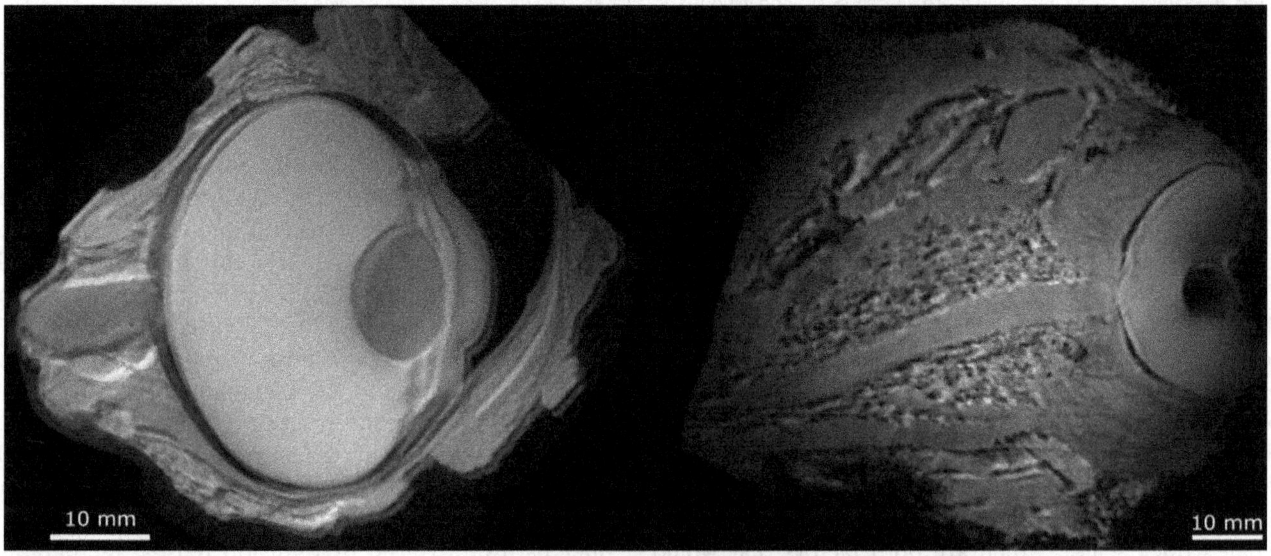

Fig. 6 *Left* pig eye scan showing optic nerve, lens, lens suspension, iris and cornea. *Right* whale eye scan showing optic nerve, lens, and lack of internal structures in the eye. Deterioration of the cornea is evident in whale eye

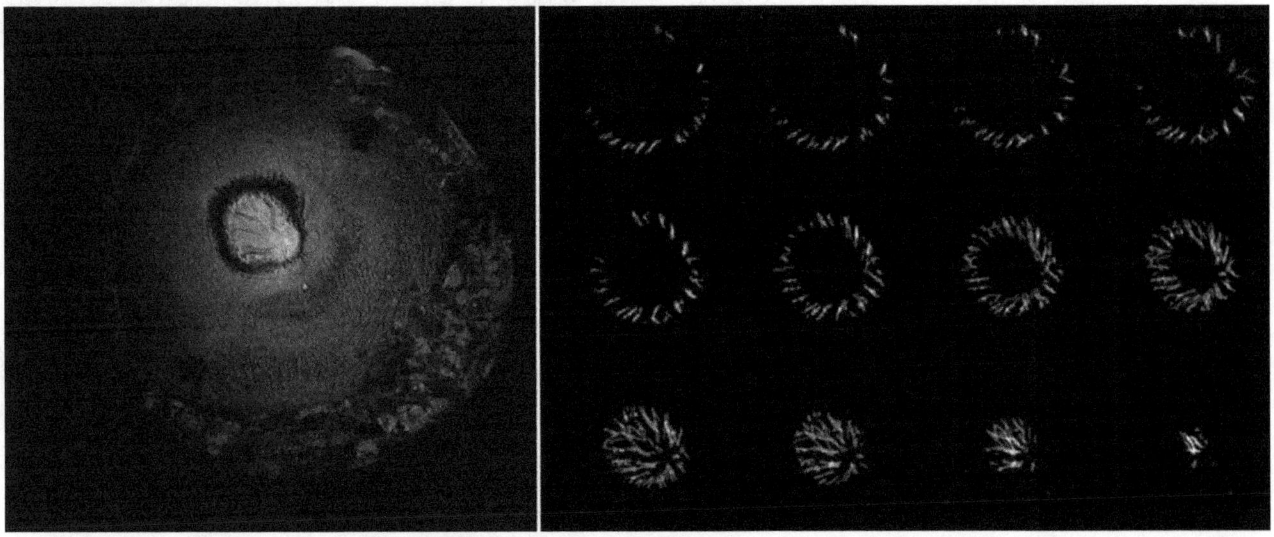

Fig. 7 *Left* an example of the visualization of the eye vasculature (elongated dark structures in the *central bright area*) of the whale. *Right* the vascular components isolated by manual segmentation over 12 image planes

dissection of the eye while leaving the sample intact. Modern scanning techniques could offer methods for non-destructive investigation of the musculature allowing such retraction mechanism.

Conclusions

The use of modern scanning techniques in marine mammal research offers detailed studies of anatomical structures in situ that can increase our knowledge of e.g. anatomical adaptations to an aquatic lifestyle. Even though age could not be estimated based on tooth growing lines, the scanning techniques provided insight into tooth anatomy without the need to cut into the teeth which can be highly desirable for e.g. museum specimens. However, ZTE MRI techniques are continuously being improved and may soon provide sufficient resolution for age estimation. It was possible to get anatomical details of retina vasculation in situ with MRI. However, in soft tissues the state of the sample is the determining factor for successful use of high resolution MRI scanning in marine biology.

Authors' contributions

AKOA, OLM, THJ, LFJ, AH and BH designed the study. AKOA, THJ, LFJ and AH collected the organs. OLM and BH performed the scans and prepared Figs. 1, 2, 3, 4, 5, 6 and 7 and method details. AKOA, OLM, and BH wrote the main manuscript text. All authors read and approved the final manuscript.

Author details

[1] Department of Nuclear Medicine and PET Center, Institute of Clinical Medicine, Aarhus University Hospital, Nørrebrogade 44, 10C, 8000 Aarhus, Denmark. [2] Department of Chemistry and Bioscience, Aalborg University/Aalborg Zoo, Mølleparkvej 63, 9000 Aalborg, Denmark. [3] Fisheries and Maritime Museum, Tarphagevej 2, 6710 Esbjerg, Denmark. [4] Natural History Museum of Denmark, University of Copenhagen, Universitetsparken 15, 2100 Copenhagen, Denmark. [5] Center of Functionally Integrative Neuroscience, Aarhus University Hospital, Nørrebrogade 44, 10G, 8000 Aarhus, Denmark.

Acknowledgements

We thank Mia Hougaard Christiansen, Rikke Nielsen, and Niels Jorgen Rosenkrants, Department of Neuroradiology, Aarhus University Hospital, Aarhus, Denmark for scanning and reconstructing the whale teeth on the Siemens Somatom Definition Flash CT scanner.

Competing interests

The authors declare that they have no competing interests.

Funding

External funding was not used in this study. The authors performed the scans in their spare time.

References

1. Diguardo G, Agrimi U, Morelli L, Cardeti G, Terracciano G, Kennedy S. Post-mortem investigations on cetaceans found stranded on the coasts of Italy between 1990 and 1993. Vet Rec. 1995;136:439–42.
2. Mass AM, Supin AY, Abramov AV, Mukhametov LM, Rozanova EI. Ocular anatomy, ganglion cell distribution and retinal resolution of a killer whale (*Orcinus orca*). Brain Behav Evol. 2013;81:1–11. doi:10.1159/000341949.
3. Moore MJ, Knowlton AR, Kraus SD, McLellan WA, Bonde RK. Morphometry, gross morphology and available histopathology in North Atlantic right whale (*Eubalaene glacialis*) mortalities (1970–2002). J Cetac Res Managem. 2004;6:199–214.

4. Alstrup AKO, Hedayat A, Jensen TH, Hammer AS, Munk OL, Jensen HE. Necropsy report of a fin whale (*Balaenoptera physalus*) stranded in Denmark in 2010. Aquat Mammals. 2013;39:385–8.
5. Lauridsen H, Hansen K, Wang T, Agger P, Andersen JL, Knudsen PS, et al. Inside out: modern imaging techniques to reveal animal anatomy. PLoS ONE. 2011;6:e17879. doi:10.1371/journal.pone.0017879.
6. Flint JJ, Lee CH, Hansen B, Fey M, Schmidig D, Bui JD, et al. Magnetic resonance microscopy of mammalian neurons. NeuroImage. 2009;46:1037–40. doi:10.1016/j.Neuroimage.2009.03.009.
7. Flint JJ, Hansen B, Fey M, Schmidig D, King MA, Vestergaard-Poulsen P, et al. Cellular-level diffusion tensor microscopy and fiber tracking in mammalian nervous tissue with direct histological correlation. NeuroImage. 2010;52:556–61. doi:10.1016/j.neuroimage.2010.04.031.
8. Hansen B, Flint JJ, Heon-Lee C, Fey M, Vincent F, King MA, et al. Diffusion tensor microscopy in human nervous tissue with quantitative correlation based on direct histological comparison. NeuroImage. 2011;57:1458–65. doi:10.1016/j.neuroimage.2011.04.052.
9. Flint JJ, Hansen B, Portnoy S, Lee CH, King MA, Fey M, et al. Magnetic resonance microscopy of human and porcine neurons and cellular processes. NeuroImage. 2012;60:1404–11. doi:10.1016/j.neuroimage.2012.01.050.
10. Goldman LW. Principles of CT and CT technology. J Nucl Med Technol. 2007;35:115–28. doi:10.2967/jnmt.107.042978.
11. Gignac P, Kley NJ, Clarke JA, Colbert MW, Morhardt AC, Cerio D, et al. Diffusible iodinebased contrastenhanced computed tomography (diceCT): an emerging tool for rapid, high-resolution, 3D imaging of metazoan soft tissues. J Anat. 2016;228:889–909.
12. Hendee WR, Ritenour ER. Medical imaging physics. 4th ed. Hoboken: Wiley; 2002.
13. Bernstein MA, King KF, Zhou ZJ. Handbook of MRI pulse sequences. Cambridge: Academic Press; 2004.
14. Brown RW, Cheng YCN, Haacke EM, Thompson MR, Venkatesan R. Magnetic resonance imaging: physical principles and sequence design. 2nd ed. Cambridge: Wiley; 2014.
15. Glover GH, Pauly JM, Bradshaw KM. Boron-11 imaging with a three-dimensional reconstruction method. J Magn Reson Imag. 1992;2:47–52.
16. Rahmer J, Bornert P, Groen J, Bos C. Three-dimensional radial ultrashort echo-time imaging with T2 adapted sampling. Magn Reson Med. 2006;55:1075–82. doi:10.1002/mrm.20868.
17. Hafner S. Fast imaging in liquids and solids with the back-projection low angle shot (BLAST) technique. Magn Reson Imag. 1994;12:1047–51.
18. Madio DP, Lowe IJ. Ultra-fast imaging using low flip angles and FIDs. Magn Reson Med. 1995;34:525–9.
19. Weiger M, Pruessmann KP, Hennel F. MRI with zero echo time: hard versus sweep pulse excitation. Magn Reson Med. 2011;66:379–89. doi:10.1002/mrm.22799.
20. Weiger M, Pruessmann KP, Bracher AK, Köhler S, Lehmann V, Wolfram U, et al. High-resolution ZTE imaging of human teeth. NMR Biomed. 2012;25:1144–51. doi:10.1002/nbm.2783.
21. Soldevilla MS, McKenny MF, Wiggins SM, Shadwick RE, Cranford TW, Hildebrand JA. Cuvier's beaked whale (*Ziphius cavirostris*) head tissues: physical properties and CT imaging. J Exp Biol. 2005;208:2319–32. doi:10.1242/jeb.01624.
22. Cranford TW, Krysl P, Hildebrand JA. Acoustic pathways revealed: simulated sound transmission and reception in Cuvier's beaked whale (*Ziphius cavirostris*). Bioinspir Biomim. 2008. doi:10.1088/1748-3182/3/1/016001.
23. Cranford TW, McKenny MF, Soldevilla MS, Wiggins SM, Goldbogen JA, Shadwick RE, et al. Anatomic geometry of sound transmission and reception in Cuvier's beaked whale (*Ziphius cavirostris*). Anat Rec. 2008;291:353–78. doi:10.1002/ar.20652.
24. Cranford TW. The sperm whale's nose: sexual selection on a grand scale? Mar Mammal Sci. 1999;15:1133–57. doi:10.1111/j.1748-7692.1999.tb00882.x.
25. Marino L, Murphy TL, Deweerd AL, Morris JA, Fobbs AJ, Humblot N, et al. Anatomy and three-dimensional reconstructions of the brain of the white whale (*Delphinapterus leucas*) from magnetic resonance images. Anat Rec. 2001;262:429–39.
26. Marino L, Sudheimer K, Pabst DA, McLellan WA, Johnson JI. Magnetic resonance images of the brain of a dwarf sperm whale (*Kogia simus*). J Anat. 2003;203:57–76.
27. Pyenson ND, Goldbogen JA, Vogl AW, Szathmary G, Drake RL, Shadwick RE. Discovery of a sensory organ that coordinates lunge feeding in rorqual whales. Nature. 2012;485:498–501. doi:10.1038/nature11135.
28. Bow JM, Purday C. A method of preparing sperm whale teeth for age determination. Nature. 1966;210:437–8.
29. Ganss C, Lussi A, Schlueter N. The histological features and physical properties of eroded dental hard tissues. Monogr Oral Sci. 2014;25:99–107. doi:10.1159/000359939).
30. Bjerager P, Heegaard S, Togaard J. Anatomy of the eye of the sperm whale (*Physeter macrocephalus L.*). Aquat Mamm. 2003;29:31–6.
31. Mass AM, Supin AY. Adaptive features of aquatic mammals' eye. Anat Rec (Hoboken). 2007;290:701–5. doi:10.1002/ar.20529.
32. Basser PJ, Pajevic S, Pierpaoli C, Duda J, Aldroubi A. In vivo fiber tractography using DT-MRI data. Magn Reson Med. 2000;44:625–32.

3

Puberty in female wild boar (*Sus scrofa*) in Sweden

Anna Malmsten* and Anne-Marie Dalin

Abstract

Background: Since the re-appearance of wild boars in Sweden in the 1970s, the population has increased. Besides having large litter sizes, puberty at an early age is considered as an important factor contributing to the high reproductive potential of wild boar. Although controversial, supplemental feeding is applied to varying extent throughout the wild boar range in Sweden, and its effect on wild boar reproduction is debated. The aim of this study was to investigate the proportion of post-pubertal female wild boar gilts in a population subjected to supplemental feeding, in relation to age, weight, and season. Also, the effect of another definition of puberty (based upon follicular size) on the outcome of the proportion of female wild boar gilts considered to be able to reproduce in a population was illustrated. Between Jan 2013 and Dec 2015 reproductive organs from 592 female wild boars, were collected. Ovaries and uterus were macroscopically examined, and reproductive stage was determined by the presence of ovarian structures and uterus characteristics. Age was estimated using tooth eruption and tooth replacement, and weight was noted. A subset of 175 female wild boars, aged 5–15 months, was included in this study. An animal was considered to be post-pubertal if the ovaries contained one or more *corpora lutea* (CL) or if the uterus showed signs of previous pregnancy (presence of enlarged blood vessels in the cut surface between the mesometric ligament and the uterus).

Results: In total, 29 (16.6 %) animals were classified as post-pubertal. Field dressed weight ranged from 20.6 to 65.3 kg. Season, weight, and age class significantly influenced the variation in proportion of post-pubertal females. Post-pubertal animals were found in autumn, winter, and spring, but not in the summer season. Another definition of puberty, based on follicle size, lead to different result on proportions of animals considered to have passed puberty.

Conclusions: Season, weight, and age significantly influenced the variation in proportion of post-pubertal wild boar females. The proportion of post-pubertal animals increased with age and weight. However, weight is probably a better proxy for puberty than age group is. The proportion of post-pubertal females also increased from summer to spring suggesting a seasonal reproductive pattern. Different definitions of puberty will result in various outcomes, which high-lights the importance of using adequate definition of puberty.

Keywords: Ovaries, Uterus, Follicles, Corpora lutea, Wildlife management, Reproduction

Background

From the 1980s to the 2010s populations of wild boar (*Sus scrofa*) have increased remarkably in Europe [1, 2], and this increase has had widespread ecologic and economic consequences. In forested areas, the increase can affect plant diversity and vegetation composition [3]. In cultivated areas, crop damage of varying severity is frequent [4, 5]. Moreover, the wild boar is also considered a reservoir of various pathogens (e.g. *Mycobacterium bovis* and Hepatitis E virus) that may infect other wildlife, domestic animals, and humans [6, 7].

In addition to the behavior of wild boar (flexible nutrition, and habitat selection etc.), the main reason for the rapid population increase is thought to be due to high reproductive potential [8]. Besides having large litter sizes, puberty at an early age is another important factor contributing to the high reproductive potential. In domestic pigs, lifetime reproductive success and longevity is dependent on several factors such as age at

*Correspondence: Anna.Malmsten@slu.se
Division of Reproduction, Department of Clinical Sciences, Swedish University of Agricultural Sciences, Box 7054, SE-750 07 Uppsala, Sweden

puberty and first mating [9, 10] as well as subsequent factors affecting body condition [11]. The sooner in life reproduction starts, the higher the lifetime offspring production may be. However, there are also disadvantages related to the start of reproduction at an early age because the female may be less physically robust.

In Sweden, since the wild boar reappeared in the 1970s when few individuals escaped enclosures, the population has increased. In 2012 and 2013, 84,000–97,000 animals were culled, per year during hunting [12]. Although controversial, supplemental feeding is applied to a varying extent throughout the wild boar range in Sweden, and its effect on wild boar reproduction is debated. Hunters and farmers claim that supplemental feeding make wild boar gilts pubertal at an earlier age than what is considered to be natural. Other statements include the ability of young gilts to reach puberty throughout the year, which also is considered to be atypical for a short day breeder such as the wild boar [13].

In domestic female animals the definition used for an animal to be able to reproduce, i.e. having attained puberty, is that it should show external signs of oestrous and ovulate [14]. Once puberty has been reached the female should be able to show regular oestrous cycles if not pregnant. In Swedish domestic crossbreed pigs, gilts usually reach puberty at 6–7 months of age [15, 16]. Season can influence reproduction of domestic pigs [17–20], e.g. puberty [21] and age at first mating [22].

In free-ranging wild boar it is difficult to monitor if a gilt shows oestrus and exhibits regular oestrus cycles. Therefore, the majority of studies of puberty in free-ranging female wild boar gilts are based on post-mortem macroscopic examinations of the reproductive organs. Yet, the definition of puberty in these studies varies, which make comparisons difficult. Most commonly signs of ovulation, which is presence of one or more *corpora lutea* (CL), is used to define if the female wild boar has reached puberty [4, 23]. However, others declare that 'puberty is assumed in individuals with follicles more than 3 mm in diameter [24], i.e. without the necessity of the presence of one or more CL. In addition, wild boar females below 1 year of age have been categorized as being cyclic, i.e. having passed puberty, if found with follicles of 6 mm in diameter or larger [25]. The exact timing of when a female passes puberty cannot be detected by macroscopic examination of reproductive organs. This method can only result in proportions of animals in a population that have passed puberty. If the exact timing of puberty needs to be studied, other methods such as repeated fecal [26] or blood [27, 28] sampling for progesterone analyses of fenced animals can be used. These methods are harder, or impossible to apply in free-ranging animals.

The aim of this study was to investigate the proportion of post-pubertal female wild boar gilts in a population subjected to supplemental feeding, in relation to age, weight, and season based on ovarian structures (presence of CL) and uterus characteristics. Also, the effect of another definition of puberty (based upon follicular size) on the outcome of the proportion of female wild boar gilts considered to be able to reproduce in a population were investigated.

Methods

As part of a larger study of female wild boar reproduction, data were collected from hunter-harvested wild boars in seven hunting estates in the southern and middle part of Sweden. Information of habitat composition, feeding practices, estimated population sizes (wild boar and other ungulates) was collected from each estate. The area of the estates varied between 10 and 87 km^2, the density of wild boars were estimated at 5–40 per km^2, and the amount of supplemental feeding was 125,000–300,000 kg/year distributed throughout the year. All estate data was sampled between January 2013 and December 2015, during which culled female wild boar samples were collected. Hunting methods used were drive hunts and stalking. In drive hunts, the hunters are posted at stands around a tracked area. The wild boars are driven towards the hunters by beaters with dogs. This method was used during the main hunting season between October and February and often resulted in a big hunting bag (30–100 animals per day). Stalking was used during spring and summer and the animals were most often shot while feeding on an open field.

In Sweden, wild boar hunting is allowed 24 h and hunting with dogs is allowed between 1 of August and 31 January. The hunting season of adult wild boars is between 16 April and 15 February. Hunting of yearlings is allowed the year around but females with dependent piglets are protected. The sampling effort was for practical reasons biased towards the main hunting season (October–February).

Whole body weight (BW) and field dressed weight (FDW, weight of the eviscerated animal with skin) were noted. In animals where only BW was noted, FDW was estimated using the relationship $FDW = -1.855 + 0.810*BW$ [Pers. comm. N. Lundeheim]. Date of harvest was noted and the year was divided into seasons; spring (March–May), summer (June–August), autumn (September–November), and winter (December–February).

Age was estimated using tooth eruption and tooth replacement [29]. In this study, animals between the ages of 5 and 15 months were included. The age span used was based on previous studies of puberty in domestic pig [16]. Animals where divided into three age classes according to Matschke [29]; 5–8 months, 7.5–12 months, and 12–15 months. The uterus and ovaries were macroscopically examined. The uterus was cut open and the color and thickness of the endometrium was examined. Signs of pregnancy (embryos/fetuses) or signs of previous pregnancy were noted. Presence of enlarged blood vessels in the cut surface between the mesometric ligament (*ligamentum mesometrium*) and the uterus indicated previous pregnancy [Pers. comm. E. Persson; 30]. Luteal structures (*corpora hemorrhagica*, active CL, and regressing CL) were cut open, counted and the diameter was measured to the nearest millimeter. The number and diameter of luteal structures, and follicles (≥4 mm) found in the ovaries was noted. An animal was considered to be post-pubertal if the ovaries contained one or more CL [4, 23], or if the uterus showed signs of previous pregnancy [30]. In order to illustrate how another definition of puberty may influence the outcome of the study, we compared the proportions of post-pubertal animals (according to the definition above) with the proportion of animals found with CL or follicles ≥4 mm [24].

Statistical analyses

Because the response variable is binary, data were analyzed using as generalized linear models (see e.g. [31]) with a binomial distribution and a logistic link function. The Glimmix procedure of the SAS (2009) package was used [32]. The relation between probability of puberty and age, weight and season was of primary interest. Weight was available as a continuous variable, while age was assessed roughly into three classes based on dental status.

In the model building process, models were compared based on the Alailke Information Criterion, AIC [33]. Preliminary analyses suggested that weight, but not age class, should be used as a continuous covariate. In a first model, all interactions were included, but they could all be removed from the model, in a stepwise fashion, based on the AIC. Thus, the final model can be written as

$$\mathrm{logit}(p_{ijk}) = \mu + \alpha_i + \gamma_j + \beta x_k$$

where α_i denotes season *i*, γ_j denotes age class *j*, and x_k is the weight of boar *k*.

The assumptions used were checked by preparing appropriate residual plots; no apparent deviations from the assumptions could be detected. Pairwise comparisons were adjusted for multiplicity using Tukey's method.

Fisher's exact test in R [34] was used to compare the proportion of post-pubertal female wild boars and the proportion of animals found with CL or follicles ≥4 mm, in different age classes.

Results

During the sampling period, 592 female wild boars of different ages were culled and sampled. Of these, 175 individuals met the requirements to be included in this study, which were complete sets of reproductive organs, age span 5–15 months, and weight information. Field dressed weight ranged from 20.6 to 65.3 kg.

In total, 29 (16.6 %) of the examined animals were considered as post-pubertal, and one or more CL were found in all but one of these animals. Of these, 15 were pregnant, nine were cyclic, and four had regressed CL and uterus with signs of previous pregnancy. One animal had no CL structure but the uterus showed signs of previous pregnancy. The mean number of CL in cyclic animals ($n = 9$) was 4.7 (range 2–8) and in pregnant animals ($n = 15$) 5.6 (range 2–9). The mean number of embryos/fetuses was 4.8 (range 2–9) in 13 pregnant animals in which pregnancy had proceeded more than 3 weeks. Counting the exact number of embryos before 3 week of pregnancy ($n = 2$) is difficult at only macroscopic examination. Post-pubertal females were found all seasons but the summer (Fig. 1).

In a first statistical analysis, age class, weight and season were analyzed separately. All of them showed significant relations to puberty: weight ($P < 0.0001$); season ($P = 0.0079$) and age class ($P = 0.0006$). In the joint model, season ($P = 0.0395$) and weight ($P = 0.0002$) were significant, but not age class ($P = 0.7398$). This is because age and weight are highly correlated, and weight is probably a better proxy for puberty than age class is. In Fig. 2, the fitted values from the model are plotted against body weight, with one curve for each season.

There were significant differences of proportions of post-pubertal animals and animals found with CL or follicles ≥4 mm, in different age classes ($P < 0.001$). The different proportions are presented in Table 1.

Discussion

As expected, this study shows that the weight of the female wild boar and as well as the season influenced the variation in proportion of post-pubertal females. The body composition (fat content) has been shown to affect age at puberty in various species [30, 35, 36], including wild boar [25]. To start reproducing, females of most mammal species need to pass a body mass and composition threshold. Females that pass this threshold early, due to favorable conditions such as high feed availability, will thus start reproducing at a young age.

In this study, we found higher proportions of gilts that had passed puberty in the winter and spring months than during the summer and the autumn. No post-pubertal animal was found in the summer season. However, females, regardless of age, accompanied by piglets are

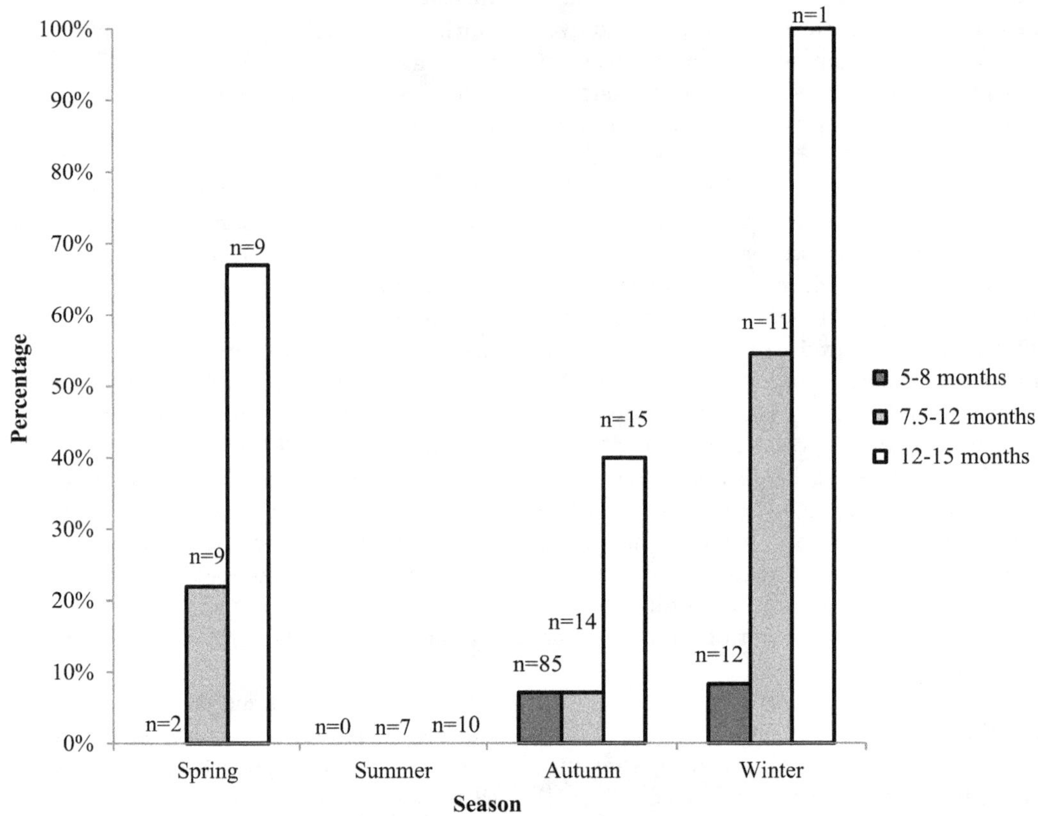

Fig. 1 The proportion of post-pubertal female wild boars according to age class and culling season

prohibited to hunt which might have affected the result. Moreover, the examined animals were culled during hunting and the sampling effort was biased towards the main hunting season October–February which might have influenced the results. Still, the wild boar is a "short day breeder" [13], and we believe that the result mostly are explained by the stimulatory effect of the short days of autumn and winter.

In wild boar, as in most other game species, population growth is dependent on the proportion of females that are able to reproduce. In a species where reproductive capability is reached at a young age, the population growth will be fast, especially in pluriparous species. Because of hunting constraints (not culling females accompanied by piglets), animals included in this study cannot be considered as a random sample. Thus, an underestimation of the proportion post-pubertal animals is possible. Only 11.4 % of the animals aged <12 months were classified as post-pubertal. In southern and middle part of Sweden, the feed availability (excluding supplemental feeding) is high for wild boar, both as crops and natural feed. During periods of natural feed shortage, as in winter, supplemental feeding is extensive. Considering the food availability, one would suspect that the proportion of post-pubertal animals would have been higher and more in accordance to other studies [4, 23] of wild boars using the same definition of puberty (occurrence of ovarian CL) as in present study. Extensive supplemental feeding has earlier been discussed as one of the main causes of passing puberty at a young age [23]. Cellina [23] reported that in Luxemburg, 24 % of supplementary fed wild boar females aged <12 months were post-pubertal, and the youngest was four months old. No females younger than 5 months of age were investigated in the present study, but based on the low proportion (7.1 %) of post-pubertal gilts aged 5–8 months it is unlikely that younger females had passed puberty to a significant extent. However, due to the wide age category (months), it is impossible to know whether pregnant animals in this study had reached puberty within the noted age category or at a younger age.

Ahmad et al. [4] showed a very high proportion (25/32) of gilts aged 4–7 months in Pakistan with CL, which differ from wild boars in this study as well as from a study in Luxemburg [23]. Thus, wild boars in Pakistan seem to be more similar to domestic pigs than Swedish wild boar. Therefore, the genetic background of wild boars may be of importance for the pubertal age as seen in the domestic pigs [32] and need to be studied in different regions/

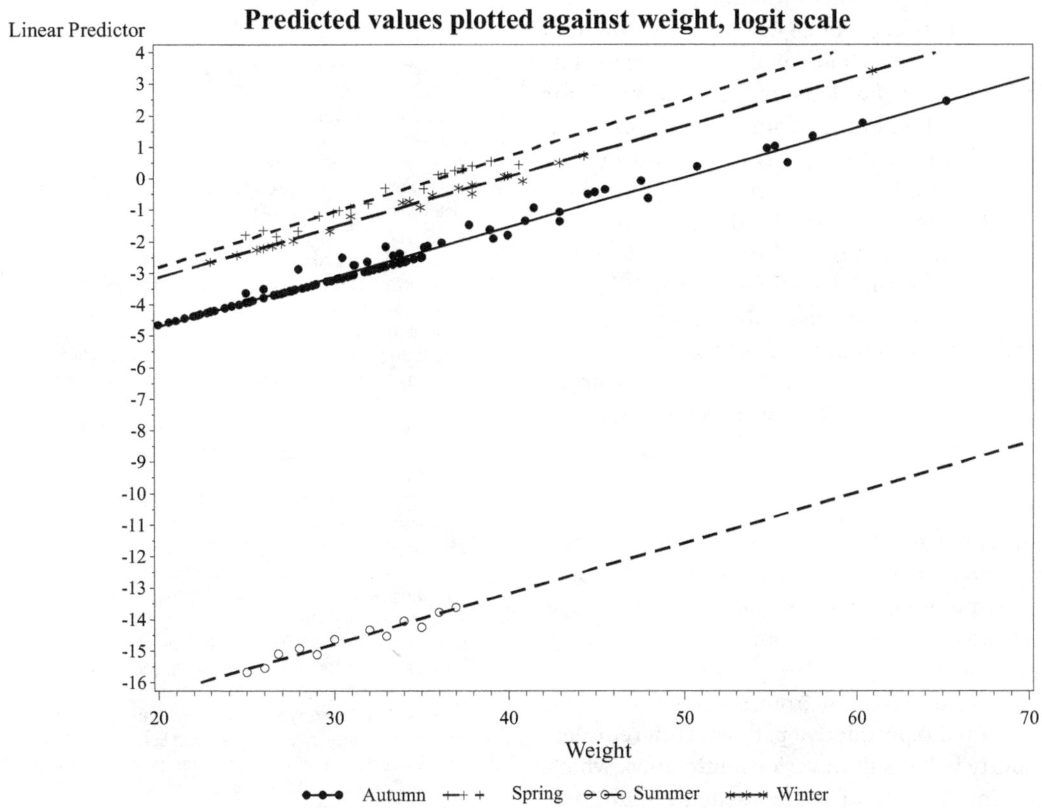

Fig. 2 Predicted values of puberty in female wild boars, plotted against body weight and divided by season

Table 1 Numbers and proportion of Swedish female wild boars in puberty in different age classes, according to two previously used definitions

Age class (months)	N	Females attained puberty (%) according to definition A[a]	Females attained puberty (%) according to definition B[b]
5–8	99	7 (7.1)	79 (79.8)
7.5–12	41	9 (22.0)	37 (90.2)
12–15	35	13 (37.1)	34 (97.1)
Total	175	29 (16.6)	150 (85.7)

[a] Presence of corpus luteum or previous signs of pregnancy in uterus [4, 23]

[b] Presence of corpora luteum or ovarian follicles ≥4 mm [24]

countries. Domestic, crossbred pigs normally reach puberty at 6–7 months of age [15, 16] and if gilts have not reached puberty at the age of 8 months they are considered to have delayed puberty [16]. This illustrates one substantial difference between domestic European pig breeds and wild boar. As presented in Table 1, different definitions of puberty have a major effect on the result of the proportion of female wild boar gilts considered to have passed puberty in a population as well as in different age classes. In the present study, 79.8 % of the examined wild boars aged 5–8 months was found with follicles ≥4 mm only or with CL and would have reached puberty according to this definition. This result is similar to the one of Gethöffer et al. [24] who found an 80 % chance of juveniles having attained sexual maturity at 8 months of age using that definition. Gethöffer et al. [24] based their definition of puberty on studies on the viability of the oocyte in various follicle sizes. A great caution must be taken when using such definition of puberty because a large number of follicles will become atretic before the animal has reached puberty, with no regards to whether the oocyte is viable or not at a certain stage. When using only follicle size, the proportion of wild boar females considered being capable to reproduce will be overestimated.

Presence of CL shows that ovulation indeed has occurred. This is the definitions of puberty used for domestic pigs [16, 37] and other domestic species when examining reproductive organs. It is also important to include uterus characteristics when evaluating if an animal has reached puberty or not. In the present study one of the animals that had passed puberty had no CL (being anoestral) and would have been 'missjugded' as non-pubertal using definitions that only consider ovarian findings. In addition, by examining the uterus it is possible to distinguish gilts in anoestrous from sows in anoestrus (passed pregnancy), as well as pregnant females (>2 weeks of pregnancy) from females that are cyclic.

Conclusions

Season, weight and age significantly influenced the variation in proportion of post-pubertal females. The proportion of post-pubertal animals increased with age and weight. However, weight is probably a better proxy for puberty than age group is. The proportion of post-pubertal females also increased from summer to spring suggesting a seasonal reproductive pattern. Different definitions of puberty will result in various outcomes, which high-lights the importance of using adequate definition of puberty.

Authors' contributions

AM and AMD were involved in the design and coordination of the study, data collection, organ examination, and drafting the manuscript. Both authors read and approved the final manuscript.

Acknowledgements

We thank all of the wildlife managers and hunters who assisted in data collection. We are most thankful to Ulf Olsson and Nils Lundeheim for their statistical guidance. The study was supported financially by the Swedish Environmental Protection Agency and the Swedish Association for Hunting and Wildlife Management.

Competing interests

The authors declare that they have no competing interests.

References

1. Boitani L, Trapanese P, Mattei L. Methods of population estimates of a hunted wild boar (*Sus scrofa* L.) population in Tuscany (Italy). IBEX J Mt Ecol. 1995;3:204–8.
2. Ježek M, Štípek K, Kušta T, Červený J, Vícha J. Reproductive and morphometric characteristics of wild boar (*Sus scrofa*) in the Czech Republic. J For Sci. 2011;57:285–92.
3. Welander J. Spatial and temporal dynamics of wild boar (*Sus scrofa*) rooting in a mosaic landscape. J Zool. 2000;252:263–71.
4. Ahmad E, Brooks JE, Hussain I, Khan MH. Reproduction in Eurasian wild boar in central Punjab Pakistan. Acta Theriol. 1995;40:163–73.
5. Geisser H, Reyer HU. The influence of food and temperature on population density of wild boar *Sus scrofa* in the Thurgau (Switzerland). J Zool. 2005;267:89–96.
6. Naranjo V, Gortázar C, Vicente J, de la Fuente J. Evidence of the role of European wild boar as a reservoir of Mycobacterium tuberculosis complex. Vet Microbiol. 2008;127:1–9.
7. Ruiz-Fons F, Segalés J, Gortázar C. A review of viral diseases of the European wild boar: effects of population dynamics and reservoir role. The Vet J. 2008;176:158–69.
8. Servanty S, Gaillard JM, Allaine D, Brandt D, Baubet E. Litter size and fetal sex ratio adjustment in a highly polytocous species: the wild boar. Behav Ecol. 2007;18:427–32.
9. Tummaruk P, Lundeheim N, Einarsson S, Dalin AM. Effect of birth litter size, birth parity number, growth rate, backfat thickness and age at first mating of gilts on their reproductive performance as sows. Anim Rep Sci. 2001;66:225–37.
10. Bortololozzo FP, Bernhard ML, Kummer R, Wentz I. Growth, body state and breeding performance in gilts and primiparous sows. Soc Reprod Fertil Suppl. 2009;66:281–91.
11. Engblom L, Lundeheim N, Strandberg E, del Schneider M, Dalin AM, Andersson K. Factors affecting length of productive life in Swedish commercial sows. J Anim Sci. 2007;86:432–41.
12. Svenska Jägareförbundet. 2016. http://jagareforbundet.se/aktuellt/forbundsnyheter/2015/07/rapport-fran-vildsvinssasongen-201314/. Accessed 4 Apr 2016.
13. Mauget R. Seasonality of reproduction in the wild boar. In: Cole DJA, Foxcroft GR, editors. Control of pig reproduction. London: Butterworths; 1982. p. 509–26.
14. Evans ACO, O'Doherty JV. Endocrine changes and management factors affecting puberty in gilts. Livest Prod Sci. 2001;68:1–12.
15. Hughes PE. Factors affecting the natural attainment of puberty in the gilt. In: Cole DJA, Foxcroft GR, editors. Control of pig reproduction. London: Butterworths; 1982. p. 117–38.
16. Dalin AM, Eliasson L. Clinical, morphological and endocrinological studies in gilts with delayed puberty. Acta Vet Scand. 1987;28:263–9.
17. Love RJ, Evans G. Kluoiec C. Seasonal effects on fertility in gilts and sows. J Reprod Fertil Suppl. 1993;48:191–206.
18. Peltoniemi OAT, Love RJ, Heinonen M, Tuovinen V, Saloniemi H. Seasonal and management effects on fertility of the sow: a descriptive study. Anim Rep Sci. 1999;55:47–61.
19. Tummaruk P, Lundeheim N, Einarsson S, Dalin AM. Reproductive performance of purebred Swedish Landrace and Swedish Yorkshire sows I. Seasonal variation and parity influence. Acta Agric Scand. 2000;50:205–16.
20. Tast A, Peltoniemi OAT, Virolainen JV, Love RJ. Early disruption of pregnancy as a manifestation of seasonal infertility in pigs. Anim Reprod Sci. 2002;74:75–86.
21. Paterson AM, Pearce GP. D'AntuònoMF. Seasonal variation in attainment of puberty in isolated and boar-exposed domestic gilts. Anim Reprod Sci. 1991;24:323–33.
22. Tummaruk P, Lundeheim N, Einarsson S, Dalin AM. Factors influencing age at first mating in purebred Swedish Landrace and Swedish Yorkshire gilts. Anim Reprod Sci. 2000;63:241–53.
23. Cellina S. Effects of supplemental feeding on the body condition and reproductive state of wild boar *Sus scrofa* in Luxembourg. Dissertation, University of Sussex. 2008.
24. Gethöffer F, Sodeikat G, Pohlmeyer K. Reproductive parameters of wild boar (*Sus Scrofa*) in three different parts of Germany. Eur J Wildl Res. 2007;53:287–97.
25. Gaillard JM, Jullien JM. Body weight effect on reproduction of young wild boar (*Sus Scrofa*) females: a comparative analysis. Folia Zool. 1993;42:204–12.
26. Hultén F, Zang BR, Forsberg M, Dalin AM. Applying a progesterone assay to faecal samples collected from sows during the oetrous cycle. Reprod Dom Anim. 1995;30:101–5.
27. Delcroix I, Mauget R, Signoret JP. Existence of synchronization of reproduction at the level of the social group of the European wild boar (*Sus scrofa*). J Reprod Fert. 1990;89:613–7.

28. Tast A, Hälli O, Peltoniemi OA. A practical method for non-surgically inserting intra arterial catheters in European wild boars (*Sus scrofa*). Vet Res Commun. 2000;24:25–30.
29. Matschke GH. Aging European wild hogs by dentition. J Wildl Manag. 1967;31:109–10.
30. Malmsten J. Söderquist, Thulin CG, Gavier Widén D, Yon L, Dalin AM. Reproductive characteristics in female Swedish moose (*Alces alces*), with emphasis on puberty, timing of oestrus, and mating. Acta Vet Scand. 2014;56:1–10.
31. Olsson U. Generalized linear models—an applied approach. Lund: Studentlitteratur; 2002.
32. SAS Institute Inc. (2011): SAS/Stat User's Guide. Version 9. Cary, N. C., SAS Institute Inc.
33. Akaike H. Prediction and entropy. In: Atkinson AC, Fienberg SE, editors. A celebration of statistics. New York: Springer; 1985. p. 1–24.
34. R Core Team. 2013. R: a language and environment for statistical computing. r foundation for statistical computing, Vienna, http://www.R-project.org/. ISBN 3-900051-07-0.
35. Hutchens LK, Hintz RL, Johnson RK. Breed comparison for age and weight at puberty in gilts. J Anim Sci. 1982;55:60–6.
36. Eliasson L, Rydhmer L, Einarsson S, Andersson K. Relationship between puberty and production traits in the gilt: 1 age at puberty. Anim Reprod Sci. 1991;25:143–54.
37. Andersson AM, Einarsson S, Edqvist LE. Prepubertal LH, oestradiol-17β and progesterone pattern in gilts. Zbl Vet Med A. 1983;30:438–46.

4

The effect of dexmedetomidine on cerebral perfusion and oxygenation in healthy piglets with normal and lowered blood pressure anaesthetized with propofol-remifentanil total intravenous anaesthesia

Mai Louise Grandsgaard Mikkelsen[1*], Rikard Ambrus[2], Rune Rasmussen[3], James Edward Miles[1], Helle Harding Poulsen[1], Finn Borgbjerg Moltke[4,5] and Thomas Eriksen[1]

Abstract

Background: During anaesthesia and surgery, in particular neurosurgery, preservation of cerebral perfusion and oxygenation (CPO) is essential for normal postoperative brain function. The isolated effects on CPO of either individual anaesthetic drugs or entire anaesthetic protocols are of importance in both clinical and research settings. Total intravenous anaesthesia (TIVA) with propofol and remifentanil is widely used in human neuroanaesthesia. In addition, dexmedetomidine is receiving increasing attention as an anaesthetic adjuvant in neurosurgical, intensive care, and paediatric patients. Despite the extensive use of pigs as animal models in neuroscience and the increasing use of both propofol-remifentanil and dexmedetomidine, very little is known about their combined effect on CPO in pigs with uninjured brains. This study investigates the effect of dexmedetomidine on CPO in piglets with normal and lowered blood pressure during background anaesthesia with propofol-remifentanil TIVA. Sixteen healthy female Danish pigs (crossbreeds of Danish Landrace, Yorkshire and Duroc, 25–34 kg) were used. Three animals were subsequently excluded. The animals were randomly allocated into one of two groups with either normal blood pressure (NBP, $n = 6$) or with induced low blood pressure (LBP, $n = 7$). Both groups were subjected to the same experimental protocol. Intravenous propofol induction was performed without premedication. Anaesthesia was maintained with propofol-remifentanil TIVA, and later supplemented with continuous infusion of dexmedetomidine. Assessments of cerebral perfusion obtained by laser speckle contrast imaging (LSCI) were related to cerebral oxygenation measures ($P_{br}O_2$) obtained by an intracerebral Clark-type Licox probe.

Results: Addition of dexmedetomidine resulted in a 32% reduction in median $P_{br}O_2$ values for the LBP group ($P = 0.03$), but no significant changes in $P_{br}O_2$ were observed for the NBP group. No significant changes in LSCI readings were observed in either group between any time points, despite a 28% decrease in the LBP group following dexmedetomidine administration. Caval block resulted in a significant ($P = 0.02$) reduction in median MAP from

*Correspondence: mailo@sund.ku.dk
[1] Department of Veterinary Clinical Sciences, Faculty of Health and Medical Sciences, University of Copenhagen, 16 Dyrlægevej, 1870 Frederiksberg C, Denmark
Full list of author information is available at the end of the article

68 mmHg (range 63–85) at PCB to 58 mmHg (range 53–63) in the LBP group, but no significant differences in either $P_{br}O_2$ or LSCI were observed due to this intervention ($P = 0.6$ and $P = 0.3$ respectively).

Conclusions: Addition of dexmedetomidine to propofol-remifentanil TIVA resulted in a significant decrease in cerebral oxygenation ($P_{br}O_2$) measurements in piglets with lowered blood pressure. Cerebral perfusion (LSCI) did not decrease significantly in this group. In piglets with normal blood pressure, no significant changes in cerebral perfusion or oxygenation were seen in response to addition of dexmedetomidine to the background anaesthesia.

Keywords: Cerebral perfusion, Cerebral oxygenation, Swine, Propofol, Remifentanil, Dexmedetomidine, Laser speckle contrast imaging, Licox

Background

During anaesthesia and surgery, in particular neurosurgery, preservation of cerebral perfusion and oxygenation (CPO) is essential for normal postoperative brain function [1, 2]. Choice of anaesthetic protocol, cerebral pathology, the patient's haemodynamic stability, and their interaction can influence the CPO response [3, 4]. Studies in rabbits have shown significant differences in the cerebral perfusion responses to anaesthetics in normal and injured brains [5, 6], so CPO results from neurocritical studies cannot be definitively translated to patients with normal brain physiology. In humans over 60 years, both short and long-term postoperative cognitive disorders can be seen following anaesthesia in relation to both non-cardiac and non-neurologic major surgery [7]. In this context, understanding of the anaesthetic effect on CPO in the healthy brain must be considered a prerequisite for understanding the pathology and anaesthetic influence in the diseased brain [3]. Total intravenous anaesthesia (TIVA) with a combination of propofol and remifentanil is extensively used during ambulatory surgery, paediatric surgery and neurosurgery in humans [8–11]. This combination of anaesthetics has several characteristics that preserve cerebrovascular reactivity to CO_2 and autoregulatory mechanisms [11–14], and can be a suitable basis anaestesia in experimental CPO studies.

In this context, alpha$_2$-adrenergic-agonists, in particular dexmedetomidine, are receiving increasing attention as sedatives and as anaesthetic adjuvants for neurosurgical, intensive care and paediatric human patients [15–19]. In veterinary anaesthesia, α_2-adrenergic-agonists have been used widely for sedation and as part of general anaesthesia for many years [20–22]. Dexmedetomidine potentiates propofol and opioids and has been shown to reduce cerebral blood flow (CBF), possess neuroprotective properties, and to be suitable for continuous infusion in TIVA and conscious sedation in humans [17, 23–26]. In spite of this, the use of dexmedetomidine in patients with cardiovascular disease or cerebral pathology is still debated primarily with regards to systemic hypotension, bradycardia and potential cerebral vasoconstriction [27].

Both in human and veterinary anaesthesia it is recommended that these patients need individually tailored neuroanaesthesia in order to maintain optimal CPO [21, 28, 29]. Due to ethical concerns regarding clinical studies in humans, strategies for individually tailored neuroanesthesia are often explored in experimental animals. Porcine animal models are well described in neuroscience and are often preferred over smaller animals due to the closer resemblance to the human brain in anatomy, growth, and development [30]. Despite the extensive use of pigs as animal models and the abundant use of propofol-remifentanil in human neuroanaesthesia and dexmedetomidine in veterinary anaesthesia in general, very little is known about their combined effect on CPO in anaesthetized pigs with uninjured brains. Guidelines for anaesthesia in experimental animal trials studying CPO are, therefore, poorly established [31].

The objective of this study was to investigate the effect of dexmedetomidine on CPO in piglets with normal and lowered blood pressure during background anaesthesia with propofol-remifentanil TIVA.

Methods

Study design

This study was designed as a non-blinded, two-arm parallel group, experimental animal trial. Animals were allocated into one of two groups with either normal blood pressure (NBP) or with low blood pressure (LBP) by a computerized lottery draw randomization schedule (www.random.org). Figure 1 illustrates the experimental protocol; additional data will be reported separately. Full details and data regarding the entire study are presented in Additional file 1. The Danish Animal Experiments Inspectorate approved the study (licence no. 2013-15-2934-00909), and all procedures were performed in accordance with national legislation and The Council of Europe Convention ETS 123. All animals were acquired through, and housed by, the Department of Animal Experimental Medicine at the University of Copenhagen. The piglets were inspected and considered healthy on reception at the housing facility by the veterinarian

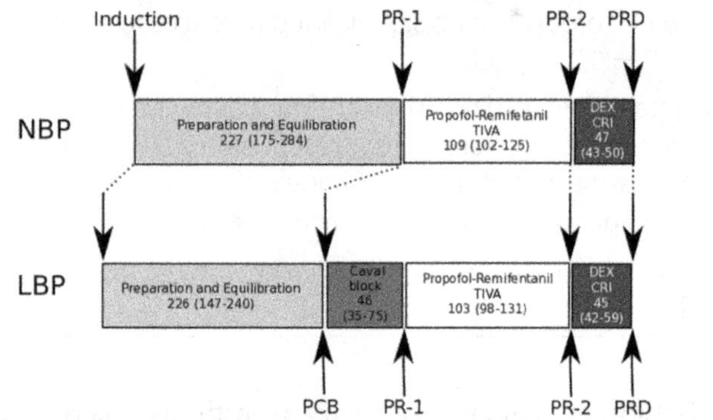

Fig. 1 Experimental design. The experimental flow for the two groups (*NBP* normal blood pressure group, *LBP* low blood pressure group), with the median duration of each period (min–max range in brackets). Key time points are marked (*arrows*), and corresponding time points between groups are joined by *dotted lines*. *PCB* Pre-caval Block, *PR-1* Propofol-remifentanil experimental start, *PR-2* Propofol-remifentanil end–immediately prior to dexmedetomidine infusion, *PR-D* following dexmedetomidine infusion

responsible for the trial. The piglets were allowed to acclimatize to the facility for at least 1 week before the experiment began. The piglets were housed in groups of 3–4 (in the same group as they arrived) in cement-floored pens measuring 5.5 m^2 with fine wood chip and straw bedding. Environmental enrichment with toys and music were supplied through the daytime. A 7:17 light:dark cycle was used and the room temperature were kept at 19–20 °C. The piglets were fed a commercial finisher diet (Svinefoder 5, Nordsjællands Andels Grovvareforening Amba, Helsinge, Denmark), given according to weight twice daily (0800 and 1500), and the piglets had free access to water. Food, but not water, was withheld overnight prior to the experiment.

The results of this study are reported in accordance with ARRIVE guidelines [32].

Animals and anaesthesia

Sixteen healthy female Danish pigs (crossbreeds of Danish Landrace, Yorkshire and Duroc) with a median weight of 27 kg (range 25–34) were used. Venous access for propofol induction was secured the day prior to the experiment under sedation (see Additional file 2), using catheters (Arrow® arterial catheterization set, SAC-00822: 20 ga × 8 cm, Teleflex, Ireland) placed in the auricular vein of both ears.

All 16 animals were subjected to the same anaesthetic protocol: no premedication was given on the day of the experiment. General anaesthesia was induced by an intravenous (iv) bolus of 4–8 mg/kg propofol (10 mg/ml Propofol "B. Braun", B. Braun Melsungen, Germany), while the animals were still in their pen to minimise stress. After transport to the experimental area, they were placed in ventral recumbency on a padded operating table and mechanically ventilated following endotracheal intubation. A mechanical ventilator (Bag-in-bottle respirator, Type no. 86,298, Dameca A/S, Roedovre, Denmark) was used to maintain end tidal CO_2 ($EtCO_2$) between 35 and 50 mmHg by regulation of the respiration rate (RR) (11–21/min) and tidal volume (10–15 ml/kg) to keep the inflation pressure below 20 cm H_2O using an inspiration:expiration ratio of 1:2 and a set PEAK pressure of 20 cm H_2O. The circuit used was a co-axial circle-system.

General anaesthesia was maintained by propofol (10 mg/ml Propofol "B. Braun", B. Braun Melsungen, Germany) and remifentanil (1 mg/ml Ultiva®, GlaxoSmithKline Pharma, Denmark, diluted with sterile water to 100 μg/ml) TIVA using separate syringe pumps (Terumo, Terufusion Syringe Pump TE-331, Belgium). Doses were based on our pilot studies, with a propofol dose range of 12–20 mg/kg/h and a remifentanil dose range of 20–45 μg/kg/h. Doses were individually regulated to accomplish unresponsiveness to noxious stimuli (dewclaw pinching). Propofol doses were adjusted to control anaesthetic depth (assessed as lack of movement) and remifentanil doses were adjusted to eliminate responses to noxious stimuli. Propofol and remifentanil doses were not altered after animal preparation was completed. Dexmedetomidine (0.5 mg/ml Dexdomitor®, Orion Pharma Animal Health, Sollentuna, Sweden) was added following time point PR2 (Fig. 1) with an iv bolus of 1 μg/kg administrated over 10 min, followed by a fixed dose of 0.7 μg/kg/h iv (5 μg/ml solution).

Surgical preparation and instrumentation

All invasive procedures were conducted after local infiltration with a mixture of lidocaine (20 mg/ml Xylocain® AstraZeneca, Copenhagen, Denmark) and bupivacaine (5 mg/ml Marcain® AstraZeneca, Copenhagen, Denmark).

A circular craniotomy (20–30 mm) was performed over the right parietal lobe with a 5 mm craniotome (Midas Rex, Medtronic, Heerlen, The Netherlands). After dural excision, cerebral perfusion was directly measured semi-quantitatively (laser speckle perfusion units—LSPU) using a laser speckle contrast imaging (LSCI) camera (moorFLPI-2, Moor Instruments, Devon, UK) placed perpendicular to and 25 cm from the region of interest. The position of the head of the animal remained unchanged throughout the experiment. An intracerebral Clark-type probe connected to a Licox® Brain Tissue Oxygen Monitoring System (Integra LifeSciences, New Jersey, USA) was placed in the periphery of the craniotomy, in white matter 25 mm subdurally and secured to the craniotomy edge with bone wax for recording of cerebral oxygenation (partial pressure of oxygen in brain tissue—$P_{br}O_2$).

The femoral artery was cannulated (Arrow® arterial catheterization set, SAC-01620: 20 ga × 16 cm, Teleflex, Ireland) for invasive blood pressure monitoring and intermittent blood collection for blood gas analysis (GEM Premier 3000, Instrumentation Laboratory, Lexington MA, USA). The femoral vein was cannulated for placement of an 8 French balloon-tipped catheter (MILA International Inc., Kentucky, USA) in all animals but only used for induction of caval block in the LBP group. The catheter was premeasured to position the balloon in the caudal vena cava just caudal to the heart. Caval block was induced by injecting sterile isotonic NaCl into the catheter balloon to partially obstruct the vena cava.

A urinary catheter with a closed collecting bag was placed to prevent bladder distension. Fluids were administered throughout the experiment at 2.5 ml/kg/h iv (glucose 50 mg/ml, B. Braun Melsungen. Germany).

A multiparametric bedside monitor (Datex-Ohmeda S/5, Helsinki, Finland) was used to record cardiovascular and pulmonary variables every 30 s: data were transferred to a personal computer using Datex-Ohmeda S/5™ Collect software (GE Healthcare, Helsinki, Finland). Recorded variables were pulse rate, invasive mean arterial blood pressure (MAP), body temperature by oesophageal probe, fraction of inspired oxygen (FiO_2) and $EtCO_2$. The electrocardiogram and peripheral oxygen saturation by pulse oximetry (SpO_2) measured on the tail or the lower lip were monitored for continuous assessment.

Experimental protocol

After instrumentation the Licox probe was equilibrated for up to 2 h or until $P_{br}O_2$ exceeded 25 mmHg before baseline data were collected (PR-1–NBP and PCB–LBP) for all animals (Fig. 1). In the LBP group, MAP was then lowered by caval block until a stable MAP of 50–60 mmHg was reached, and data recording was repeated (PR1–LBP). The caval block was maintained unadjusted throughout the experiment. Data were collected at all key time points (Fig. 1), with time point PRD placed following 30 min of dexmedetomidine infusion. Arterial blood gas samples for analysis of pH, P_aCO_2, P_aO_2, bicarbonate (HCO_3^-), base excess (BE), blood glucose, lactate, total haemoglobin concentration (THbc) and haematocrit (Hct) were obtained at each time point.

Between PR-1 and PR-2, and following PRD, vasopressor challenges were made using norepinephrine and phenylephrine. A 30-min washout period was allowed before time point PR2. Data collected during these periods of vasopressor challenge will be reported separately.

At the end of the experiments, the animals were euthanized with pentobarbital sodium iv (400 mg/ml, Euthasol vet., Virbac, Denmark).

Statistics

Statistical per protocol analysis was performed using SPSS 24.0 software (IBM® SPSS® Statistics for Mac, IBM Corp. ©, Armonk, NY, USA), and Microsoft® Excel® for Mac 2011 version 14.3.9 (2010 Microsoft Corporation). Normal distribution of data could not be assumed due to the sample size and non-parametric statistical analyses were used. Data are reported as median values with either range (min–max) or 95% confidence intervals (95% CI) obtained using Hodges–Lehmann estimates given where appropriate. P-values ≤ 0.05 were considered statistically significant. Comparisons between time-points PCB and PR-1 (LBP group) were made using Wilcoxon's signed rank test. Comparisons between LBP and NBP were made using the independent-samples median test. Comparisons of primary outcome measures ($P_{br}O_2$ and LSPU) and secondary explanatory variables (haemodynamics and blood gas) across time points PR-1 to PR-2 and PR-2 to PRD were made using Friedman's ANOVA with post hoc Bonferroni corrected pairwise comparisons when Friedman's ANOVA was significant. Comparisons between selected time point medians and literature-derived cut-off values were made using the one-sided, one-sample Wilcoxon signed rank test to determine if medians lay above the cut-off. A sample size of 16 animals, divided into two groups of 8, was calculated using conservative estimates based on earlier studies [33] with expected power of 80% in detecting a minimum of 30% difference in MAP with a two-tailed significance level of 5% after supplementation of dexmedetomidine.

Results

All 16 animals completed the experimental protocol. Data from three (NBP group n = 2, LBP group n = 1) piglets were excluded from analysis. One piglet developed signs of brain oedema with a severe reduction in CPO following craniotomy (LBP group). In the NBP group, one pig had persistently and unexplainably high pulse rate, $EtCO_2$, P_aCO_2 and a low pH, which were expected to produce an atypical CPO response. The other pig was excluded due to technical difficulties.

Anaesthesia time, preparation time, anaesthetic doses and baseline CPO measurements were not statistically different between NBP and LBP groups. Both groups reached normal cerebral oxygenation levels following animal preparation and equilibration of the Licox probe (Table 1) [8, 34].

Caval block resulted in a significant (P = 0.02) reduction in median MAP from 68 mmHg (range 63–85) at

Table 1 Baseline data. Data were recorded at time points PR1 (normal blood pressure group—NBP) and PCB (low blood pressure group—LBP), prior to induction of caval block in the LBP group

	Propofol-remifentanil 1 (PR-1) NBP (n = 6)	Pre-caval block (PCB) LBP (n = 7)	P value
Preparation time (min)	227 (175–284)	226 (147–240)	0.63
Propofol dose (mg/kg/h)	15 (12–20)	15 (12–18)	1.00
Remifentanil dose (µg/kg/h)	30 (20–40)	25 (20–45)	0.53
Cerebral oxygenation ($P_{br}O_2$ mmHg)	25.6 (19.9–55.7)	29.6 (20.3–32.2)	0.45
Cerebral perfusion (LSPU)	1033.9 (730.4–1251.5)	1090.7 (845.5–1762.0)	0.53

Data are reported as median and range (min–max)

$P_{br}O_2$, partial pressure of oxygen in brain tissue; LSPU, laser speckle perfusion unit

PCB to 58 mmHg (range 53–63) at PR1 in the LBP group (Fig. 2), but no significant differences in either $P_{br}O_2$ or LSPU were observed due to this intervention ($P = 0.6$ and $P = 0.3$ respectively) (Fig. 3).

A significant difference in the intra-group distributions of $P_{br}O_2$ readings was observed between time points PR-1, PR-2 and PRD for group LBP ($P = 0.05$), but not for NBP ($P = 0.5$). Post-hoc Bonferroni corrected pairwise comparisons showed a significant ($P = 0.03$) 32% reduction in median $P_{br}O_2$ values (−7 mmHg, 95% CI −2; −17) for LBP between PR-2 and PRD. Median $P_{br}O_2$ readings for both groups were significantly ($P < 0.03$, one-tailed) higher than the threshold value of 15 mmHg for cerebral ischaemia at all time points [35, 36]. No significant changes in the distributions of LSPU readings were observed for either group between time-points PR-1, PR-2 and PRD, despite a 28% fall in LSPU values (median difference −186 LSPU, 95% CI −7; −478) in the LBP group following dexmedetomidine administration. No significant between-group differences were detected at any time point.

In the LBP group, median MAP was significantly ($P < 0.03$, one-tailed) greater than the lower limit for cerebral autoregulation (LLCA) of 50 mmHg at all time points except PRD, but in the NBP group median MAP was consistently above this limit ($P = 0.01$, one-tailed).

No statistically significant intra-group changes in MAP over time points PR-1, PR-2 and PRD were observed, despite a trend to an increase from PR-1 to PR-2 (median 6 mmHg, 95% CI −10; 13 and 9 mmHg, 95% CI −4; 25 for LBP and NBP, respectively) and a decrease from PR-2 to PRD (median −10 mmHg, 95% CI −1; −22 and −6 mmHg, 95% CI −18; 5). This corresponds to a 19% reduction of median MAP in the LBP group following dexmedetomidine infusion. At all time points, median MAP values were significantly ($P = 0.03$) lower for the LBP group than for the NBP group, with median differences of 8−25 mmHg.

In the LBP group, there was a significant ($P = 0.02$) increase in median pulse rate following initiation of caval block (median increase 10, 95% CI 2; 47). No significant differences were found between time points PR1, PR2 and PRD for either group, or between groups at any time point.

For both LBP and NBP groups, a significant ($P = 0.02$ for both) intra-group change in $EtCO_2$ distributions was observed. Pairwise testing showed a significant decrease in median values of 5 mmHg (95% CI 2; 11) for LBP ($P = 0.02$) and 4 mmHg (95% CI 2; 5) for NBP ($P = 0.01$) between time points PR-2 and PR-D. This was associated in the LBP group, but not the NBP group, with a significant ($P = 0.03$) decrease in median $PaCO_2$ readings of 5 mmHg (95% CI 2.5; 9) from PR-2 to PR-D. A trend to increasing $EtCO_2$ levels in the LBP group between PR-1 and PR-2 was associated with a significant ($P = 0.03$) increase in P_aCO_2 levels (median increase 6, 95% CI 1; 11). Median P_aCO_2 values were 0-3.5 mmHg higher, and median $EtCO_2$ values 0.6–2 mmHg higher, in the LBP group than the NBP group, but this was not statistically significant at any time point.

Median body temperature was 0.8–1.5 °C higher in the LBP group than the NBP group across time points PR-1, PR-2 to PRD, but this was not statistically significant (Table 2). No significant intra-group changes in distribution were observed.

Additional physiological parameters are reported in Table 2.

Discussion

The key finding in this study was the significant fall in cerebral oxygenation following supplementation with dexmedetomidine to propofol-remifentanil TIVA in piglets with lowered blood pressure but not in piglets with normal blood pressure.

Cerebral perfusion and oxygenation response to dexmedetomidine

In the piglets with normal blood pressure neither cerebral perfusion nor oxygenation changed significantly after addition of dexmedetomidine to propofol-remifentanil TIVA. This supports previous findings that

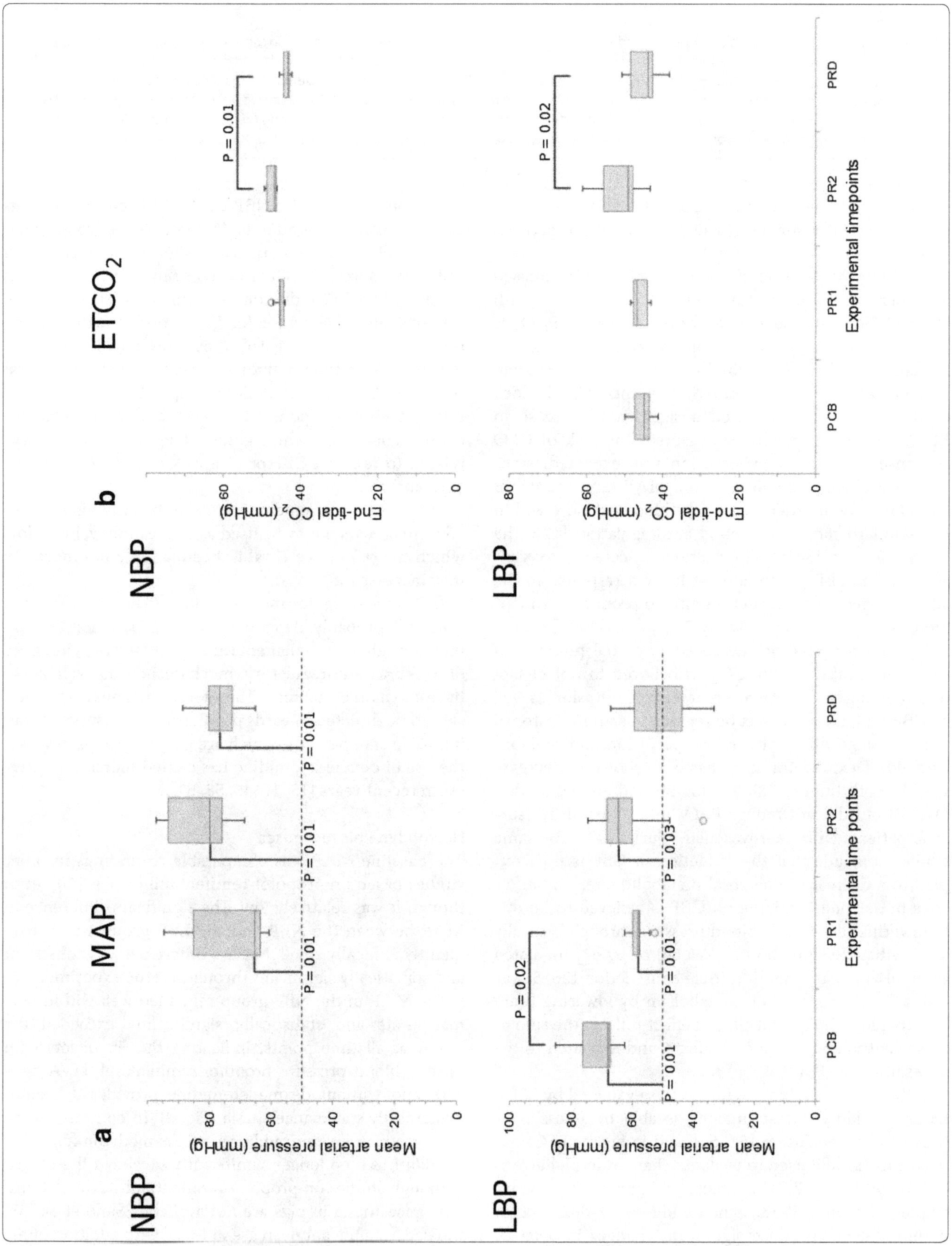

a
MAP
NBP
LBP
Mean arterial pressure (mmHg)
P = 0.01
P = 0.01
P = 0.01
P = 0.02
P = 0.01
P = 0.01
P = 0.03
PCB
PR1
PR2
PRD
Experimental time points
b
ETCO2
NBP
LBP
End-tidal CO2 (mmHg)
P = 0.01
P = 0.02
PCB
PR1
PR2
PRD
Experimental timepoints

(See figure on previous page.)

Fig. 2 *Boxplots* of mean arterial blood pressure and end-tidal carbon dioxide at the different timepoints. *Box* and *whisker* plots showing median (line), interquartile range (*shaded*) and outliers (*circles*) for mean arterial pressure (in mmHg) (**a**), and end-tidal carbon dioxide ($ETCO_2$, in mmHg) (**b**) in the normal blood pressure group (NBP) and low blood pressure group (LBP). *Whiskers* extend a maximum of 1.5× the interquartile range. The lower mean arterial pressure limit for cerebral autoregulation is shown (*dashed line*). Experimental timepoints: *PCB* pre-caval block, *PR-1* initial baseline for propofol-remifentanil TIVA, *PR-2* immediately before dexmedetomidine administration, *PRD* following propofol-remifentanil-dexmedetomidine TIVA. Significant differences from either the autoregulation limit (*vertical bars*) or between timepoints (*horizontal bars*) are shown

dexmedetomidine does not affect $P_{br}O_2$ in patients with normal blood pressure and healthy brains [19] or patients with neurovascular injuries [43].

Cerebral oxygenation measured by Licox decreased after dexmedetomidine supplementation in piglets with lowered blood pressure. The normal range for $P_{br}O_2$ is 25–30 mmHg in pigs [34], which is comparable to the human normal range of 25–50 mmHg [8]. Our median baseline results were within these limits. Caval block in the LBP group produced a significant decrease in MAP, but not in the CPO measures. The lack of CPO response to induced hypotension was expected, since the caval block was adjusted to a MAP target range of 50–60 mmHg in order to keep the blood pressure within the standard range of cerebral autoregulation [12]. The subsequent significant 32% decrease in cerebral oxygenation in the LBP group is most likely a response to the additive effect of dexmedetomidine to propofol-remifentanil TIVA.

Cerebral oxygenation measured as partial pressure of oxygen in brain tissue ($P_{br}O_2$) is believed to reflect factors affecting both oxygen cerebral tissue diffusion as well as CBF [35] and may thus be regarded as an indicator of the combined effect of cerebral perfusion and metabolism [44]. Dexmedetomidine has been shown to decrease CBF in both human [25, 26, 45, 46] and animal studies [47, 48] but did not reduce $P_{br}O_2$ in a series of five surgical patients with neurovascular injuries [43]. The same studies conclude that the reduction in CBF is not coupled to a decrease in cerebral metabolic rate. The influence of dexmedetomidine on CBF is believed to be due to lowering of systemic blood pressure through centrally α_{2A}-mediated sympatholysis [49, 50] or by α_{2B}-mediated cerebral vascular smooth muscle constriction [26, 51] as well as lowering cerebral metabolism by lowering brain activity [26]. The overall clinical effect reflects the sum of these central and peripheral effects, and is related to the doses used [52, 53].

In this study, cerebral perfusion was evaluated by LSCI. Laser speckle contrast imaging is able to assess real-time cerebral perfusion [54–56], and in piglets LSCI has been successfully used to evaluate changes in pial arteriolar blood flow [57]. Our results disagree with previous studies [25, 26, 45–48], since addition of dexmedetomidine did not produce significant changes in cerebral perfusion in either the NBP or the LBP group. The significant decrease found in $P_{br}O_2$ in the latter group, could not be related to a statistically significant decrease in LSPU measures, despite a decrease in 6 out of 7 piglets resulting in a 30% reduction of median LSPU. A post hoc power analysis (G*power for Mac, version 3.19.2) based on our LSPU data revealed a low power (0.47), increasing the risk of Type II error, so that an effect on cerebral perfusion by dexmedetomidine might have been falsely rejected. Since we did not assess cerebral metabolism, we cannot conclude if the significant $P_{br}O_2$ reduction was related to reduced CBF or to a lack of reduction in cerebral metabolism.

All $P_{br}O_2$ measurements were significantly higher than 15 mmHg, which may be used as a threshold value below which the risks of cerebral ischaemia [35], and mortality may increase [36].

The clinical significance of reduced cerebral oxygenation will probably depend on the $P_{br}O_2$ prior to dexmedetomidine supplementation and to the integrity of cerebral autoregulatory mechanisms, as well as to haemodynamic stability. Therefore, particular attention should be directed towards paediatric, neurosurgical, and intensive care patients, which are patient groups in which the use of dexmedetomidine has gained increasing interest in recent years [15, 17, 45, 58, 59].

Haemodynamic responses

The baseline MAP was comparable to findings in other studies based on propofol-remifentanil in pigs [60], even though it was relatively low. The significant difference in MAP between the NBP and the LBP group was consequently clinically small, but the difference was consistent and statistically significant throughout the experiment.

The MAP in the NBP group remained well within normal limits and statistically significantly exceeded the LLCA at all time points, indicating that in piglets with normal blood pressure propofol-remifentanil TIVA both with and without dexmedetomidine provides a haemodynamically stable anaesthesia (Fig. 2). In contrast, in the LBP group following addition of dexmedetomidine the median MAP no longer significantly exceeded the LLCA. Although studies on propofol-remifentanil-dexmedetomidine anaesthesia in pigs are not available, Sano et al. [33] showed a significant decrease in MAP with addition of the

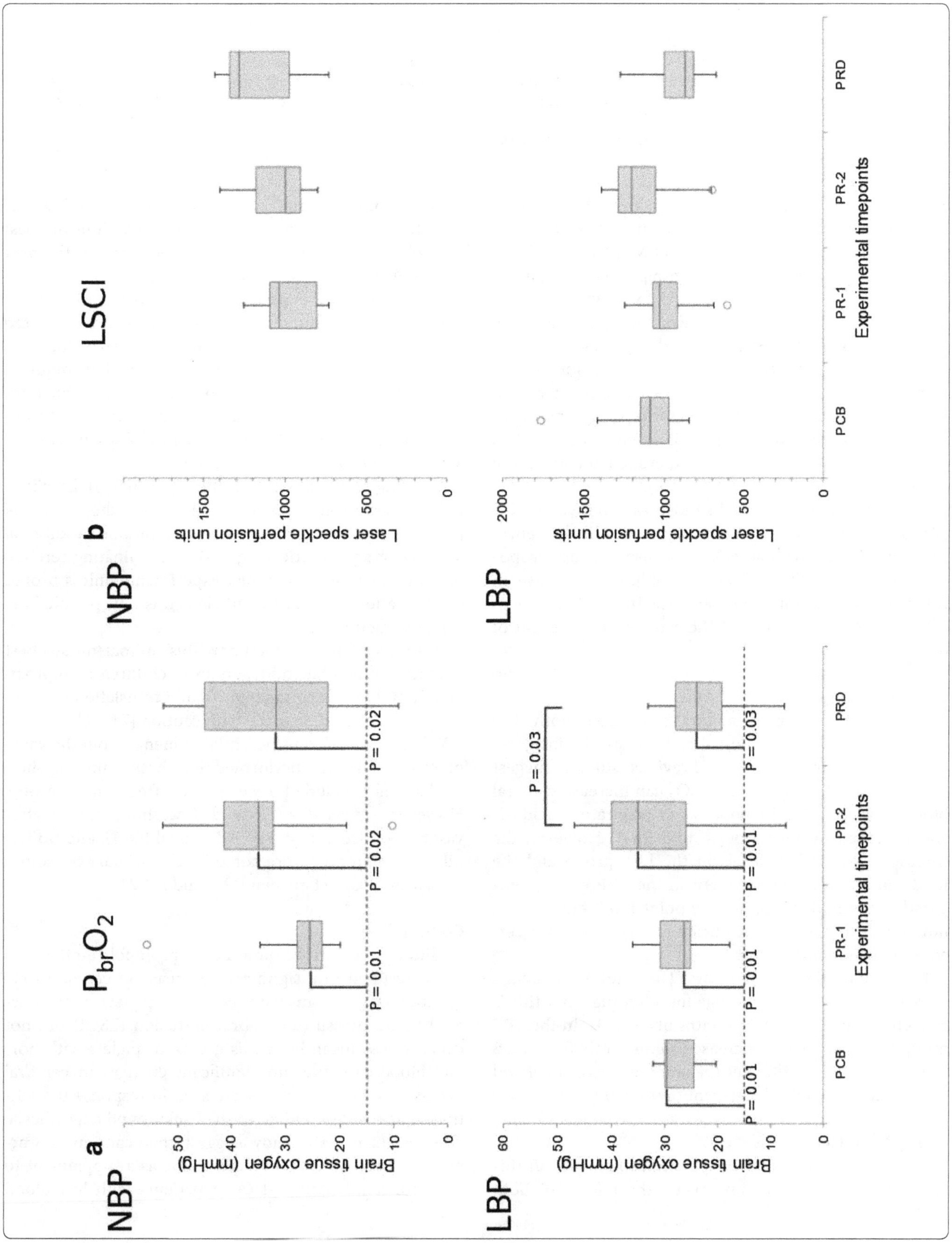
a
b
NBP
LBP
$P_{br}O_2$
LSCI
Brain tissue oxygen (mmHg)
Laser speckle perfusion units
Experimental timepoints
PCB
PR-1
PR-2
PRD
P = 0.01
P = 0.02
P = 0.03

(See figure on previous page.)

Fig. 3 *Boxplots* of cerebral perfusion and oxygenation at the different time points. *Box* and *whisker plots* showing median (*line*), interquartile range (*shaded*) and outliers (*circles*) for partial pressure of tissue oxygen ($P_{br}O_2$, in mmHg) (**a**) and laser speckle perfusion units (**b**) in the normal blood pressure group (NBP) and low blood pressure group (LBP). *Whiskers* extend a maximum of 1.5× the interquartile range. The value for ischaemic threshold is shown (*dashed line*). Experimental time points: *PCB* pre-caval block, *PR-1* initial baseline for propofol-remifentanil TIVA, *PR-2* immediately before dexmedetomidine administration, *PRD* following propofol–remifentanil–dexmedetomidine TIVA. Significant differences from either the ischaemia limit (*vertical bars*) or between timepoints (*horizontal bars*) are shown

same dose of dexmedetomidine to background anaesthesia of propofol alone, in contrast to our findings in the NBP group. The observed 19% decrease in MAP after addition of dexmedetomidine in the LBP group, even though not statistically significant, corresponds to previous reports in humans [50, 61, 62] and is mediated by activation of central α_2-adrenergic receptors and subsequent attenuation of sympathetic activity [63]. Thus, individuals with compromised cardiovascular function may be at risk of experiencing an additional decrease in MAP when dexmedetomidine is added to propofol-remifentanil TIVA, which may be a concern in both experimental and clinical settings.

The significant increase in pulse rate between PCB and PR-1 observed in the LBP group likely represents an intact sympathetic response during propofol-remifentanil TIVA. The lack of pulse increase in response to the apparent decrease in MAP between PR-2 and PRD could reflect the sympatholytic effect of dexmedetomidine.

Background physiology

Mild to moderate hypercapnia was observed in both NBP and LBP groups, with minimal and statistically insignificant inter-group differences. Previous studies suggest that even small increases in P_aCO_2 can increase cerebral blood flow [26]. Mild compensated respiratory acidosis was observed in both groups until PR-1. However, the slightly higher P_aCO_2 levels in the LBP group and the mild acidosis was more evident in the LBP group compared to the NBP group at time point PR-2, but this did not appear to have any significant consequences for cerebral perfusion in our study.

Throughout the study, both THbc and haematocrit were below the reference range for adult pigs, but this is expected in piglets of 2–3 months of age [64]. In the LBP group both parameters increased significantly from PCB to PR1 and PR1 to PR2, but the amounts were small and not considered clinically relevant to this study.

Strengths and limitations

The model, experimental design and sample size in this study, were selected to investigate the effects of both dexmedetomidine and hypotension and to follow the 3 Rs tenet for the use of animals in research in the best possible way [65]. Some power was lost due to the post hoc exclusion of three animals.

The porcine model presented here was technically feasible, effectively inducing hypotension, which persisted throughout an experimental time period exceeding 7 h. The craniotomy was technically simple, but required careful preparation and the only complication encountered was a small haematoma in one animal. This complication represents the main methodological concern about LSCI recording in this model.

Avoiding premedication on the experimental day eliminates interference from other drugs on the effects of propofol, remifentanil and dexmedetomidine. Additional sedative or anaesthetic drugs risk contaminating cerebral outcome measures in animal experiments unless proper consideration is given to sufficient washout periods and drug interactions [8, 66–68].

In terms of neural maturity, this animal model best mirrors cerebral haemodynamics in children of approximately 10 months of age [69, 70] and translation to other age groups should be made with caution [71, 72].

We cannot exclude a potential influence from the vasopressor challenges performed on these animals, since we have not included a vasopressor-free control group. However, we used an extended washout period after vasopressor treatment (see Additional file 1), and no significant differences were noted for the primary outcomes measures of CPO between PR-1 and PR-2.

Conclusions

Addition of dexmedetomidine to propofol-remifentanil TIVA resulted in a significant decrease in cerebral oxygenation ($P_{br}O_2$) measurements in piglets with lowered blood pressure. Cerebral perfusion (LSCI) did not decrease significantly in this group. In piglets with normal blood pressure, no significant changes in cerebral perfusion or oxygenation were seen in response to addition of dexmedetomidine to the background anaesthesia. The results of this study suggest that caution is warranted when using dexmedetomidine as a supplement to propofol-remifentanil TIVA in patients with low blood

Table 2 Physiologic, anaesthetic and blood gas data for the two experimental groups (low blood pressure—LBP and normal blood pressure—NBP) at key study time points

Group	Pre-caval block (PCB)	Propofol-remifentanil 1 (PR-1)		Propofol-remifentanil 2 (PR-2)		Propofol-remifentanil-dexmedetomidine (PRD)		Reference ranges
	LBP	NBP	LBP	NBP	LBP	NBP	LBP	
Body temperature (°C)	38.6 (37.5–40.0)	37.9 (37.3–38.9)	38.7 (37.5–39.9)	38.3 (37.7–39.3)	39.7 (38.0–40.9)	38.3 (37.2–39.3)	40 (38.1–40.1)	38.7–39.8 [37]
FIO_2 (%)	84 (82–87)	83 (78–85)	85 (82–87)	84 (80–85)	86 (83–87)	84 (79–85)	85 (83–87)	–
Pulse rate (beats/min)	80 (54–104)	67 (57–85)	87[a] (58–137)	80 (68–85)	114 (67–179)	78 (51–111)	111 (71–153)	70–120 [37]
$ETCO_2$ (mmHg)	45 (41–50)	45 (44–47)	47 (43–48)	47 (46–49)	49 (43–61)	43[a] (42–45)	44[a] (38–51)	35–50 mmHg [41]
pH[1]	7.4 (7.34–7.46)	7.43 (7.38–7.47)	7.41 (7.35–7.46)	7.41 (7.31–7.46)	7.32[b] (7.25–7.46)	7.46[a] (7.39–7.49)	7.37[a] (7.29–7.48)	7.4–7.43[38];7.4–7.53 [39]
pCO_2 (mmHg)[1]	49 (48–56)	51 (48–52)	50 (45–55)	53 (49–60)	56[a] (45–68)	51 (48–52)	52[a] (44–55)	41.8–49.1 [38]
pO_2 (mmHg)[1]	443 (432–482)	449 (431–507)	463 (411–487)	452 (433–485)	447 (426–498)	455 (422–497)	480 (434–498)	18.8–39.1 [38]
HCO_3^- (mmol/l)	31 (28–34)	33 (30–35)	30 (28–34)	33 (30–37)	29 (25–32)	35 (31–38)	30[b] (24–33)	24.9–30.3 [38] 22–33 [39]
Base excess (mmol/l)	6 (3–11)	9 (5–12)	5 (3–10)	10 (4–14)	4 (−1– 9)	11 (7–15)	5[b] (−2–10)	1.3–5.1(+) [38]
Glucose (mmol/l)	4.9 (3.9–5.6)	5.4 (4.8–6.9)	5.5[a] (4.8–8.0)	7.2 (4.9–8.4)	9.6 (4.4–14.7)	5.2 (3.7–5.9)	6.4 (4.3–9.5)	2.6–6.5 [39]
Lactate (mmol/l)	0.5 (0.4–2.1)	0.9 (0.7–1.0)	0.9[a] (0.4–2.4)	0.7 (0.3–1.4)	1.2 (0.7–3.0)	0.5 (0.3–0.9)	1.3 (0.5–3.9)	0.5–1.5 [39]; 0.5–5.5 [40]
Total haemoglobin (mmol/l)	4.6 (4.6–5.6)	4.6 (4.6–6.1)	5.0[a] (4.6–6.1)	4.9 (4.6–6.1)	5.6[a] (5.0–7.0)	4.7 (4.2–6.1)	5.2 (4.6–6.0)	6.21–9.93 [37]
Haematocrit (%)	24 (24–29)	24 (24–32)	26[a] (24–32)	26 (24–32)	29[a] (26–36)	25 (22–32)	27 (24–31)	29.5–45.9 [42]

Median values are shown with range (min–max)

For the LBP group, statistically significant differences were pulse rate (P = 0.02, median increase 10, 95% CI 2; 47), $ETCO_2$ (P = 0.02, median decrease 5 mmHg, 95% CI 2; 11), pH (P = 0.05, median increase 0.04, 95% CI 0.01; 0.08), pCO_2 (P = 0.03, median increase 6 mmHg, 95% CI 1; 11, and P = 0.03, median decrease 5 mmHg, 95% CI 3; 9), glucose (P = 0.05, median increase 1.2 mmol/l, 95% CI 0.0; 2.7, and P = 0.02, median increase 3.5 mmol/l, 95% CI 0.8; 7.1), lactate (P = 0.04, median increase 0.2 mmol/l, 95% CI 0.0; 1.0), total haemoglobin (P = 0.05, median increase 0.4 mmol/l, 95% CI 0.0; 0.8 and P = 0.02, median increase 0.5, 95% CI 0.2; 1.2), and haematocrit (P = 0.05, median increase 2%, 95% CI 0; 4, and P = 0.02 (median increase 3%, 95% CI 1; 6). For the NBP group, statistically significant differences were $ETCO_2$ (P = 0.01, median decrease 4 mmHg, 95% CI 2; 5) and pH (P = 0.01, median increase 0.05, 95% CI 0.02; 0.08). Significant intergroup differences were pH (P = 0.03, median difference 0.09, 95% CI 0.01; 0.15), HCO_3^- P = 0.03 (median difference 6 mmol/l, 95% CI 2; 9) and base excess (P = 0.03, median difference 7 mmol/l, 95% CI 2; 12)

[1] Temperature corrected values

[a] Statistically significant differences from the previous study time point

[b] Statistically significant differences from the other experimental group within the same time point

pressure, since it could result in decreased cerebral oxygenation. Further and larger studies are required for confirmation of these results.

Additional files

Additional file 1. Illustration of experimental flow and data-set of the main experiment. Cerebral perfusion and oxygenation readings, physiological and haemodynamic data, blood gas data, and anaesthesia time at all time points throughout the experiment. PCB, PR-1, PR-2 and PRD are the reported time points used for statistical analysis in the manuscript entitled: *The effect of dexmedetomidine on cerebral perfusion and oxygenation in healthy piglets with normal and lowered blood pressure anaesthetized with propofol-remifentanil TIVA.* Analysis of the data collected at the remaining time points will be reported in later manuscript. NIRS: Near infra red spectroscopy; LSCI: Laser speckle contrast imaging; MAP: mean arterial pressure; EtCO2: End-tidal carbon dioxide; FiO2: Fraction of inspired oxygen; (T): data corrected for body temperature; PaCO2: Partial pressure of arterial carbon dioxide; PaO2: Partial pressure of arterial oxygen; HCO3: Hydrogen bicarbonate; Hct: Haematocrit; THbc: Total haemoglobin concentration; NA: data not available.

Additional file 2. Sedation protocols. Sedation protocols for intravenous catheter placement on the day prior to the main experiment. One of two intramuscularly injected (im) sedation protocols were used Animal no. 1-11 received protocol 1 (NBP: n = 5, LBP: n = 6), and animal no. 12-16 received protocol 2 (NBP: n = 3, LBP: n = 2).

Abbreviations

CPO: cerebral perfusion and oxygenation; CRI: constant rate infusion; CSF: cerebrospinal fluid; $EtCO_2$: end tidal CO_2; FiO_2: fraction of inspired O_2; im: intramuscular; iv: intravenous; LBP: low blood pressure group; LLCA: lower limit of cerebral autoregulation; LSCI: laser speckle contrast imaging; LSPU: laser speckle perfusion unit; MAP: mean arterial pressure; Max: maximum; Min: minimum; NBP: normal blood pressure group; P_aCO_2: partial pressure of arterial CO_2; P_aO_2: partial pressure of arterial O_2; $P_{br}O_2$: partial pressure of oxygen in brain tissue; PCB: pre-caval block (time point); PR: pulse rate; PR-n: propofol/remifentanil TIVA (n: time-point number); PRD: propofol/remifentanil TIVA + dexmedetomidine CRI (time point); TIVA: total intravenous anaesthesia.

Authors' contributions

MLGM, TE, HHP and FBM conceived the overall objective, study design and experimental protocol for this study. MLGM was the primary license holder and responsible for the ethical approvals and the overall experimental execution. MLGM, TE and RA were present at all experiments. TE performed all surgeries and RA performed all laser speckle contrast imaging. Data analysis and statistical revision was done in collaboration with FBM, JEM and RA. HHP supervised anaesthesia and RR contributed with substantial intellectual guidance and interpretations of data, as well as critical revision of the manuscript. All authors read and approved the final manuscript.

Author details

[1] Department of Veterinary Clinical Sciences, Faculty of Health and Medical Sciences, University of Copenhagen, 16 Dyrlægevej, 1870 Frederiksberg C, Denmark. [2] Department of Surgical Gastroenterology C, Rigshospitalet, Faculty of Health and Medical Sciences, University of Copenhagen, 9 Blegdamsvej, 2100 Copenhagen Ø, Denmark. [3] Department of Neurosurgery, The Neuroscience Centre, Rigshospitalet, Faculty of Health and Medical Sciences, University of Copenhagen, 9 Blegdamsvej, 2100 Copenhagen Ø, Denmark. [4] Department of Neuroanaesthesia, Rigshospitalet, University of Copenhagen, 9 Blegdamsvej, 2100 Copenhagen Ø, Denmark. [5] Department of Anaesthesia, Bispebjerg and Frederiksberg Hospitals, Faculty of Health and Medical Sciences, University of Copenhagen, 23 Bispebjerg Bakke, 2400 Copenhagen NV, Denmark.

Competing interests

The authors declare that they have no competing interests.

Funding

This study was funded by a Ph.D. scholarship granted by the University of Copenhagen.

References

1. Venkatesh B. Monitoring cerebral perfusion and oxygenation: an elusive goal. Crit Care Resusc. 2005;7:195–9.
2. Pasternak JJ, Lanier WL. Neuroanesthesiology update. J Neurosurg Anesthesiol. 2015;27:87–122.
3. Dagal A, Lam AM. General considerations in neuroanaesthesia. In: Matta BF, Menon DK, Smith M, editors. Core topics in neuroanaesthesia and neurointensive care. edn. New York: Cambridge University Press; 2011. p.147–61.
4. Engelhard K, Werner C. The effects of general anesthesia and variations in hemodynamics on cerebral perfusion. Appl Cardiopulm Pathophysiol. 2009;13:157–9.
5. Ramani R, Todd M, Warner D. A680 The CBF response to isoflurane following brain injury in the rabbit. Anesthesiology. 1990;73:A680.
6. Van Aken H, Van Hemelrijck J. An overview of the influence of anesthesia on cerebral blood flow and cerebral metabolism. Minerva Anestesiol. 1993;59:615–20.
7. Goettel N, Burkhart CS, Rossi A, Cabella BC, Berres M, Monsch AU, et al. Associations between impaired cerebral blood flow autoregulation, cerebral oxygenation, and biomarkers of brain injury and postoperative cognitive dysfunction in elderly patients after major noncardiac surgery. Anesth Analg. 2017;124:934–42.
8. Cole CD, Gottfried ON, Gupta DK, Couldwell WT. Total intravenous anesthesia: advantages for intracranial surgery. Neurosurgery. 2007;61(Suppl 2):369–78.
9. Eikaas H, Raeder J. Total intravenous anaesthesia techniques for ambulatory surgery. Curr Opin Anaesthesiol. 2009;22:725–9.
10. Coles JP, Leary TS, Monteiro JN, Brazier P, Summors A, Doyle P, Matta BF, Gupta AK. Propofol anesthesia for craniotomy: a double-blind comparison of remifentanil, alfentanil, and fentanyl. J Neurosurg Anesthesiol. 2000;12:15–20.
11. Lauder GR. Total intravenous anesthesia will supercede inhalational anesthesia in pediatric anesthetic practice. Paediatr Anaesth. 2015;25:52–64.
12. Dagal A, Lam AM. Cerebral autoregulation and anesthesia. Curr Opin Anaesthesiol. 2009;22:547–52.
13. Conti A, Iacopino DG, Fodale V, Micalizzi S, Penna O, Santamaria LB. Cerebral haemodynamic changes during propofol-remifentanil or sevoflurane anaesthesia: transcranial Doppler study under bispectral index monitoring. Br J Anaesth. 2006;97:333–9.
14. Engelhard K, Werner C, Mollenberg O, Kochs E. Effects of remifentanil/propofol in comparison with isoflurane on dynamic cerebrovascular autoregulation in humans. Acta Anaesthesiol Scand. 2001;45:971–6.
15. Mahmoud M, Mason KP. Dexmedetomidine: review, update, and future considerations of paediatric perioperative and periprocedural applications and limitations. Br J Anaesth. 2015;115:171–82.
16. Chrysostomou C, Schmitt CG. Dexmedetomidine: sedation, analgesia and beyond. Expert Opin Drug Metab Toxicol. 2008;4:619–27.
17. Rozet I. Anesthesia for functional neurosurgery: the role of dexmedetomidine. Curr Opin Anaesthesiol. 2008;21:537–43.
18. Cormack JR, Orme RM, Costello TG. The role of α2-agonists in neurosurgery. J Clin Neurosci. 2005;12:375–8.
19. Bekker A, Sturaitis MK. Dexmedetomidine for neurological surgery. Neurosurgery. 2005;57(Suppl 1):1–10; discussion 11–10.
20. Murrell JC, Hellebrekers LJ. Medetomidine and dexmedetomidine: a review of cardiovascular effects and antinociceptive properties in the dog. Vet Anaesth Analg. 2005;32:117–27.
21. Flaherty D. Alpha(2)-adrenoceptor agonists in small animal practice 1. Why they do what they do. In Pract. 2013;35:513–7.
22. Grimm KA, Lamont LA, Tranquilli WJ, Greene SA, Robertson SA. Veterinary anesthesia and analgesia. 5th ed. Ames: Wiley Blackwill; 2015.
23. Degos V, Charpentier TL, Chhor V, Brissaud O, Lebon S, Schwendimann L, Bednareck N, Passemard S, Mantz J, Gressens P. Neuroprotective effects of dexmedetomidine against glutamate agonist-induced neuronal cell death are related to increased astrocyte brain-derived neurotrophic factor expression. Anesthesiology. 2013;118:1123–32.

24. Kang WS, Kim SY, Son JC, Kim JD, Muhammad HB, Kim SH, Yoon TG, Kim TY. The effect of dexmedetomidine on the adjuvant propofol requirement and intraoperative hemodynamics during remifentanil-based anesthesia. Korean J Anesthesiol. 2012;62:113–8.
25. Drummond JC, Dao AV, Roth DM, Cheng CR, Atwater BI, Minokadeh A, Pasco LC, Patel PM. Effect of dexmedetomidine on cerebral blood flow velocity, cerebral metabolic rate, and carbon dioxide response in normal humans. Anesthesiology. 2008;108:225–32.
26. Prielipp RC, Wall MH, Tobin JR, Groban L, Cannon MA, Fahey FH, Gage HD, Stump DA, James RL, Bennett J. Dexmedetomidine-induced sedation in volunteers decreases regional and global cerebral blood flow. Anesth Analg. 2002;95:1052–9.
27. Tsaousi GG, Lamperti M, Bilotta F. Role of dexmedetomidine for sedation in neurocritical care patients: a qualitative systematic review and meta-analysis of current evidence. Clin Neuropharmacol. 2016;39:144–51.
28. Tsaousi GG, Bilotta F. Is dexmedetomidine a favorable agent for cerebral hemodynamics? Indian J Crit Care Med. 2016;20:1–2.
29. Farag E, Argalious M, Sessler DI, Kurz A, Ebrahim ZY, Schubert A. Use of alpha(2)-agonists in neuroanesthesia: an overview. Ochsner J. 2011;11:57–69.
30. Lind NM, Moustgaard A, Jelsing J, Vajta G, Cumming P, Hansen AK. The use of pigs in neuroscience: modeling brain disorders. Neurosci Biobehav Rev. 2007;31:728–51.
31. Alstrup AK, Smith DF. Anaesthesia for positron emission tomography scanning of animal brains. Lab Anim. 2013;47:12–8.
32. Kilkenny C, Browne WJ, Cuthill IC, Emerson M, Altman DG. Improving bioscience research reporting: the ARRIVE guidelines for reporting animal research. PLoS Biol. 2010;8:e1000412.
33. Sano H, Dot M, Mimuro S, Yu S, Kurita T, Sato S. Evaluation of the hypnotic and hemodynamic effects of dexmedetomidine on propofol-sedated swine. Exp Anim. 2010;59:199–205.
34. Maas AI, Fleckenstein W, de Jong DA, van Santbrink H. Monitoring cerebral oxygenation: experimental studies and preliminary clinical results of continuous monitoring of cerebrospinal fluid and brain tissue oxygen tension. Acta Neurochir Suppl (Wien). 1993;59:50–7.
35. Rohlwink UK, Figaji AA. Methods of monitoring brain oxygenation. Childs Nerv Syst. 2010;26:453–64.
36. Bratton S, Bullock, MR, Carney N, Chesnut RM, Coplin W, Ghajar J, et al. Brain oxygen monitoring and thresholds. In: Bullock MR, Povlishock JT. Guidelines for the management of severe traumatic brain injury. J Neurotrauma. 2007;24(Suppl 1):S65–S70. doi:10.1089/neu.2007.9986.
37. Aiello SE, editor. The Merck veterinary manual. 8th ed. Whitehouse Station, New Jersey: Merck and Co. Inc; 1998.
38. Harris WH. Hemoglobin, blood gases and serum electrolyte values in swine. Can Vet J. 1974;15:282–5.
39. Hannon JP, Bossone CA, Wade CE. Normal physiological values for conscious pigs used in biomedical research. Lab Anim Sci. 1990;40:293–8.
40. Hofmaier F, Dinger K, Braun R, Sterner-Kock A. Range of blood lactate values in farm pigs prior to experimental surgery. Lab Anim. 2013;47:130–2.
41. Swindle MM. Swine in the laboratory: surgery, anesthesia, imaging, and experimental techniques. 2nd ed. Boca Raton: CRC Press; 2007.
42. Poole TB, English P, Universities Federation for Animal Welfare. The UFAW handbook on the care and management of laboratory animals. 7th ed. Malden: Oxford, Blackwell Science; 1999.
43. Drummond JC, Sturaitis MK. Brain tissue oxygenation during dexmedetomidine administration in surgical patients with neurovascular injuries. J Neurosurg Anesthesiol. 2010;22:336–41.
44. Lang EW, Jaeger M. Systematic and comprehensive literature review of publications on direct cerebral oxygenation monitoring. Open Crit Care Med J. 2013;6:1–24.
45. Wang X, Ji J, Fen L, Wang A. Effects of dexmedetomidine on cerebral blood flow in critically ill patients with or without traumatic brain injury: a prospective controlled trial. Brain Inj. 2013;27:1617–22.
46. Arulvelan A, Manikandan S, Easwer HV, Krishnakumar K. Cerebral vascular effects of loading dose of dexmedetomidine: a Transcranial Color Doppler study. Indian J Crit Care Med. 2016;20:9–13.
47. Zornow MH, Fleischer JE, Scheller MS, Nakakimura K, Drummond JC. Dexmedetomidine, an alpha 2-adrenergic agonist, decreases cerebral blood flow in the isoflurane-anesthetized dog. Anesth Analg. 1990;70:624–30.
48. Karlsson BR, Forsman M, Roald OK, Heier MS, Steen PA. Effect of dexmedetomidine, a selective and potent alpha 2-agonist, on cerebral blood flow and oxygen consumption during halothane anesthesia in dogs. Anesth Analg. 1990;71:125–9.
49. Talke P, Richardson CA, Scheinin M, Fisher DM. Postoperative pharmacokinetics and sympatholytic effects of dexmedetomidine. Anesth Analg. 1997;85:1136–42.
50. Weerink MA, Struys MM, Hannivoort LN, Barends CR, Absalom AR, Colin P. Clinical pharmacokinetics and pharmacodynamics of dexmedetomidine. Clin Pharmacokinet. 2017. doi:10.1007/s40262-017-0507-7.
51. Zornow MH, Maze M, Dyck JB, Shafer SL. Dexmedetomidine decreases cerebral blood flow velocity in humans. J Cereb Blood Flow Metab. 1993;13:350–3.
52. Bekker A, Jorden V. Alpha-2 agonists in neuroanesthesia. Semin Anesth Perioper Med Pain. 2004;23:181–91.
53. Kamibayashi T, Maze M. Clinical uses of alpha2 -adrenergic agonists. Anesthesiology. 2000;93:1345–9.
54. Parthasarathy AB, Weber EL, Richards LM, Fox DJ, Dunn AK. Laser speckle contrast imaging of cerebral blood flow in humans during neurosurgery: a pilot clinical study. J Biomed Opt. 2010;15:066030. doi:10.1117/1.3526368.
55. Hecht N, Woitzik J, Dreier JP, Vajkoczy P. Intraoperative monitoring of cerebral blood flow by laser speckle contrast analysis. Neurosurg Focus. 2009;27:E11.
56. Richards LM, Towle EL, Fox DJ, Dunn AK. Intraoperative laser speckle contrast imaging with retrospective motion correction for quantitative assessment of cerebral blood flow. Neurophotonics. 2014;1:015006. doi:10.1117/1.NPh.1.1.015006.
57. Domoki F, Zolei D, Olah O, Toth-Szuki V, Hopp B, Bari F, Smausz T. Evaluation of laser-speckle contrast image analysis techniques in the cortical microcirculation of piglets. Microvasc Res. 2012;83:311–7.
58. Peng K, Wu S, Liu H, Ji F. Dexmedetomidine as an anesthetic adjuvant for intracranial procedures: meta-analysis of randomized controlled trials. J Clin Neurosci. 2014;21:1951–8.
59. Gerlach AT, Murphy CV, Dasta JF. An updated focused review of dexmedetomidine in adults. Ann Pharmacother. 2009;43:2064–74.
60. Mikkelsen ML, Ambrus R, Miles JE, Poulsen HH, Moltke FB, Eriksen T. Effect of propofol and remifentanil on cerebral perfusion and oxygenation in pigs: a systematic review. Acta Vet Scand. 2016;58:42.
61. Roberts DJ, Haroon B, Hall RI. Sedation for critically ill or injured adults in the intensive care unit: a shifting paradigm. Drugs. 2012;72:1881–916.
62. Ganjoo P, Farber NE, Hudetz A, Smith JJ, Samso E, Kampine JP, Schmeling WT. In vivo effects of dexmedetomidine on laser-Doppler flow and pial arteriolar diameter. Anesthesiology. 1998;88:429–39.
63. Coursin DB, Coursin DB, Maccioli GA. Dexmedetomidine. Curr Opin Crit Care. 2001;7:221–6.
64. Miller ER, Ullrey DE, Ackermann I, Schmidt DA, Luecke RW, Hoefer JA. Swine hematology from birth to maturity. II. Erythrocyte population, size and hemoglobin concentration. J Anim Sci. 1961;20:890–7.
65. Burden N, Chapman K, Sewell F, Robinson V. Pioneering better science through the 3Rs: an introduction to the national centre for the replacement, refinement, and reduction of animals in research (NC3Rs). J Am Assoc Lab Anim Sci. 2015;54:198–208.
66. Loscher W, Ganter M, Fassbender CP. Correlation between drug and metabolite concentrations in plasma and anesthetic action of ketamine in swine. Am J Vet Res. 1990;51:391–8.
67. Lacoste L, Bouquet S, Ingrand P, Caritez JC, Carretier M, Debaene B. Intranasal midazolam in piglets: pharmacodynamics (0.2 vs 0.4 mg/kg) and pharmacokinetics (0.4 mg/kg) with bioavailability determination. Lab Anim. 2000;34:29–35.
68. Veselis RA, Reinsel RA, Beattie BJ, Mawlawi OR, Feshchenko VA, DiResta GR, Larson SM, Blasberg RG. Midazolam changes cerebral blood flow in discrete brain regions: an H2(15)O positron emission tomography study. Anesthesiology. 1997;87:1106–17.
69. Conrad MS, Dilger RN, Johnson RW. Brain growth of the domestic pig (Sus scrofa) from 2 to 24 weeks of age: a longitudinal MRI study. Dev Neurosci. 2012;34:291–8.
70. Conrad MS, Johnson RW. The domestic piglet: an important model for investigating the neurodevelopmental consequences of early life insults. Annu Rev Anim Biosci. 2015;3:245–64.

5

C-kit receptor immunopositive interstitial cells (Cajal-type) in the porcine reproductive tract

Malgorzata Domino[1,2], Bartosz Pawlinski[1,2], Romuald Zabielski[1,2] and Zdzislaw Gajewski[1,2*]

Abstract

Background: Interstitial Cajal cells have been suspected as being the pacemaker cells of smooth muscle motor activity and discharging slow triggering waves in the gut as well as in other organs containing smooth muscles where they are known as interstitial Cajal-like cells (ICLC). The present study describes ICLC localization and density in the porcine oviduct and uterus. Differences in ICLC density were examined using histological, immunohistochemical and immunofluorescent methods and c-kit expression was determined.

Results: interstitial Cajal-like cells with characteristic morphological and immunological phenotypes were found. Star-like or spindle-shaped cells with very long, moniliform processes were localized in the muscle layers of the oviduct and uterine walls at variable densities that decreased progressively from high in the oviduct to low in the uterus.

Conclusions: The detailed description of ICLC in the porcine reproductive tract may lead to a better understanding of reproductive tract motility. Our approach is inexpensive and effective for ICLC evaluation and may in the future be applied to clinical diagnosis.

Keywords: Myometrium, Oviduct, C-kit/CD 117, Interstitial Cajal-like cell, ICLC, Sow

Background

Interstitial Cajal cells (ICC) are the pacemaker cells of gut motor activity [1]. They have been found in the wall of the gastrointestinal tract of several species, including humans [2, 3]. The ICC may be essential for smooth muscle contractility in the gastrointestinal tract and probably also in the urinary and reproductive tracts by discharging slow triggering waves [4]. More recently, cells with morphology and antigenicity similar to ICC have been found outside the gastrointestinal tract, i.e., in the vas deferens [5], urethra [6], bladder [7], prostate gland [8], lymphatic vessels [9], uterus [10], blood vessels [11], fallopian tube [12, 13], mammary gland [14] and pancreas [15] of mice, rats and humans. These cells are most commonly known as interstitial Cajal-like cells (ICLC). The defining features of ICLC were indicated by examination of hematoxylin and eosin (HE) stained sections, characterized by immunohistochemistry and confirmed by transmission electron microscopy (TEM) [13]. Ultrastructural criteria were proposed by Huizinga et al. [16] for the enteric ICC and by Popescu et al. [13] for extra-intestinal ICLC. ICLC ultrastructure provides valuable morphological hints for ICLC identification. TEM identifies mainly qualitative characteristics so Popescu et al. [13] performed immunohistochemical studies to specifically identify ICLC. They observed cells with typical interstitial localization and phenotype more or less similar to those of ICC. The discovery of the c-kit receptor as a marker for ICLC allows easier recognition of these cells at the light microscopic level. The type III tyrosine kinase receptor (c-kit; Kit protein; CD117) present on the cell surface is one of the criteria for specific identification of ICLC [17]. Because c-kit expression can also be detected in mast cells [18], morphological evaluation based on live-tissue methylene blue staining or HE staining of fixed tissues and assessment of

*Correspondence: zgajewski@supermedia.pl
[1] Department of Large Animal Diseases with Clinic, Faculty of Veterinary Medicine, Warsaw University of Life Sciences (WULS-SGGW), Nowoursynowska 100, 02-797 Warsaw, Poland

ultrastructure by TEM or scanning electron microscopy (SEM) is crucial for proper identification of ICLC. The ICLC morphology is characterized as a triangular, spindle-shaped or star-like body, a distinct nucleus, and two or more, very long, moniliform processes [13, 18]. The ICLC display on TEM images as a slender cell body with a thin rim of cytoplasm around the nucleus and long cytoplasmic processes that suddenly emerge from the cellular body. Organelles are distributed near the nuclear pole and in the dilated regions of cell prolongations [13, 16].

The morphological and functional roles of ICLC in the reproductive tract have also been the subject of interest recently and c-kit positive cells have been identified in the human uterus [10]. Subsequently, ICLC have been described in the human uterus and fallopian tube [13]. Finally, re-investigation of cells originally regarded as being ICLC in the male and female reproductive tracts of mice, rats, rabbits and humans has identified them as 'myometrial Cajal-like interstitial cells' (m-ICLC) to describe their ultrastructural similarities with ICC [19]. These m-ICLC again seemed to be located mainly in the boundaries of smooth muscle bundles throughout the myometrium, forming a network between smooth muscle cells, nerves and capillaries [18], and were present in myometrial biopsies taken throughout reproductive life [19, 20]. A further study supported the observation that m-ICLC are c-kit positive [20]. Popescu's team tested many markers and concluded that the positive reaction of markers differs between organs and species [14]. On the other hand, there is a lack of morphological and physiological evidence of ICLC in livestock species, especial within the reproductive tract.

The aim of the present study was to localize and identify ICLC in the porcine reproductive tract and describe their morphology in order to help understanding of reproductive tract motility. This may have clinical implications by explaining infertility in sows without any proven uterine and fallopian tube abnormalities.

Methods

Myometrial tissue samples

Full-thickness tissue samples of porcine myometrium were obtained at a slaughterhouse from 12 mature sows aged 10–24 months, body weight 80–140 kg. The animals were clinically healthy and their reproductive tracts did not show any gross pathology. To avoid endometrial contamination, parts of the external muscular layer of the uterus (body, middle of the horn, horn tip) and oviducts (isthmus, infundibulum) were excised from areas free of macroscopically visible abnormalities. All tissue samples were obtained in accordance with a protocol approved by the local Ethics Committee (No 10/2011), in accordance to generally accepted international practice.

Histology

Unless otherwise indicated, all reagents were purchased from Sigma-Aldrich (Sigma-Aldrich, Poland). Tissue samples were fixed in 4% neutral buffered paraformaldehyde, processed, embedded in paraffin and 5 μm sections were prepared using standard histology procedures. Sections were mounted on glass slides, de-paraffinized and rehydrated in a series of xylene and decreasing concentrations of ethanol. Slides were then stained with HE using a standard protocol and mounted under Canadian balsam resin for histological evaluation. Immunohistochemical and immunofluorescence labeling against CD117 (c-kit) was performed using a staining protocol modified from Ciontea et al. [18]. For the assessment of immunohistochemical and immunofluorescence reactions for CD117 specificity, porcine ileum paraffin blocks were used as a positive control (PC) and staining protocols with the primary antibody omitted were used as a negative control (NC).

Electron microscopy

Tissue samples were also frozen in liquid nitrogen using standard procedures. Afterwards, samples were cut using a cryostat to 15 μm sections. Sections were mounted on aluminum pin stubs using double-sided carbon adhesives. Fresh sections were examined under a SEM Phenom XL (Phenom-World, Netherlands).

Immunohistochemistry

Prior to immunolabeling, slides were boiled in citrate buffer for antigen-retrieval, then washed in phosphate-buffered saline (PBS) and permeabilized in PBS containing 1% bovine serum albumin (BSA) for 30 min. Primary antibodies (CD117/c-kit, Dako, USA) were applied in a 1:100 dilution for 1 h at 4 °C. A HRP-labelled polymer conjugated with secondary antibodies and 3,3′-diaminobenzidine (DAB)+ substrate-chromogen [EnVision+ System-HRP (DAB), Dako, USA] were used to detect the primary immune reaction. Following incubation steps, slides were rinsed three times in PBS. After labeling, the coverslips were mounted with Canadian balsam. The slides were examined under a light microscope BX-61 (Olympus, Poland) using MicroImage, v. 4.0 software (Olympus, Poland). Negative controls were prepared following the same protocol, but omitting the primary antibodies.

Immunofluorescence

Polyclonal Alexa Fluor 488 (Molecular Probes, USA) labeled chicken anti-mouse antibodies (dilution 1:500 for 2 h at 4 °C) were used to detect the primary immune reaction (the first part of the protocol was identical to the IHC protocol). Finally, nuclei were counterstained with 1 mM 7-Aminoactinomycin D (7-AAD, 250 μl/ml, Sigma

Aldrich, Poland). Following incubation steps, samples were rinsed three times in PBS. After labeling, the coverslips were mounted using mounting medium for fluorescence microscopy. Immunofluorescence labeled cells were examined under a confocal microscope (FV-500, Olympus, Poland). Quantitative evaluation was performed under a scanning cytometer (SCAN^R, Olympus, Poland).

Statistical analyses

The immunohistochemical and immunofluorescence data were statistically analyzed by Graph-Pad InStat software (San Diego, USA). A one-way analysis of variance (ANOVA) was performed, followed by the Tukey–Kramer Multiple Comparisons Test, with $P < 0.005$ considered significant and $P < 0.0001$ as highly significant.

Results

The characteristics of ICLC in the porcine reproductive tract were demonstrated by histology, immunohistochemistry, immunofluorescence and scanning electron microscopy (Fig. 1). ICLC were defined as c-kit-immunopositive nucleated cells with a triangular, spindle-shaped or star-like body and two or more, very long, moniliform processes. Such cells were also found in the positive control samples (porcine ileum) while they were absent in the negative controls (Fig. 2).

ICLC evaluation

C-kit-positive ICC-like cells with dendritic processes and large and oval nuclei were identified in the uterine body, uterine horns (middle and tip) and oviducts (isthmus and infundibulum). They were distinguishable from the c-kit-negative and non-branching smooth muscle cells and from the c-kit-positive non-branching mast cells by confocal microscopy (Fig. 3). In the wide-field microscope, the basophil cytoplasm and large oval nucleus allowed ICLC to be distinguished from eosinophil myocytes and fibroblasts.

In both light and confocal microscopy, most ICLC displayed a characteristic morphology, i.e., a triangular, spindle-shaped or star-like body with two or more, very

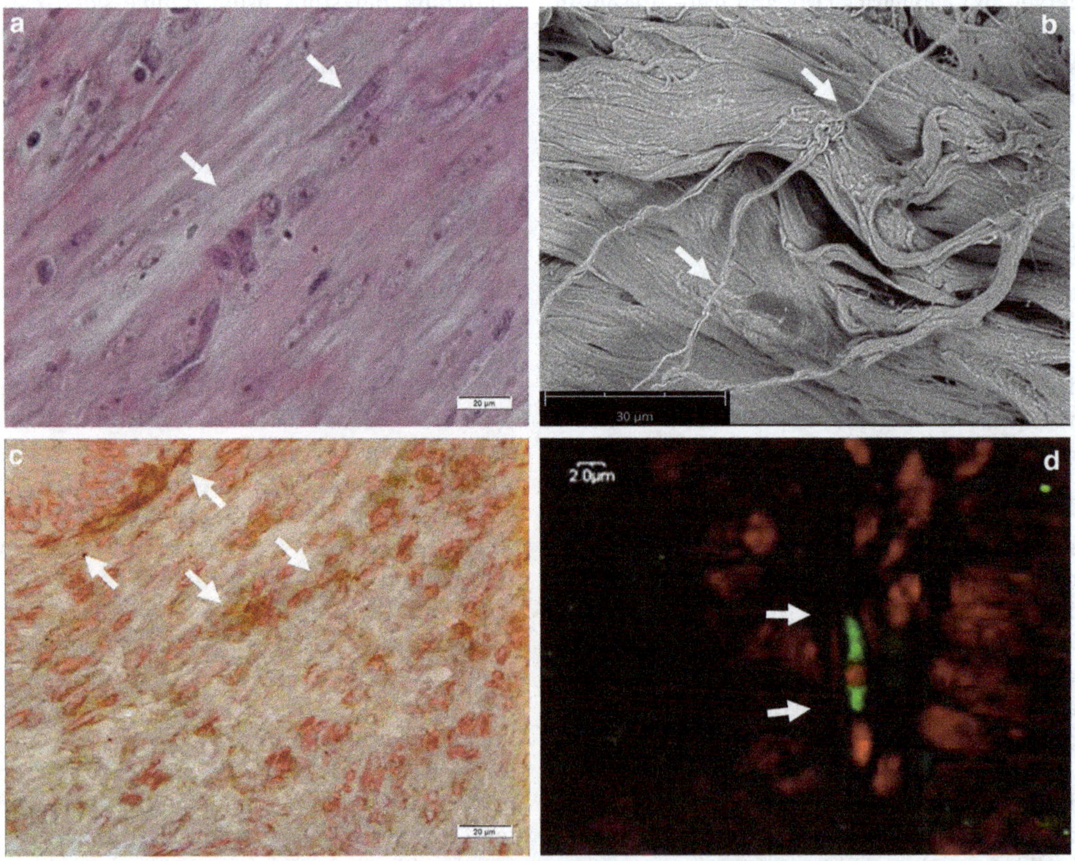

Fig. 1 Muscular layer of the uterine body. Fusiform cells with long processes and oval nucleus show morphology typical for ICLC (*arrows*). **a** Wide-field microscopy of a HE stained tissue section, original magnification 400x. **b** Scanning electron microscopy, original magnification 1500x; **c** wide-field microscopy following IHC labeling, original magnification 400x; **d** confocal microscopy following IF labeling, original magnification 3000x

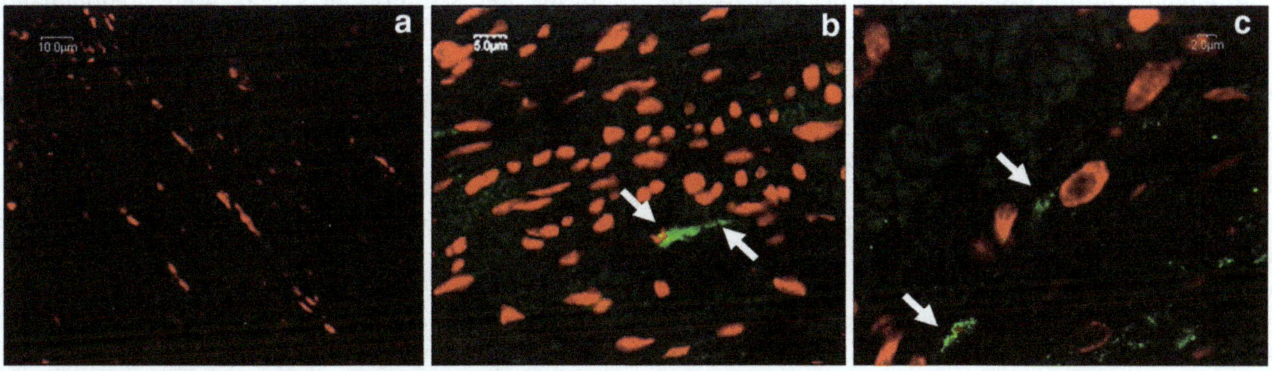

Fig. 2 Confocal microscopy following IF labeling, emission spectra of AF 488 and 7AAD. **a** Muscular layer of corpus uteri—negative control (NC), original magnification 600x; **b** muscular layer of ileum—positive control (PC), original magnification 1500x; **c** muscular layer of corpus uteri—study group, original magnification 3000x

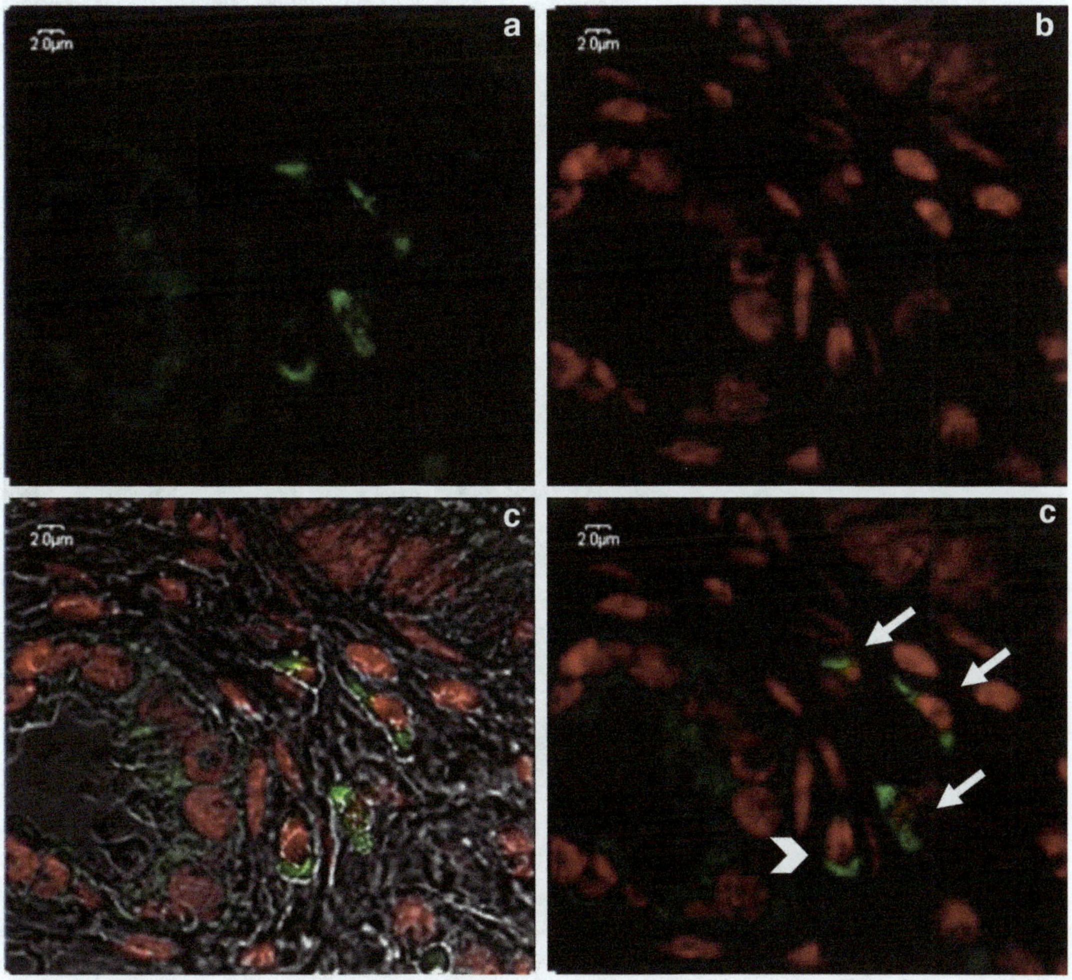

Fig. 3 Muscular layer of oviduct infundibulum. A group of the fusiform and trigonal c-kit-positive cells (*arrows*) laid in close proximity, were distinguished from the c-kit-positive nonbranching mast cells (*arrowhead*). **a** Emission spectra of AF 488, **b** emission spectra of 7AAD, **c** emission spectra of AF 488 and 7AAD as well as tissue structure, **d** emission spectra of AF 488 and 7AAD. Confocal microscopy following IF labeling, original magnification 3000x

long, moniliform processes and a distinct nucleus. The typical ultrastructure of a triangular-shaped cell located between smooth muscle cells with electron dense cytoplasm, numerous mitochondria and tips of ICLC prolongations was demonstrated by SEM.

The morphology of ICLC varied between different parts of the porcine reproductive tract. In the infundibulum and isthmus of the oviduct, ICLC consisted of fusiform cells with an oval nucleus and two cytoplasmic processes. In the uterine wall, however, the predominant type of ICLC were spindle-shape cells and triangular cells with three cytoplasmic processes. Star-like or pentagonal shaped cells were observed sporadically dispersed in the connective tissue layer, especially in the tip of the uterine horn adjacent to the oviduct (Fig. 4).

In the uterus and oviducts, ICLC were predominantly located between smooth muscle cells of both longitudinal and circular muscle layers. Their processes formed a network connecting smooth muscle cells, nerve cells and capillaries (Fig. 5).

ICLC density

The ICLC density differed among different parts of the reproductive tract (Tables 1 and 2).

The highest density of ICLC was found in the isthmus of the oviduct and the uterine horn tip, while a relatively low density of ICLC was found in the uterus (horns and body). The ICLC density was on average 22–34% higher in the isthmus and the tip of the uterine horn adjacent to the oviduct than in the uterine horns

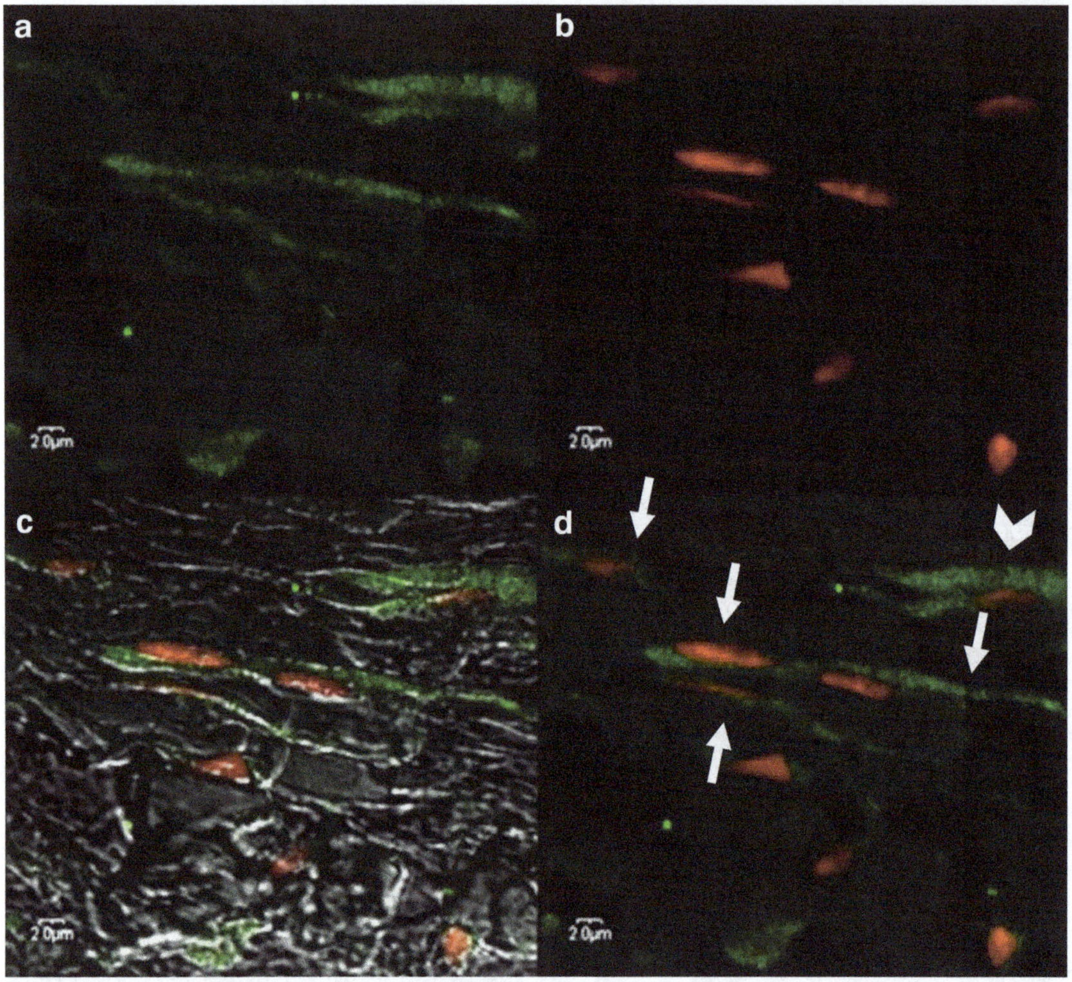

Fig. 4 Muscular layer of tip of the uterine horn adjacent to the oviduct. Fusiform and trigonal c-kit-positive ICLC (*arrows*) as well as star-like shape ICLC (*arrowhead*) forming a network through the long cellular processes. **a** Emission spectra of AF 488, **b** emission spectra of 7AAD, **c** emission spectra of AF 488 and 7AAD as well as tissue structure, **d** emission spectra of AF 488 and 7AAD. Confocal microscopy following IF labeling, original magnification 3000x

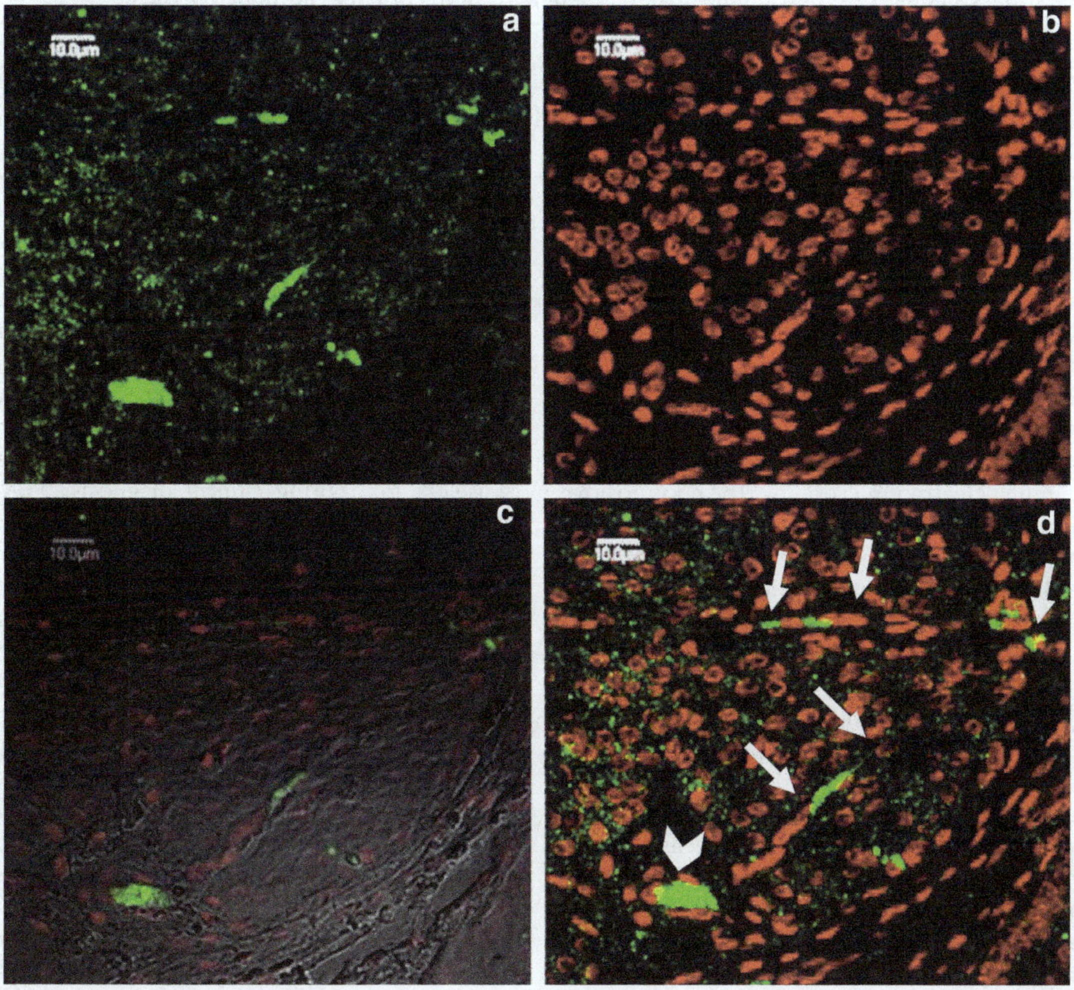

Fig. 5 Muscular layer of tip of the uterine horn adjacent to the oviduct. Fusiform and trigonal c-kit-positive ICLC (*arrows*). The long, moniliform cellular processes formed a network contacting smooth muscle cells, nerve cells and capillaries (*arrowhead*). **a** Emission spectra of AF 488, **b** emission spectra of 7AAD, **c** emission spectra of AF 488 and 7AAD as well as tissue structure, **d** emission spectra of AF 488 and 7AAD. Confocal microscopy following IF labeling, original magnification 600x

Table 1 Interstitial Cajal-like cell density (mean ± SD) in segments of the porcine reproductive tract

Staining method	Oviduct (infundibulum)	Oviduct (isthmus)	Uterine horn (tip)	Uterine horn (middle)	Corpus uteri
HE	2.22 ± 0.09^{a}	5.35 ± 0.80^{b}	6.78 ± 0.76^{c}	3.89 ± 0.44^{d}	4.43 ± 0.79^{d}
IHC	4.13 ± 0.35^{A}	5.21 ± 0.31^{B}	5.25 ± 0.24^{B}	3.92 ± 0.25^{A}	4.20 ± 0.45^{A}
IF	2.16 ± 0.82^{x}	4.12 ± 1.01^{y}	3.10 ± 0.92^{z}	3.17 ± 1.04^{z}	1.22 ± 0.38^{v}

HE hematoxylin-eosin staining, *IHC* immunohistochemical labeling, *IF* Immunofluorescent labeling

Kolmogorow-Smirnow test ($\alpha = 0.05$). Density defined as cell numbers in 20 fields of view

Different letters indicate statistically significant differences independently in row HE, ICH, IF ($P < 0.0001$)

and corpus, and the density decreased with increasing distance from the oviduct. However, in the oviduct itself, the ICLC density in the infundibulum was about 38% less than in the isthmus. A significantly higher ($P < 0.0001$) density of ICLC was found in the isthmus of the oviduct (5.21 ± 0.3; 99.3%) and in the uterine horn tip (5.25 ± 0.24; 100.0%) by immunofluorescence microscopy, while a lower density of ICLC was observed in the uterine horn (3.92 ± 0.25; 74.7%) and body (4.20 ± 0.45; 79.9%).

Table 2 Interstitial Cajal-like cells percentage (mean) in segments of the porcine reproductive tract

Staining method	Oviduct (infundibulum) (%)	Oviduct (isthmus) (%)	Uterine horn (tip) (%)	Uterine horn (middle) (%)	Corpus uteri (%)
HE	32.7^{a}	79.0^{b}	100.0^{c}	57.4^{d}	65.4^{d}
IHC	78.6^{A}	99.3^{B}	100.0^{B}	74.7^{A}	79.9^{A}
IF	52.4^{x}	100.0^{y}	75.3^{z}	77.1^{z}	29.6^{v}

HE hematoxylin-eosin staining, *IHC* immunohistochemical labeling, *IF* immunofluorescence labeling

One-way ANOVA test with multiple comparisons Tukey test ($P < 0.0001$). Different letters indicate statistically significant differences

Discussion

This study describes for the first time the occurrence and density of c-kit-positive ICLC in different parts of the porcine reproductive tract. Changes in ICLC density were estimated by histological, immunohistochemical and immunofluorescence methods and confirmed especially by scanning electron microscopy. The c-kit positive fusiform or spindle-shaped cells with multiple, long, thin, moniliform processes in a characteristic location (outside the epithelium) are in agreement with previous results [18, 19]. However, we did not find that routine HE staining was sufficient for identification of ICLC, as found also by Popescu et al. [13]. In our experience, the main problem remains the difficulty of differentiating between the cell processes and collagen fibers [12]. Hutchings et al. [19] assembled criteria that allowed the differentiation of m-ICLC from fibroblasts based on close contact with target nerve bundles and smooth muscle cells, characteristic cytoplasmic processes, and gap junctions with smooth muscle cells or with each other. Evaluation of these criteria in porcine tissues was possible when they were examined by immunofluorescence. Therefore, the HE approach was used only for initial screening and to examine tissue architecture.

The specificity of immunoreactions was confirmed in the positive control—porcine ileum used as reference material and the negative control—lack of signal. We confirmed similar immunophenotypes of ICC and ICLC in porcine specimens and ruled out detected signals as being from specific secondary antibody binding. Furthermore, the porcine ICLC immunophenotype was obtained by correlating morphology with immunohistochemistry and immunofluorescence. The specificity of the primary antibody (CD117/c-kit) was confirmed in porcine specimens using commercial antibody (Dako, USA). Popescu et al. [13] referred this method as the most effective. Those authors assessed the intensity of ICLC reactivity in tissues from the human uterus and fallopian tube and stated that the anti CD117/c-kit polyclonal antibody (Dako, USA) in 1:100 dilution demonstrated a strong reaction (i.e., strikingly positive even at low magnification). We adopted the published staining protocol for porcine tissues using both immunohistochemical and immunofluorescence labeling.

Interstitial Cajal-like cells have specific ultrastructural morphological features evident in transmission electron microscopy (TEM) that together with morphology and c-kit expression are considered the 'gold' [16] and 'platinum standard' [13] for identification of these cells. TEM of ultra-thin myometrium sections is not effective and is useless for routine clinical diagnosis. TEM requires extensive sample preparation in which the thickness of the specimens should be less than 100 nm. In comparison, sample preparation for SEM is not that difficult. SEM focuses on the sample's surface and its composition whereas TEM provides details about internal composition. Therefore, TEM can show many more characteristics of the sample, such as morphology, crystallization, stress or even magnetic domains. On the other hand, SEM shows only the morphology of samples, which is enough for ICLC confirmation in screening sections but insufficient for detailed cell research (e.g., verifying multicontact synapses, distances between membranes, conformation of the endoplasmic reticulum). The SEM is a better tool for surface characterization compared to TEM which is better for internal structure analysis but it is still hardly effective for routine clinical use. Thus, we were looking for a simple, quick, relatively inexpensive and effective ICLC evaluation protocol that would be useful in clinical diagnosis of reproductive disorders in livestock animals. The protocols described in this study are easy to perform and permits general characterization of myometrial ICLC.

In agreement with other reports [20–23], the m-ICLC observed in porcine reproductive tract were c-kit positive. In all porcine oviductal and uterine slides the ICLC were located mainly on the boundaries of smooth muscle bundles throughout the myometrium, similar to human tissues [19], but the morphology and density were slight different, depending on cell localization. Similar to the human fallopian tube [12, 19] and myometrium [18, 19], cells with very long, moniliform cytoplasmic processes predominantly exhibiting fusiform and spindle-shaped or triangular cell bodies, respectively.

At the same time, a large number of ICLC was localized near small blood vessels which corroborates earlier findings [10, 12, 13, 23]. Shafic et al. [10] suggested that the ICC themselves are under the control of excitatory or inhibitory transmitters. Their close contact with blood vessels suggests that ICLC may be particularly responsive to humoral stimuli, which is supported by the presence of ICLC ovarian steroid hormone receptors. It was reported that human myometrial ICLC express estrogen and progesterone receptors [23, 24]. However, more studies are needed to fully elucidate the function of ICLC in the porcine reproductive tract.

Furthermore, in the present study, the highest density of ICLC was found in the isthmus of the oviduct and the tip of the uterine horn, while a lower density of ICLC was found in the uterus proper (horns and corpus). Therefore, based on quantitative analysis, we suggest the uterine horn tip as the place with the highest ICLC density. Shafic et al. [10] reported that uterine electric activity appears to be controlled through ICC, whose continuous pacemaker activity is conducted to the smooth muscle cells of the uterus. We speculate that ICLC accumulation in the isthmus of the oviduct and the tip of the uterine horn may be connected with ICLC functional activity. However, the role of ICLC as the "primary" pacemakers, which initiate slow waves in the myometrium and oviduct muscle layers, needs to be determined in future investigations.

Conclusions

The results confirm the presence of ICLC in the porcine reproductive tract and indicate that a combination of light and confocal microscopy techniques is a viable approach to identify ICLC in clinical diagnostics. These methods are inexpensive and effective in ICLC evaluation. We believe that in the future our approach can be applied to clinical diagnosis. The detailed description of ICLC in the porcine reproductive tract may lead to a better understanding of reproductive tract motility and have clinical implications by explaining infertility in sows without any proven uterine and fallopian tube abnormalities.

Authors' contributions

ZG and RZ designed the research and contributed the analytical tools. BP took part in planning the experimental study and contributed to the provision of the materials and methods. MD and BP performed the research. MD analyzed the data and drafted the manuscript. All authors read and approved the final manuscript.

Author details

[1] Department of Large Animal Diseases with Clinic, Faculty of Veterinary Medicine, Warsaw University of Life Sciences (WULS-SGGW), Nowoursynowska 100, 02-797 Warsaw, Poland. [2] Veterinary Research Centre and Center for Biomedical Research, Warsaw University of Life Sciences (WULS-SGGW), Nowoursynowska 100, 02-797 Warsaw, Poland.

Acknowledgements

This work was supported by the State Committee for Research Investigation Grant NN308 077439. The study was conducted in the Veterinary Research Centre WULS (WCB) and the Center for Biomedical Research (CBB) supported by EFRR RPO WM 2007–2013. We thank Dr. Barry Bavister for his professional editing of the manuscript.

Competing interests

The authors declare that they have no competing interests.

References

1. Garcia-Lopez P, Garcia-Marin V, Martínez-Murillo R, Freire M. Updating old ideas and recent advances regarding the interstitial cells of Cajal. Brain Res Rev. 2009;61:154–69.
2. Cajal SR. Sur les ganglions et plexus nerveux de l'intestin. Soc Biol. 1983;45:213–23.
3. Torihashi S, Horisawa M, Watanabe Y. C-Kit immunoreactive interstitial cells in the human gastrointestinal tract. J Auton Nerv Syst. 1999;75:38–50.
4. Kito Y, Suzuki H. Properties of pacemaker potentials recorded from myenteric interstitial cells of Cajal distributed in the mouse small intestine. J Physiol. 2003;553:803–18.
5. Burton LD, Housley GD, Salih SG, Jaeenwood D. P2X2receptor expression by intestinal cells of Cajal in vas deferens implicated in semen emission. Auton Neurosci Basic Clin. 2000;84:147–61.
6. Sergenat GP, Hollywood MS, McCloskey KD, Thornbury KD, McHale MG. Specialized peacemaking cells in the rabbit urethra. J Physiol. 2000;526:356–66.
7. Shafik A, El-Sibai O, Shafik AA, Shafik I. Identification of interstitial cells of Cajal in human urinary bladder: concept of vesical pacemaker. Urology. 2004;64:809–13.
8. Exintaris B, Klemm MF, Lang RJ. Spontanous slow wave and contractile activity of guinea pig prostate. J Urol. 2002;168:315–22.
9. McCloskey KD, Hollywood MA, Thornbury KD, Ward SM, McHale NG. Kit-like immunopositive cells in sheep mesenteric lymphatic vessels. Cell Tissue Res. 2002;310:77–84.
10. Shafik A, El-Sibai O, Shafik I. Identification of c-kit-positive cells in the uterus. Int J Gynaecol Obstet. 2004;87:254–5.
11. Harhun MI, Pucovský V, Povstyan OV, Gordienko DV, Bolton TB. Interstitial cells in the vasculature. J Cell Mol Med. 2005;9:232–43.
12. Popescu LM, Ciontea SM, Cretoin D, Hinescu ME, Radu E, Ionescu N, et al. Novel type of interstitial cell in human fallopian tube. J Cell Mol Med. 2005;9:479–523.
13. Popescu LM, Ciontea SM, Cretoiu D. Interstitial Cajal-like cells in human uterus and fallopian tube. Ann NY Acad Sci. 2007;1101:139–65.
14. Popescu LM, Andrei F, Hinescu ME. Snapshots of mammary gland interstitial cells: methylene blue vital staining and c-kit immunopositicity. J Cell Mol Med. 2005;9:476–7.
15. Popescu LM, Hinescu ME, Ionescu N, Ciontea SM, Cretoiu D, Ardelean C. Interstitial cells of Cajal in pancreas. J Cell Mol Med. 2005;9:169–90.
16. Huizinga JD, Thuneberg L, Vanderwinden JM, et al. Interstitial cells of Cajal as targets for pharmacological intervention in gastrointestinal motor disorders. Trends Pharmacol Sci. 1997;18:393–403.
17. Maeda H, Yamagata A, Nishikawa S, Yoshinaga K, Kobayashi S, Nishi K, et al. Requirement of c-kit for development of intestinal pacemaker system. Development. 1992;116:369–75.
18. Ciontea SM, Radu E, Regalia T, Ceafalan L, Cretoiu D, Gherghiceanu M, et al. C-kit immunopositive interstitial cells (Cajal-type) in human myometrium. J Cell Mol Med. 2005;9:407–20.
19. Hutchings G, Williams O, Cretoiu D, Ciontea SM. Myometrial interstitial cells and the coordination of myometrial contractility. J Cell Mol Med. 2009;13:4268–82.
20. Hutchings G, Gevaert T, Deprest J, Nilius B, De Ridder D. Effect of prolonged c-kit receptor inhibition by imatinib mesylate on the uterine contractility of pregnant rabbits. Gynecol Obstet Invest. 2008;65:108–11.
21. Kilianczyk R, Domino M, Gajewski Z, Zabielski R, Godlewski M, Pawlinski B. Localization of the Interstitial Cajal-like Cells in the porcine reproductive tract. Reprod Domest Anim. 2015;50:43–4.
22. Pawlinski B, Domino M, Kilianczyk R, Godlewski M, Zabielski R, Gajewski Z. Identification of interstitial Cajal-like cells in the sow uterus and oviduct. Reprod Domest Anim. 2012;47:488–9.

6

Veterinarians' role in clients' decision-making regarding seriously ill companion animal patients

Stine Billeschou Christiansen[1*], Annemarie Thuri Kristensen[2], Jesper Lassen[3] and Peter Sandøe[1,3]

Abstract

Background: When companion animals become seriously ill clients may have doubts about treatment choices, if any, and turn to veterinarians for help. But how should veterinarians reply? Influence on clients' decision-making may or may not be acceptable—depending on one's attitude to principles such as 'paternalism', 'respect for autonomy' and 'shared decision-making'. This study takes as a starting point a situation where the animal is chronically ill, or aged, with potentially reduced animal welfare and client quality of life, and thus where clients need to consider treatment options or euthanasia. It is assumed throughout that both veterinarians and clients have the animals' best interest at heart. The purpose of the study was to explore the challenges these situations hold and to investigate how clients experience veterinary influence. A second aim was to reflect on the ethical implications of the role of veterinarians in these situations. Qualitative interviews were conducted with 12 dog owners considering treatment or euthanasia of their chronically ill or aged dogs.

Results: Challenges relating to the dog and to the client were identified. Some situations left the interviewees hesitant, e.g. if lacking a clear cut-off point, the dog appeared normal, the interviewee felt uncertain about treatments or animal welfare, or experienced conflicting concerns. Some interviewees found that veterinarians could influence their decisions. Such influence was received in different ways by the interviewees. Some interviewees wanted active involvement of the veterinarian in the decision-making process, and this may challenge a veterinarian's wish to respect client autonomy.

Conclusions: Different preferences are likely to exist amongst both veterinarians and clients about veterinary involvement in clients' decision-making, and such preferences may vary according to the situation. It is suggested, that one way to handle this challenge is to include respect for client preference on veterinary involvement under a wider understanding of respect for autonomy, and to apply models of shared decision-making to veterinary practice. In any case there is a need to further explore the challenges these situations raise, and for the veterinary profession to engage in more formal and structured deliberation over the role of veterinarians in relation to clients' decision-making.

Keywords: Veterinary ethics, Paternalism, Autonomy, Informed consent, Shared decision-making, Euthanasia, Companion animals, Dogs, Animal welfare, Human-animal bond

*Correspondence: sbc@sund.ku.dk
[1] Department of Large Animal Sciences, Faculty of Health and Medical Sciences, University of Copenhagen, Grønnegårdsvej 8, 1870 Frederiksberg C, Denmark
Full list of author information is available at the end of the article

Background

When a companion animal becomes seriously ill the client may be faced with difficult decisions. In some cases the answer is obvious. In others, however, the client may have doubts about which treatment to choose, whether to initiate treatment at all, or whether perhaps euthanasia is the better option. In such situations clients may turn to the veterinarian for help, asking 'What would you do if it was your animal?' Assuming that the situation leaves room for different lines of action, which are all in compliance with the law and can all be defended from a plausible ethical point of view, how should the veterinarian reply? Share his or her preferred option in similar situations? Offer an opinion on the best decision for the animal and the client? Inform the client of the options but refuse to offer any guidance on decision-making? Or initiate a dialogue with the client about what to do?

At a first glance 'What would you do?' is a straightforward question. Providing an answer backed by the relevant medical information may seem a relatively easy task. In reality, however, the situation often presents more complex issues. First of all, the circumstances of the veterinarian and client may differ, so the veterinarian's preferred option may not be relevant to the client. Secondly, the client and veterinarian may have different ethical values, so what seems the right choice to the veterinarian may not be ethically acceptable to the client. It is, however, worth noting that the question may not really be about what the veterinarian would do, but rather be an appeal to the veterinarian to relieve the client of responsibility for the decision. But if the veterinarian feels that the decision needs to be made by the client alone, all he or she can and should do is to provide the necessary factual information which can serve as part of the basis for the client's decision. Providing this information does, however, involve both a selection process (which information is relevant?) and communication with the client which may (unintentionally and non-verbally) convey the veterinarian's personal views [1]. On the other hand, if the veterinarian engages in the decision-making, he or she may influence the outcome in a very direct way [2–6].

Veterinarians may have different ideas about how they should respond, which again may reflect different ethical points of view. For example, influence on a client's decision-making may or may not be acceptable—depending on one's attitude to ethical issues and principles such as 'paternalism', 'respect for autonomy', 'informed consent' and 'shared decision-making'. In human medical ethics these topics have been discussed for a number of years. Paternalism may be understood as the view that it is acceptable to make decisions on behalf of patients with their best interests in mind. Respect for autonomy, by contrast, emphasizes that patients have the right to make their own choices. Truly autonomous decisions require the person to understand what the situation involves in order not to be manipulated. Respect for autonomy is therefore closely linked to the idea of informed consent. Informed consent, in turn, may be understood as given only if a person is competent to act, receives and comprehends full information about the options available, and voluntarily chooses one of those options. Together, respecting patient autonomy and obtaining informed consent thus aims at reducing the risk of undue influence on the patient's decision-making. These principles have been widely debated within human medicine when it comes to guidance in doctor-patient relationships and decision-making. In recent years the paternalistic approach has been downplayed and instead patient autonomy and procedures for obtaining informed consent have been encouraged. Shifting the approach in this way, it is hoped, will better protect the patient's right to decide on the care of his or her body and reduce the doctor's risk of being blamed for carrying out procedures against a patient's wish or interests (see [7–9] for thorough discussion of these principles). However, it has proved difficult to reach a consensus on the definitions of these key concepts and their applications, and the concepts have been challenged and have evolved over time.

Paternalism, where all decision-making is left to the doctor, and patient autonomy, where it is all left to the patient, may be seen as two extremes along a continuum of possibilities in the decision-making process. Intermediate alternatives, referred to as shared decision-making, may as a matter of fact reflect more accurately the way decisions are often made in practice. Shared decision-making is also discussed as an ideal—i.e. normatively, as the best way of handling the decision process in some cases [10]. Shared decision-making is described as a situation involving at least two participants, typically doctor and patient, who exchange information and preferences and reach an agreement on how to proceed. Agreement is understood as a readiness to proceed with a certain decision, not necessarily as agreement that this decision was the best option [11, 12]. Shared decision-making may be considered appropriate in cases when there are at least two reasonable medical options, and the choice between them is based on patient values and life circumstances [13].

The concepts of autonomy and informed consent can also provide guidance in veterinarian-client relationships. Inspired by human medical ethics, a similar development has taken place in veterinary medical ethics, where the ethical and communicative challenges, as well as the obligations veterinarians have when dealing with animals and clients, have been discussed. Issues include both how to respect client autonomy and how to handle conflicts when such autonomy poses risks to animal welfare. In a veterinary context, the situation differs from that of human medicine in several ways. Instead of normally just two parties to consider in the decision-making (doctor and patient) there are here three: the veterinarian, the animal and the client. The animal patient is the client's property and is generally considered unable to participate in the decision-making. As a consequence legal issues have been raised, as well as concerns about decision-making on behalf of others, like those prompted by proxy decision-making on behalf of children and the mentally impaired [14–18]. Also, the perception of animals as unable to participate in decision-making has been challenged as animals can express preferences, and it has been argued that these preferences should be taken into account [17]. Concerns about autonomy and informed consent include considerations about the veterinarian's obligations to the animal versus the client and issues arising from veterinary and client differences in assessing animal welfare [1–5, 17–33].

It has been argued, that veterinarians should promote client autonomy by providing information on the options and leaving clients to reach decisions even if the veterinarian finds the decision to be morally problematic [2]. One reason for this is for the veterinarian to avoid blame for the decisions made [2, 10, 26, 27]. Another reason is that the decision-making may give the client an opportunity for personal growth [34]. However, reasons have also been given in favour of a more active role. One relates to the protection of an animal's welfare when the client is hesitating to make a decision that would end the animal's suffering [1, 4, 29]. Another relates to respect for client preferences about the role of the veterinarian. Here, a client in doubt or emotionally overwhelmed may want the veterinarian to take an active role [1]. It has thus been argued, that the veterinarian-client relationship should be more of a two-way process [23].

Returning to the situation described in the beginning of this paper and the 'What would you do?' question, it ought to be obvious already that although this is well known amongst veterinarians in companion animal practice, there is no simple right way to respond, but rather conflicting principles underpinned by different reasons. Although a better understanding of the challenges such situations present would be helpful when supporting clients in decision-making, this scenario has received relatively little scholarly attention. Thus, one way forward is to take a closer look at situations where decision-making becomes challenging, and at the questions to which these situations give rise.

This study takes as a starting point a situation where the animal is chronically ill, or aged, with potentially reduced animal welfare and client quality of life. The client thus needs to consider treatment options or euthanasia, and it is supposed that both the veterinarian and client have the animal's best interests at heart. The purpose of the study was first to explore the challenges these situations hold, and the way clients experience veterinary influence. A second aim was to reflect on the ethical implications of the role of the veterinarian in these situations.

This paper thus addresses three questions relating to situations when decision-making becomes difficult. First of all, in what kind of situations do clients find it difficult to make a decision on their own? Here the qualitative study identifies challenges for clients considering treatment or euthanasia of their chronically ill or aged dog. Next, in cases where the animal is neither suffering nor curable, how do veterinarians respond to clients' hesitation to decide, and requests for advice? The qualitative study here analyses the way in which clients find that veterinarians have facilitated or influenced their decision-making. Finally, if a veterinarian takes a more active role, how should he or she engage in decisions about the initiation or continuation of treatments, or about euthanasia? Drawing on the results from the qualitative study, the role of veterinarians and the ethical implications when clients seek advice on treatment or euthanasia is addressed.

Methods

In order to obtain detailed descriptions of a variety of client-experiences, individual in-depth qualitative interviews with dog owners were carried out. The dog owners were recruited among the clients of the University Hospital for Companion Animals at the University of Copenhagen, and a privately owned companion animal practice in Copenhagen.

Initially, searches were run in electronic patient records systems for diagnoses and choices of treatment that allowed potential interviewees to be identified. The results reported in this paper are part of a series of interviews which also concerned client quality of life. Both aspects relating to client quality of life and aspects relating to the sharing of concerns with the veterinarian therefore framed the selection of interviewees. Two initial recruitment criteria for the selection of dog owners for further screening were applied: (1) that the owner had engaged with treatments and care that could be expected to affect his or her own life; and (2) that where the dog had died, this was no longer than 8 months ago. Furthermore, the selection process focused on cases where notes were made in the patient records of clients expressing worries about animal welfare, treatment choices, euthanasia and/or their own quality of life, as these clients had obviously shared these concerns with the veterinarians.

The dog owners identified were then contacted and asked about their interest in, and consent to, participation and further screening. Given that this was a qualitative study exploring the different kinds of situation and challenge clients face when they need to make decisions about treatment and euthanasia, it was important to recruit a diverse group of interviewees. The purpose of the screening was therefore to ensure that interviewees were selected to cover, between them, a variety of factors that could reasonably be expected to influence the clients' situation in various ways. Factors directly connected with the animal patient included diagnoses, medication needs and other forms of patient care, and the age of the dog and whether it was still alive. Client-related factors revolved primarily around the client's circumstances and included composition of the household and the perceived economic burden of the veterinary treatment. The interviewees were thus selected with the goal of covering the diversity of the questions to be explored—not as a representative group reflecting the frequency, or distribution, of the relevant phenomena in clients in general [35]. Ten interviews had been conducted when only minor new nuances emerged. Two more interviews were then conducted to ensure that the point of saturation regarding the issues to be explored had been reached [36], i.e. twelve interviews were conducted in total. Results of the interviews regarding client quality of life and a table presenting the screening details and the diversity of the interviewees' screening profiles have been published previously [37].

All interviews took place at the clients' homes in 2008. In some households the legal owner of the dog was not its primary caregiver. In these cases, the primary caregiver was chosen for interview. The interviews were semi-structured and followed an interview guide. The interview guide ensured that all interviews would cover the same themes (although not necessarily in the same order), and also allowed interviews to follow issues that had emerged as important. The themes of the interview guide that were relevant to this paper were: client concerns about animal welfare and euthanasia (with the aim of uncovering the kind of concerns experienced and challenges faced in client decision-making); and client experiences of veterinary visits (with the aim of uncovering how clients found that veterinarians had or could have helped them make decisions). The questions in the interview guide were open so as to stimulate fuller replies, which were explored further: for example, 'Did you worry about anything?' and 'Do you think the vet did something to help you through this?' (The interview guide is available as Additional file 1). Beyond what was requested by the interviewer, interviewees were encouraged to add information they considered relevant. The interviews lasted 2 h on average. They were recorded and transcribed verbatim.

The transcribed interviews were analysed qualitatively by the first author using the software ATLAS.ti 5.0 to code and retrieve relevant text. The construction of codes and initial data analysis followed the template organizing style [38], with codes based on key points from the interview guide as well as additional aspects raised in the interviews. The text relating to each code was then analysed for features illuminating that aspect: for example, for the code 'euthanasia decision' issues relating to both challenges of the situation and to decision-making then emerged, which in turn triggered a closer examination of the aspects that made it harder or easier to make decisions about euthanasia. Abductive reasoning, allowing dynamic interaction between data and the generation of ideas [39], thus inspired further analysis and interpretation.

The study was approved by the Ethical and Administrative Committee of the Department of Veterinary Clinical and Animal Sciences, University of Copenhagen, as well as by the Danish Data Protection Agency. Interview excerpts appearing in this paper were translated from Danish by the first author. In some cases text has been omitted, which is indicated by "...(...)...", and text in [...] has sometimes been added for clarity.

When reporting the results and considering the ethical implications the term "interviewee" is used when reference is made to the interviews in this study, and the term "client" is used for general discussion. The term "owner" is used in the short dog-owner description placed at the end of each interview quote.

Results

The interviews generated data informing the two questions aimed at the study's first purpose: exploring the situation of the client when he or she is considering further treatment or euthanasia of a chronically ill or aged dog. The first question explored the challenges these situations hold, i.e. what features of the situation ease or complicate the client's decision-making? The second question explored the clients' experiences of veterinary influence, i.e. how do clients find that veterinarians have, or could have, facilitated their decision-making? It should be noted, that in some cases the experiences shared by the interviewees related to veterinary practices other than those from which they were recruited. The second purpose—ethical reflection on the role of the veterinarian in these situations—is dealt with in the discussion.

Features easing or complicating the client's decision-making

For some interviewees the decision to euthanize the dog was easy, relatively speaking. For others, it was more difficult. Here the challenges related either mainly to the dog or mainly to the client.

Situations leaving interviewees capable and at peace with their decisions

Some conditions made the decision to euthanize the dog easier. Several related to poor welfare of the dog: for example, the dog was suffering, no longer happy, unable to function, or otherwise clearly not doing well; or episodes of illness were occurring too often. Other conditions related to the exhaustion of other options, i.e. when everything had been tried out and it was futile to pursue treatment. Clear signs of health deterioration or client fatigue tended to favour the decision to euthanize. More than one of these conditions could be present at the same time. Thus:

> *"It was the last week or so that it started going downhill, and I'd already asked if there was anything else we could do...(...)...And when there wasn't anything left to do and we could just anticipate her getting worse and worse, I felt that then it wasn't as hard to make that decision. Because it didn't work... [It worked] neither for the dog nor for us" (owner of euthanized dog with cancer).*

Situations where interviewees found decision-making more difficult

Other situations created more of a grey area and interviewee hesitation. Here dog-related challenges included the lack of a clear cut-off point in cases with slow deterioration or fluctuating levels of health. Client-related challenges included lack of knowledge, conflicts of concerns and the taking of responsibility.

Dog-related challenges

Slow deterioration A clear cut-off point was hard to identify when the dog's condition was slowly deteriorating without any major turn of events. It could be difficult to decide exactly when to stop, as the lack of a clear sign, well-defined criteria or an obvious cut-off point, could make it hard to comfortably draw a line and opt for euthanasia. For example:

> *"I think it is difficult to know when to make that decision, because, for about one and a half years she has been old and you've been saying now is the time you should consider getting it done. But I have to admit that I also think that if you are not in pain, if you can move around in the garden more or less without being anxious or afraid or such like, when you can find your water and food and you can eat and are not incontinent, and can do your business and accept patting ...then I don't have to make the decision. But exactly when you should do it, that is a bit difficult, I think" (owner of euthanized old dog with dementia).*

Fluctuating levels of health When good health alternated with bad, a clear cut-off point was also lacking, but another challenge was added when it came to deciding that enough is enough. During the bad episodes considerations in favour of ceasing treatment might emerge, but then questions might also arise why euthanasia was not chosen last time and why the dog should not be given yet another chance. Some interviewees felt torn between blaming themselves for not having euthanized the dog earlier to avoid this phase, on the one hand, and hoping that this episode would be the last and that the next course of treatment would make things better, on the other. As some conditions allow repeated treatments and perhaps also hold a seemingly endless list of additional treatment options, interviewees could find themselves caught in a pattern where they had very strong hopes that things would get better, and thus kept seeking treatments, optimistically believing that the next one would be the one that would get the condition under control. For example:

> *"It is just really hard to say, 'Okay, now it is over,' because....I mean, it's just, why now? I could allow for one more episode or I could have stopped a long time ago, but when you have gone down the road of wanting to try everything for him, it is just really difficult suddenly to put your foot down and say this is it" (owner of euthanized dog with epilepsy).*

In addition, if the dog appeared normal, and was, for instance, playing happily in the garden when the euthanasia decision was close, it could be hard to bring the dog to the veterinarian for the final visit, even if the interviewee knew that the dog was ill and had witnessed episodes when the dog was obviously not well:

> *"You feel like you walk in with a dog that you can't see or sense anything wrong with, so it makes it a bit hard to euthanize it, when you can't really see that it is ill. But I knew that he was...." (owner of euthanized dog with epilepsy).*

Client-related challenges

Lack of knowledge Knowledge was a significant factor in the decision-making process. For example:

> *"If we had known even more about it, it would probably have been easier to make the decision than it was" (owner of living dog with cancer).*

But, although finding that veterinarians took time to provide information, the interviewees could feel unable to absorb or understand all the information they had been given about the dog's medical condition, and thus doubt their own judgements about the best way forward. For example:

> *"I think they were really good at taking time to explain if you had any questions, and they also told us a lot about the disease, but to remember exactly what happens, it was...(...)...I don't know if I actually got any wiser about what goes on during such a treatment...(...)...I had to trust that it was good, what they told me to do, and that was what I had decided to do, I think" (owner of euthanized dog with cancer).*

Strong concerns about animal welfare were expressed along with the need to ensure that the dog was not suffering. But unless their dogs showed clear signs of being well or unwell, interviewees sometimes felt uncertain about their dogs' welfare. For example:

> *"If only you knew, he is old and he is tired, but he must not feel bad, and I just can't tell, and maybe it's because I close my eyes, because maybe there is small chance, right?" (owner of living old dog with diabetes).*

Uncertainty about the animal patient's welfare raised concerns about when it was time to consider euthanasia:

> *"I don't know if you can measure whether a dog is in pain or not...(...)...but it would be nice if you could be more certain that now it is time to do it, because now it is better for the dog" (owner of euthanized old dog with dementia).*

Conflicting concerns In the process of decision-making, weighing up conflicting concerns about the dog and the interviewee could be difficult. Several kinds of conflict arose when treatments and euthanasia were being considered. One set of conflicts related to the treatment of the dog only. Here, the wish to give the dog a chance by initiating or continuing treatment was in conflict with the wish to protect the dog from suffering and thus choose euthanasia. When a treatment was chosen, conflicts could arise because the desired effects of the treatment had to be weighed against unwanted potential side-effects. For example:

> *"I also considered an operation to insert a tube in her throat so she could breathe. Because that was the only operation they could offer, and considering that there was a 50 % chance, I wanted to give her the 50 %, but I really wouldn't put her through all that. The little dog had been through enough. So it wasn't worth it" (owner of euthanized dog with asthma).*

Another set of conflicts put dog interests against human interests. The risk of postponing euthanasia for too long for the interviewee's own sake (e.g. because it was hard for the interviewee to part with the dog) was one issue of this kind. Others focused on finding the right balance of sacrifice made by the interviewee when caring for the dog, and on the concern that euthanasia should not simply be an easy way out of commitments to the dog:

> *"It shouldn't be euthanasia just because it is hard for me. That's how I feel. I don't want to euthanize it just because it is hard for me. And ... I think it sounds bad, too, to euthanize an animal just because it does not fit in. I could never do that" (owner of living dog with epilepsy).*

Other conflicts arose when humans identified with the dog's condition. Here euthanasia could be postponed as it raised complex questions, too tough to deal with, about human patients in similar situations. An example:

> *"My husband was ill and he found it very difficult that we should part with the dog, because he thought, well, now she is ill and old and then you just get rid of her, and maybe he felt it was a bit like that with him too, you know" (owner of euthanized old dog with dementia).*

Finally, conflicts sometimes arose when family members disagreed over the choice of treatment or about the timing of euthanasia.

Taking responsibility Taking responsibility for ending the dog's life and the feeling of being an executioner were hard for some interviewees to bear. It could be seen as preferable for the dog to die peacefully in its sleep, or even as a result of an accident, as this would at least relieve the interviewee of responsibility for the death. Although acknowledging that decisions about euthanasia were their responsibility, making this decision sometimes felt wrong and made the interviewee feel like a bad person for taking a life:

> *"It would be easier if they were hit by a bus or something, I think. Because then it's over, or if you just woke up one day and it was lying there, dead. But that you have to make that decision yourself. I think that's horrible" (owner of living dog with allergy).*

How clients find that veterinarians had or could have facilitated their decision-making

The interviewees generally expressed a lot of concern about their dogs' welfare, and they were aware that in some cases inaction could potentially lead to the one situation they probably feared the most: one in which they had let their dogs suffer. Where there was doubt about whether to euthanize the dog, two different strategies were reported. One was: better to be safe than sorry. Here it is acknowledged that the only way to ensure that the dog does not suffer is euthanasia at a relatively early stage. But at the same time it might seem pointless to euthanize the dog while it is still well simply to avoid the risk of suffering:

> *"That would not make sense. Well, you better get it over with right away, it will be hell over the next 8 months – don't go there! Then you would be in a situation where you put down an animal that was doing fine and all. And I don't know, I mean, I don't think that is okay either" (owner of living old dog with dementia).*

The other strategy was to ask friends, family or veterinarians for opinions and help with the decision to be made. Such input, particularly from the veterinarian, could be instrumental in moving the decision-making process forward.

Interviewees gave two main reasons for wanting more involvement from veterinarians in decisions about treatment and euthanasia. The first was the feeling that they could not assess the dog's condition, or the implications of the treatment, properly; they felt they needed the veterinarian's expert opinion before making a decision. The second was that, particularly where euthanasia was concerned, they felt that the responsibility of this decision was too great for them to take on alone. The opportunity to share the decision-making, and thus the responsibility, with the veterinarian brought relief here.

How veterinarians influence decisions

Interviewees reported several ways in which veterinarians had contributed to their decision-making: by providing information and professional assessments, by supporting impending decisions, by legitimising certain considerations, and by providing specific guidance.

The provision of information and professional assessments When interviewees found that they did not have the required knowledge to assess their dog's welfare they sometimes relied on the veterinarian's evaluation. The interviewees explained how the veterinarian could provide them with the relevant information on the dog's medical condition and the treatment options; and he or she could offer a professional assessment of the situation and the dog's welfare:

> *"I spoke to the vet and the vet presented the arguments – this thing about [the fact that] it had not spread further yet, it was only in one lymph node, and we had come in at an early stage, and that he wasn't older than he was, and that despite this being an aggressive form it would make good sense to start the treatment" (owner of living dog with cancer).*

At the same time, interviewees could be aware that veterinary knowledge covered only the medical aspects of the illness and treatment, and physical aspects of dog welfare. In the assessment of the dog's mental state and functioning in its everyday life, an interviewee might well feel more competent than the veterinarian. It was mentioned that the overall assessment of the dog's welfare was best achieved through a combination of veterinary and client knowledge. For example:

> *"They know much more about the dog somehow, about the physical stuff at least, than I do, but I know more about the emotional issues than they do; they don't know my dog like I do. I think it is important to mix both" (owner of living dog with epilepsy).*

Support for impending decisions Where an interviewee was leaning towards a particular decision, such as to euthanize the dog, confirmation from someone else that this was the right decision was sometimes sought in an effort to move the decision-making on. In this situation arguments in favour of continued treatment could be less welcome. For example:

> *"But I still needed confirmation that this [euthanasia] was right, and he [the interviewee's brother] didn't at the time, and therefore he shouldn't talk about it then. But the veterinarian confirmed straight away that this was the right thing to do" (owner of euthanized dog with asthma).*

Hope was also expressed that the veterinarian would not suggest further initiatives, but in cases where the veterinarian was reluctant to euthanize, an impending decision to do just that might be reconsidered:

> *"Clearly I need advice, but not if I take him to a vet who says I think we should give him some pills and wait and see for 10 days. Then I honestly don't know what to say, because I don't think I want that...(...)... But I know what the vet will say, that is, that the vet will support that my dog should be euthanized... (...)...If the vet surprises me and says, well, your dog should have some antibiotics, I think that, because it*

is this vet, I will say 'OK, fine then, that's what we'll do,' because I trust this one" (owner of living old dog with dementia).

Veterinary legitimisation of certain considerations Certain considerations could be difficult to address for or may perhaps be suppressed by the interviewee. Such considerations could, however, be decisive either in favour of, or against, a certain course of action. Some interviewees reported that the veterinarian's sensitivity to such considerations could be important for their decision-making. For example, if the thought of euthanasia was associated with a feeling of guilt, it could be difficult to address this issue with the veterinarian, and a veterinarian engaged in a longer treatment process might on occasion seem less sensitive to a wish for dialogue about the euthanasia option. Thus, for example:

"I tried to bring up that, maybe, I was considering euthanasia, and it was really difficult for me, because I think it is wrong, I feel I'm a bad person because, well, my dog is my child, right ... It was as if they didn't really understand what I was trying to say" (owner of living dog with epilepsy).

Furthermore, interviewees might neglect the impact on their own lives resulting from their dog's needs for special care and thus jeopardize their own quality of life. It was reported how a veterinarian could legitimise concerns for the interviewee's own well-being by raising awareness of concerns and limits to further treatment other than those relating to the dog, e.g.:

"The vet reminded me that it was ... well, that it was not a decision I should feel bad about if I decided to euthanize my dog if I felt he had become too much for me. And I think it was good to get that part in as well, because I felt like I'd totally forgotten about that, because you just take care of this animal like you've always done and all..." (owner of living old dog with dementia).

The provision of guidance In some cases interviewees reported that the veterinarian had tried to bring the decision-making forward, e.g. by recommending euthanasia or giving the interviewee a deadline for final evaluation. These interviewees were unsure if they would themselves have made the decision at that particular time, but found the encouragement from the veterinarian helpful, as part of the responsibility was taken off their shoulders:

"They were the ones who said enough was enough. And then I thought that, yeah, it probably is. So I agreed that now was the time – I could see she got worse and worse the last week, you know. I mean, if she had been bad before, hopefully I would have made that decision before, because she shouldn't be. So, I believe it was right, what they said, but I'm not quite sure if I myself would also have said it at that time too" (owner of euthanized dog with cancer).

Similarly, a continued support for treatment by the veterinarian could be perceived as an indication that euthanasia, based on welfare concerns, was unnecessary:

"The vet wouldn't just say we should go on and on if it wasn't right for the dog" (owner of living dog with cancer).

Client perspectives on veterinary influence

In cases where interviewees had shared their doubts about treatment and euthanasia with the veterinarian three separate perspectives were found. One perspective was simple awareness that the veterinarian had opinions based on concerns other than just a clinical evaluation without this necessarily leading to a feeling of being influenced in the decision-making. For example:

"The vet has expressed an ethical opinion, which is fine with me. I mean, we don't have to agree about how we see things, but I want to know what the vet's opinion is. And then I can relate to everything else the vet says" (owner of living old dog with dementia).

Similarly there was awareness that the veterinarian might have his or her own interests or agenda:

"I also knew that maybe the vet was not completely unbiased in relation to a wish to get going and get some experiences. But what the vet did say was that it was a good decision, that we had chosen a different treatment, and the vet really supported it" (owner of living dog with cancer).

Another perspective involved the interviewee striving to be autonomous in the decision-making, yet acknowledging some veterinary influence on decisions made. When the interviewee felt unable to assess the dog's condition or the implications of a treatment properly, a veterinarian's opinion could be seen as necessary in order to decide, even though this asymmetry in knowledge could influence the interviewee in the decision-making process:

"I accepted the treatment anyway. I found I couldn't do anything else – I don't know these things, so I had to let them ... well, the decisions were of course my own, but it is really difficult to decide, because you don't have the knowledge needed. So, even though they were very keen about the decision being mine and tried to inform me, I think it is still difficult to

work out. So, it is more like, we will do what you believe in, because I don't really have the ability to decide one thing or the other – that's the way it is" (owner of euthanized dog with cancer).

In the third perspective there was a desire for greater veterinary involvement, or simply for straightforward reliance on the veterinarian's opinion, although these interviewees also accepted that decisions were ultimately theirs. These interviewees wanted clearer guidance in decision-making, in particular concerning euthanasia. One factor in this was difficulty assessing animal welfare. Thus:

"I'm not a vet. I have no tools to assess how he is. I can seek help and have someone look at him and tell me...(...)...because how can I assess if it's okay anymore? Have we gone too far? That's what I'm afraid of, and it would be easier for me if someone said now you need to make a decision" (owner of living dog with allergy).

Another factor was a feeling that the responsibility of the decision to euthanize was too big to bear alone, and thus the belief that the decision needed to be made together with the vet:

"The veterinarian has to tell me [when euthanasia is advisable], because I think it is a bit much for me to take on" (owner of living old dog with dementia).

This stronger kind of involvement by a veterinarian was sometimes seen in a positive light. Thus:

"It was quite a relief to leave the responsibility to the vet who said now you have a two-month deadline. And then I thought, 'Oh, that's nice, now I don't have to worry about that anymore' – I mean, when to euthanize him. Because I knew he had to be euthanized at some point. I just didn't know how far to go...(...)...so it really was a relief when the vet said that. Then it was like the vet's decision or responsibility, even though in the end the decision was of course mine" (owner of euthanized dog with epilepsy).

Thus, where interviewees felt uncomfortable about making the right clinical or ethical judgement, or unable to do so, the influence of the veterinarian could be significant – both in terms of what decision was made and when. Moreover, the veterinary influence sometimes provided emotional support to interviewees in handling the challenges they faced.

Discussion

There are few actual studies on the veterinarian-client relationship, although much literature mentions the importance of this topic (see [40] for a review). This study is (to the authors' knowledge) one of few to address the challenges in decision-making. Sanders [41, 42], Pilgram [40] and Morris [32] primarily explored the veterinarian's perspective on veterinary-client relations, and they covered several issues of relevance to the decision-making process. This study reports the challenges as experienced from a client perspective, and more specifically, what clients encounter when they are faced with treatment choices and the possible euthanasia of their dog. This study shows that some situations left interviewees feeling hesitant in their decision-making. While some challenges mainly related to the dog's medical condition, others related to the interviewee. Veterinarians could facilitate and in some cases influence the decision-making in several ways. The interviewees expressed different perspectives on this—one being a wish for the veterinarian to be (more) involved in the decision-making. These results are taken as a starting point for further discussion on the ethical implications for the role of veterinarians, when clients are faced with difficult decisions.

The interviewees were selected for this qualitative study, and the results therefore allow conclusions only about clients with dogs and with profiles matching the criteria of selection. Details of these clients' strong sense of obligation and commitment to care for their dogs have been described elsewhere [37]. Clearly, the general population of clients is much more diverse. Furthermore, not all findings apply to all interviewees. The circumstances and the interviewees' experiences differ, or the interviewees may respond differently to the challenges they encounter. However, the results can be seen to demonstrate that decisions about treatment choices and euthanasia are more difficult in some situations than others, and then to provide an overview of the nature of such situations and the various ways in which interviewees experienced or wanted veterinary influence on their decision-making.

The interviews were conducted in Denmark, and it may be worth noting two points in relation to the legal framework in this country. Firstly, according to the Danish Animal Welfare Act veterinarians have a legal obligation to intervene if they are aware of an incurably ill animal that will experience unnecessary suffering if it is allowed to go on living, e.g. to ensure that such an animal is euthanized, even if this goes against the wish of the client [43]. Secondly, there is no legal structure to guide or secure how to get informed consent from clients. None of the interviewees reported any conflicts in relation to these legal issues, though. Cultural differences, if applying these results beyond Denmark, could be worth to consider as human-animal relations may be sensitive to cultural context [44]. Also, experiences may be different for clients with other companion animals than dogs. The experiences shared in this study are, however, assumed to be similar to experiences of clients with dogs in other Western countries, who have the animal's best interest at heart and are facing difficult decisions about treatments and euthanasia. It should be noted, though, that only the interviewees' perspectives on this matter was included, and understandings of the concept of best interest were not explored.

It should be noted as well that the interviewees were in rather different phases in terms of time since their dog's diagnosis, whether their dog was still alive or had been euthanized, and—in cases in which it had been euthanized—time since the euthanasia was performed. Animals may adapt [45], and clients' perceptions and priorities may change with time and circumstances [46, 47]. The interviews reflected only the interviewee's situation at one specific point in time. Additional interviews with the same individuals at different stages in the process would have provided a fuller picture. The results thus do not provide in-depth information on the decision-making process itself.

The overall picture in this study of the difficulties and influences a client with a seriously ill or aged dog may experience is, however, still believed to be robust: that is, it sheds some light on this complex situation and can be used as a basis for further ethical deliberation.

Ethical considerations

One of the key factors in decision-making identified in this study is knowledge—about the disease, the treatment options, and animal welfare. The study showed that veterinarians play an important role as providers of such knowledge. This raises questions about what knowledge is relevant if the client is to consent to a procedure on an informed basis, about who can provide what kind of knowledge, and about what level of detail is sufficient.

The experience of veterinary influence described in this study, in turn, raises two points. The first is that veterinarians may influence decisions even when they make an effort not to do so. The second is that clients may want veterinary influence on decision-making. These points call for a closer examination of the notion of (respect for) autonomous decision-making and how decisions can be shared in practice.

Informed consent, autonomy and shared decision-making will therefore be examined more closely in light of the study's results, with a focus on the ethical issues concerning the relation between the veterinarian and the client. No attention will be paid to situations in which client autonomy can be disregarded because animal welfare is at risk. The making of decisions by proxy may, of course, give rise to a special obligation to make decisions believed to be in the interests of the animal patient in question. As no conflicts appeared, in this study, to jeopardize the interests of the animals in the decision-making, this issue will not be considered further. Nor will legal aspects be addressed.

When is informed consent, or informed choice, sufficiently informed?

Although efforts are made to present relevant information at a level of detail suited to the client's understanding, the provision of this information does not necessarily mean that the client fully comprehends the details of the treatment options being explained [25, 33, 48]. The use of consent forms in veterinary practice has been encouraged [3], but it has been pointed out that ensuring that the client is properly informed is a vital part of informed consent [27], and that a signed consent form is not necessarily evidence of informed consent [49]. In this study, although the interviewees had made their decisions themselves and had agreed to procedures, it did not automatically follow that they truly understood all of the implications at stake.

The issue of informed consent is complex, but the objective of informed consent is that clients are provided with adequate information so they can make the right decision for their animal and for themselves [25] (see [27] for a thorough discussion on informed consent). It has been argued that consent can never be fully informed, and that therefore what should be aimed for is relevantly informed consent [7]. But what is adequate informed consent [25] and what information is relevant? Clearly, veterinarians need to keep up with medical knowledge to provide the necessary information to clients [50]. But in some cases there may be limited relevant information about the medical condition and treatment which can make the disclosure task difficult for the veterinarian and require that the veterinarian also informs the client of uncertainties regarding the treatment [28]. Follow-up studies may assist veterinarians [51–53], but if he or she consults follow-up studies, the studies will typically cover clinical aspects such as treatment success and side effects, but not necessarily all relevant aspects of animal welfare (including such matters as the animal's mental state and functioning in everyday life) [51, 53]. In addition, the veterinarian will not necessarily be fully aware of the potential impact, on clients' lives, of caring for their ill animals [2, 37]. However, the veterinarian needs to address these issues too if the client is to be fully and relevantly informed about what a treatment option entails.

The information from clients complements the veterinarian's assessment of animal welfare [17, 33, 54–59]. The present study indicates that clients may in some cases feel better prepared than their veterinarians to assess certain aspects of their animal's welfare because they know their animals better and see how they are doing in everyday life. This has been argued by others too [1, 17], although it has also been pointed out that veterinarians may be better placed to assess animal welfare in other cases and are better informed about likely prognoses [17]. All of this suggests that an exchange of the veterinarian's and the client's knowledge could be the best way to move the decision-making forward.

Given that clients may not fully comprehend all of the clinical information and its implications for their animal and themselves, and given also that such information may not always be available, one could argue that the client's consent or choice—given more options—is in practice probably rarely fully informed. Perhaps a less ambitious level of information in informed choice and consent is more realistic in an everyday scenario. It may not be practically feasible to present all treatment options to clients [28], and it has been suggested that veterinarians should only offer reasonable options [33]. Furthermore, it may be argued that veterinarians should consider how much clients want to know [3, 50], and that clients do not need to understand every nuance of a proposed treatment, but the information should be sufficient for the client to reasonably make informed decisions [27]. Thus, it may suffice that all available (and reasonable) options and known implications have been presented, and that the client feels sufficiently informed and agrees to the suggestions being made. It still needs to be determined, however, what is considered reasonable.

When is an autonomous decision sufficiently autonomous?

Full autonomy in decision-making may be challenged first by the limitations of knowledge just mentioned; and second, because of the worries, doubts and sadness clients may be facing at the time of decision-making, leaving them vulnerable to influence from an authority such as the veterinarian. In human medicine it has been argued that the right to choose does not mean a duty to choose [8, 13], and in fact when they are ill it may be a relief to patients not to be making demanding autonomous decisions [7]. It appears that similar considerations, about the need to make decisions in a state of mental distress, may be relevant in veterinary medicine. This study showed that for some interviewees the influence of a veterinarian was instrumental in ending the dog's life at a time which seemed suitable to the interviewee in terms of dog welfare and in giving the interviewee some peace of mind. In addition some interviewees had appreciated the way the veterinarian had helped them bring an end to a seemingly endless series of procedures that brought little if any improvement and ultimately only postponed the inevitable.

But to what extent is this compatible with the ideal of respect for client autonomy? It has been argued that human patients should be fully entitled, but not required, to take an active role in decision-making [60]. It has also been pointed out that there are two levels of respect for autonomy: one demands respect for the patient's wish for the doctor to be involved in decision-making, the other requires respect for the patient's wishes regarding treatment [61]. One could then argue, in the veterinary context, that client-autonomy is respected if and only if both levels are considered, i.e. when a client feels that the wish for veterinary involvement as well as the possibility to choose or reject a certain treatment or euthanasia is respected. This will allow the client to delegate some (or all) of the decision-making to the veterinarian, yet continues to give the client the option to veto a decision if he or she considers it unacceptable.

Is shared decision-making the way forward?

The findings in this study support the understanding that both clients and veterinarians are sources of relevant information, and that some clients would like greater involvement in decision-making. This suggests that the concept of shared decision-making may be the way forward in some cases.

In human medicine, it has been shown that patients may have different preferences regarding the involvement of doctors in decision-making—that some want to make their own decisions, some want to share the decision-making, and some prefer to delegate responsibility to the doctor [11]. The patient's personality may also be a factor to consider, and shared decision-making, therefore, is not the best solution in all encounters [62]. In fact, the whish for shared decision-making will depend on the context—e.g. on the disease and treatment options in question—and participation may be more desirable in situations when there is no clear best option [63]. Similar observations have been made in a veterinary context, where clients may have different preferences about the veterinarian's role in decision-making [64], and different approaches may be appropriate depending on the situation [33]. These observations support the findings in this study, that in situations when there was no obviously best option, where interviewees felt hesitant about making decisions, veterinary involvement could well be both sought and appreciated by the interviewee.

Shared decision-making is not, however, a simple task in practice. Several issues have been identified in both human and veterinary medicine. Different roles have been identified: two such are the facilitative role, where the doctor/veterinarian helps the patient/client uncover what he or she considers the best option, and a more collaborative role, where the doctor's/veterinarian's own preferences are drawn into the decision-making process [64, 65]. Furthermore, the same doctor/veterinarian may assume different roles in different consultations and their roles may even change during one and the same consultation [12, 32, 65]. In addition, it has been pointed out that wanting to participate in decision-making may be different from wanting to make the final decision [66]. The risk of patients/clients being pulled away from their own preferred decisions under the influence of doctors/veterinarians has also been emphasized [27, 67, 68]. Patients/clients may in such cases find that the doctor/veterinarian has more information than they do, or they may feel insecure about taking on the responsibility of decision-making [20, 64, 69]. These concerns are very similar to those expressed by interviewees in this study.

Potential disagreements may also become an issue. The interests of the animal and the client are not always reconcilable [70], and the veterinarian may have his or her own interests [4]. Disagreements may arise over e.g. the welfare and value of an animal, responsibilities to animals, and what the role of the veterinarian should be [5, 32, 41]. Veterinarians may not be willing to leave the decision entirely with clients, as they want to protect the animals' best interest (from their point of view), and if the client requests something that the veterinarian does not agree with, the veterinarian may try to negotiate a different course of action for his or her patient [32]. End-of-life care and euthanasia decision-making can be influenced by the ability of those involved to reach consensus [71], and veterinarians thus need to handle disagreements when engaging in shared decision-making [32]. It has been suggested that perhaps veterinary practice can learn from human medicine, e.g. regarding the development of decision-aids [33].

In human medicine patients often want to share decision-making with their doctor [72]. In the veterinary context getting information about the client's perspective may promote shared decision-making [73], but some have warned against taking the principle of informed consent lightly just because clients ask for veterinary involvement [27]. Others suggest that veterinarians should inform clients of their personal view, and thus help clients even though they then risk influencing decisions made [31]. Some have argued that providing comfort for the human caregiver is a legitimate responsibility and goal in veterinary practice [74], and that it is acceptable to influence clients when they explicitly want to be influenced and animal welfare is respected [1]. Shared decision-making thus seems to offer valuable perspectives on how veterinarians can engage in decision-making, but several challenges still need to be addressed.

So, what should you do?

In addition to being a medical expert, the veterinarian may act as a support person and facilitator in decision-making [20, 42]. Veterinarians may find that they need to offer emotional as well as informational and practical support [40], and clients may indeed expect this [75]. However, veterinarians may disagree with their clients about the best way forward [76], and professional codes of conduct may be insufficient to guide veterinarians on matters such as euthanasia and end-of-life issues [77]. There may thus be a need for more emphasis on skills in communicating with clients with terminally ill animals in the veterinary education [78], and the ethical issues addressed in this paper may assist development of useful frameworks.

In human medicine it has been argued that the focus of medical ethics should be on respect for the wishes of the autonomous person, rather than respect for the autonomous choices [9, 79], and it has been suggested to ask patients first who should be involved and how decisions should be made, before obtaining informed consent regarding what decision to make [72]. Similarly, when addressing treatment options requiring difficult decisions the veterinarian could explore what level and kind of involvement the client wants in the decision-making. Next, the role of the veterinarian could be to follow these wishes until a decision on treatment has been made, keeping in mind that the client's attitude to veterinary involvement, or the client's preferred treatment option, may change in the process.

Perhaps a specifically designed consent form should be created, to clearly acknowledge that such agreements have been made. This way the client could get the help in decision-making asked for, hopefully without the veterinarian risking the criticism that he or she has failed to respect the client's own wishes in the decision-making.

The approach of shared decision-making does, however, raise additional issues. Veterinary influence on a client's decision-making is sometimes unavoidable. How can such influence be made transparent? And how can the risk of the client being moved in a direction that goes against his or her own considered preferences be minimized? Finally, the idea of shared decision-making presupposes that both the client and the veterinarian agree to participate. Therefore it is not enough that the client wants the veterinarian to be involved in the decision-making; the veterinarian also has to be willing to take on this role in order to produce the best outcome. The notion of shared decision-making, including the associated ethical issues, and a general development of the ethical framework in veterinary decision-making clearly deserve further attention.

Conclusions

This study showed that clients may encounter several challenges when they are faced with treatment choices and the possible euthanasia of their dog, and in some cases they want the veterinarian to be involved in the decision-making. The reflections presented on key ethical principles relating to clients' decision-making, suggest that there is a need to further explore the challenges these situations raise, and to develop the ethical framework around the role of veterinarians in clients' decision-making. The idea of shared decision-making deserves special consideration.

Authors' contributions

SBC conceived of the study, participated in the design, carried out the interviews, performed the main analysis of the interviews, participated in conceptualizing the ethical implications and drafted the manuscript. ATK participated in the design of the study and helped drafting the manuscript. JL participated in the design of the study and analysis of the interviews, and helped drafting the manuscript. PS participated in the design of the study and in conceptualizing its ethical implications, and helped drafting the manuscript. All authors read and approved the final manuscript.

Author details

[1] Department of Large Animal Sciences, Faculty of Health and Medical Sciences, University of Copenhagen, Grønnegårdsvej 8, 1870 Frederiksberg C, Denmark. [2] Department of Veterinary Clinical and Animal Sciences, Faculty of Health and Medical Sciences, University of Copenhagen, Dyrlægevej 16, 1870 Frederiksberg C, Denmark. [3] Department of Food and Resource Economics, Faculty of Science, University of Copenhagen, Rolighedsvej 25, 1958 Frederiksberg C, Denmark.

Acknowledgements

The authors would like to thank the interviewees for sharing their stories and the anonymous reviewers for their valuable comments on an earlier version of the manuscript.

Competing interests

The authors declare that they have no competing interests.

References

1. Yeates JW, Main DCJ. The ethics of influencing clients. J Am Vet Med Assoc. 2010;237:263–7.
2. Tannenbaum J. Veterinary ethics: animal welfare, client relations, competition and collegiality. 2nd ed. St. Louis: Mosby; 1995.
3. Stewart MF. Companion animal death—a practical and comprehensive guide for veterinary practice. Edinburgh: Butterworth Heinemann; 1999.
4. Rollin BE. The use and abuse of aesculapian authority in veterinary medicine. J Am Vet Med Assoc. 2002;220:1144–9.
5. Morgan C, McDonald M. Ethical dilemmas in veterinary medicine. Vet Clin North Am Small Anim Pract. 2007;37:165–79.
6. McGowan TW, Phillips CJC, Hodgson DR, Perkins N, McGowan CM. Euthanasia in aged horses: relationship between the owner's personality and their opinions on, and experience of, euthanasia in horses. Anthrozoös. 2012;25:261–75.
7. O'Neill O. Autonomy and trust in bioethics. Cambridge: Cambridge University Press; 2002.
8. Beauchamp TL, Childress JF. Principles of biomedical ethics. 6th ed. New York: Oxford University Press; 2009.
9. Walker RI. Medical ethics needs a new view of autonomy. J Med Philos. 2009;33:594–608.
10. Cornell KK, Kopcha M. Client-veterinarian communication: skills for client centered dialogue and shared decision making. Vet Clin N Am Small Anim Pract. 2007;37:37–47.
11. Charles C, Gafni A, Whelan T. Shared decision-making in the medical encounter: what does it mean? (Or it takes at least two to tango). Soc Sci Med. 1997;44:681–92.
12. Charles C, Gafni A, Whelan T. Decision-making in the physician-patient encounter: revisiting the shared treatment decision-making model. Soc Sci Med. 1999;49:651–61.
13. Whitney SN, McGuire AL, McGullough LB. A typology of shared decision making, informed consent, and simple consent. Ann Intern Med. 2003;140:54–9.
14. McMillan FD. Quality of life in animals. J Am Vet Med Assoc. 2000;216:1904–10.
15. Wojciechowska JI, Hewson CJ. Quality-of-life assessment in pet dogs. J Am Vet Med Assoc. 2005;226:722–8.
16. Wojciechowska JI, Hewson CJ, Stryhn H, Guy NC, Patronek GJ, Timmons V. Development of a discriminative questionnaire to assess nonphysical aspects of quality of life of dogs. Am J Vet Res. 2005;66:1453–60.
17. Morgan CA. Autonomy and paternalism in quality of life determinations in veterinary practice. Anim Welf. 2007;16(Suppl 1):143–7.
18. Gray C. Similar but not the same: the teaching of veterinary and medical ethics. Vet Rec. 2014;175:590–1.
19. Tannenbaum J. Veterinary medical ethics: a focus on conflicting interests. J Soc Issues. 1993;49:143–56.
20. Lagoni L, Butler C, Hetts S. The human-animal bond and grief. Philadelphia: Saunders Company; 1994.
21. Webster J. Animal welfare—a cool eye towards eden. Oxford: Blackwell Science; 1994.
22. Fogle B. The changing roles of animals in westerns society: influences upon and from the veterinary profession. Anthrozoös. 1999;12:234–9.
23. Hern JC. Professional conduct and self-regulation. In: Legood G, editor. Veterinary ethics: an introduction. London: Continuum; 2000. p. 63–73.
24. Mullan S, Main D. Principles of ethical decision-making in veterinary practice. In Pract. 2001;23:394–401.
25. Fettman MJ, Rollin BE. Modern elements of informed consent for general veterinary practitioners. J Am Vet Med Assoc. 2002;221:1386–93.
26. Rollin BE. Oncology and ethics. Reprod Dom Anim. 2003;38:50–3.
27. Flemming DD, Scott JF. The informed consent doctrine: what veterinarians should tell their clients. J Am Vet Med Assoc. 2004;224:1436–9.
28. Main DCJ. Offering the best to patients: ethical issues associated with the provision of veterinary services. Vet Rec. 2006;158:62–6.
29. Rollin BE. An introduction to veterinary medical ethics: theory and cases. 2nd ed. Iowa: Blackwell Publishing; 2006.
30. Rebuelto M. Ethical dilemmas in euthanasia of small companion animals. Open Ethics J. 2008;2:21–5.
31. Yeates J. Ethical aspects of euthanasia of owned animals. In Pract. 2010;32:70–3.
32. Morris P. Blue juice: euthanasia in veterinary medicine. Philadelphia: Temple University Press; 2012.
33. Yeates J. Animal welfare in veterinary practice. West Sussex: Wiley-Blackwell; 2013.
34. Guntzelman J, Riegger MH. Helping pet owners with the euthanasia decision. Vet Med. 1993;88:26–34.
35. Ritchie J, Lewis J, Elam G. Designing and selecting samples. In: Ritchie J, Lewis J, editors. Qualitative research practice. A guide for social science students and researchers. London: Sage Publications; 2003. p. 77–108.
36. Kvale S. InterView. En introduktion til det kvalitative forskningsinterview. Copenhagen: Hans Reitzels Forlag; 2002.
37. Christiansen SB, Kristensen AT, Sandøe P, Lassen J. Looking after chronically ill dogs: impacts on the caregiver's life. Anthrozoös. 2013;26:519–33.
38. Crabtree BF, Miller WL. Using codes and code manuals: a template organizing style of interpretation. In: Crabtree BF, Miller WL, editors. Doing qualitative research. 2nd ed. California: Sage Publications Inc.; 1999. p. 163–78.

39. Coffey A, Atkinson P. Making sense of qualitative data.Complementary research strategies. California: Sage Publications Inc.; 1996.
40. Pilgram MD. Communicating social support to grieving clients: the veterinarians' view. Death Stud. 2010;34:699–714.
41. Sanders CR. Annoying owners: routine interactions with problematic clients in a general veterinary practice. Qual Sociol. 1994;17:159–70.
42. Sanders CR. Killing with kindness: veterinary euthanasia and the social construction of personhood. Sociol Forum. 1995;10:195–214.
43. Ministry of Environment and Food of Denmark. Bekendtgørelse af dyreværnsloven (The Danish Animal Welfare Act), LBK no. 1150 12/09/2015, §§ 20–21. https://www.retsinformation.dk/Forms/R0710.aspx?id=174047. Accessed 29 Jan 2016.
44. Amiot CE, Bastian B. Toward a psychology of human-animal relations. Psychol Bull. 2015;141:6–47.
45. McMIllan FD. Predicting quality of life outcomes as a guide for decision-making: the challenge of hitting a moving target. Anim Welf. 2007;16(Suppl 1):135–42.
46. Levine JM, Budke CM, Levine GJ, Kerwin SC, Hettlich BF, Slater MR. Owner-perceived, weighted quality-of-life assessments in dogs with spinal cord injuries. J Am Vet Med Assoc. 2008;233:931–5.
47. Oyama MA, Rush JE, O'Sullivan ML, Williams RM, Rozanski EA, Petrie JP, Sleeper MM, Brown DC. Perceptions and priorities of owners of dogs with heart disease regarding quality versus quantity of life for their pets. J Am Vet Med Assoc. 2008;223:104–8.
48. Lidz CW. Informed consent: a critical part of modern medical research. Am J Med Sci. 2011;342:273–5.
49. Beauchamp TL. Informed consent: its history, meaning, and present challenges. Camb Q Healthc Ethics. 2011;20:515–23.
50. Jackson C, Gray C. Difficult choices: helping clients to arrive at an informed decision. In Pract. 2004;26:223–5.
51. Christiansen SB, Forkman B. Assessment of animal welfare in a veterinary context—a call for ethologists. Appl Anim Behav Sci. 2007;106:203–20.
52. Denneberg NÅ, Egenvall A. Evaluation of dog owners' perceptions concerning radiation therapy. Acta Vet Scand. 2009;51:19. doi:10.1186/1751-0147-51-19.
53. Giuffrida MA, Kerrigan SM. Measurement in prospective studies of cancer treatment in dogs and cats. J Vet Intern Med. 2014;28:1824–9.
54. Arluke A, Sanders CR. Regarding animals. Philadelphia: Temple University Press; 1996.
55. Mallery KF, Freeman LM, Harpster NK, Rush JE. Factors contributing to the decision for euthanasia of dogs with congestive heart failure. J Am Vet Med Assoc. 1999;214:1201–4.
56. Rochlitz I. The effects of road traffic accidents on domestic cats and their owners. Anim Welf. 2004;13:51–5.
57. Morton DB. A hypothetical strategy for the objective evaluation of animal well-being and quality of life using a dog model. Anim Welf. 2007;16(Suppl 1):75–81.
58. Schneider TR, Lyons JB, Tetrick MA, Accortt EE. Multidimensional quality of life and human-animal bond measures for companion dogs. J Vet Behav. 2010;5:287–301.
59. Hamilton MJ, Sarcornrattana O, Illiopoulou M, Xie Y, Kitchell B. Questionnaire-based assessment of owner concerns and doctor responsiveness: 107 canine chemotherapy patients. J Small Anim Pract. 2012;53:627–33.
60. Stirrat GM, Gill R. Autonomy in medical ethics after O'Neill. J Med Ethics. 2005;31:127–30.
61. Cribb A, Entwistle VA. Shared decision-making: trade-offs between narrower and broader conceptions. Health Expect. 2011;14:210–9.
62. Kaplan KJ, Schneiderhan M, Harrow M, Omens R. Autonomy, gender, and preference for paternalistic or informative physicians: a study of the doctor-patient relation. Ethics Med. 2002;18:49–60.
63. Müller-Engelmann M, Keller H, Donner-Banzhoff N, Krones T. Shared decision making in medicine: the influence of situational treatment factors. Patient Educ Couns. 2011;82:240–6.
64. Milani MM. The art of veterinary practice: a guide to client communication. Philadelphia: University of Pennsylvania Press; 1995.
65. White DB, Malvar G, Karr J, Lo B, Curtis JR. Expanding the paradigm of the physician's role in surrogate decision-making: an empirically derived framework. Crit Care Med. 2010;38:743–50.
66. Gillam L, Sullivan J. Ethics at the end of life: who should make decisions about treatment limitation for young children with life-threatening or lime-limiting conditions? J Paediatr Child Health. 2011;47:594–8.
67. Sanders CR. Understanding dogs—living and working with canine companions. Philadelphia: Temple University Press; 1999.
68. Brockman BK, Taylor VA, Brockman CM. The price of unconditional love: consumer decision making for high-dollar veterinary care. J Bus Res. 2008;61:397–405.
69. Gurmankin AD, Baron J, Hershey JC, Ubel PA. The role of physicians' recommendations in medical treatment decisions. Med Decis Mak. 2002;22:262–71.
70. Swabe J. Veterinary dilemmas: ambiguity and ambivalence in human-animal interaction. In: Podberscek AL, Paul ES, Serpell JA, editors. Companion animals and us: exploring the relationships between people and pets. Cambridge: Cambridge University Press; 2000. p. 292–312.
71. Shaw JR, Lagoni L. End-of-life communication in veterinary medicine: delivering bad news and euthanasia decision making. Vet Clin N Am Small Anim Pract. 2007;37:95–108.
72. Terry PB. Informed consent in clinical medicine. Chest. 2007;131:563–8.
73. Nogueira Borden LJ, Adams CL, Bonnet BN, Shaw J, Ribble CS. Use of the measure of patient-centered communication to analyze euthanasia discussions in companion animal practice. J Am Vet Med Assoc. 2010;237:1275–87.
74. McMillan FD. Comfort as the primary goal in veterinary medical practice. J Am Vet Med Assoc. 1998;212:1370–4.
75. Fernandez-Mehler P, Gloor P, Sager E, Lewis FI, Glaus TM. Veterinarians' role for pet owners facing pet loss. Vet Rec. 2013;172:555–61.
76. Yeates JW, Main DCJ. Veterinary opinions on refusing euthanasia: justifications and philosophical frameworks. Vet Rec. 2011;168:263. doi:10.1136/vr.c6352.
77. MagalhãesSant'Ana M, More SJ, Morton DB, Osborne M, Hanlon A. What do european veterinary codes of conduct actually say and mean? A case study approach. Vet Rec. 2015;176:654. doi:10.1136/vr.103005.
78. Dickinson GE, Roof KW, Roof PD, Paul ES. UK veterinarians' experiences with euthanasia. Vet Rec. 2014;175:174. doi:10.1136/vr.102636.
79. Rehbock T. Limits of autonomy in biomedical ethics? Conceptual clarifications. Camb Q Health Ethics. 2011;20:524–32.

In vitro production of bovine embryos derived from individual donors in the Corral® dish

Maaike Catteeuw[1*], Eline Wydooghe[1], Erik Mullaart[2], Hiemke M. Knijn[2] and Ann Van Soom[1]

Abstract

Background: Since the identity of the embryo is of outmost importance during commercial in vitro embryo production, bovine oocytes and embryos have to be cultured strictly per donor. Due to the rather low yield of oocytes collected after ovum pick-up (OPU) per individual cow, oocyte maturation and embryo culture take place in small groups, which is often associated with inferior embryo development. The objective of this study was to improve embryonic development in small donor groups by using the Corral® dish. This commercial dish is designed for human embryo production. It contains two central wells that are divided into quadrants by a semi-permeable wall. In human embryo culture, one embryo is placed per quadrant, allowing individual follow-up while embryos are exposed to a common medium. In our study, small groups of oocytes and subsequently embryos of different bovine donors were placed in the Corral® dish, each donor group in a separate quadrant.

Results: In two experiments, the Corral® dish was evaluated during in vitro maturation (IVM) and/or in vitro culture (IVC) by grouping oocytes and embryos of individual bovine donors per quadrant. At day 7, a significantly higher blastocyst rate was noted in the Corral® dish used during IVM and IVC than when only used during IVM (12.9% ± 2.10 versus 22.8% ± 2.67) ($P < 0.05$). However, no significant differences in blastocyst yield were observed anymore between treatment groups at day 8 post insemination.

Conclusions: In the present study, the Corral® dish was used for in vitro embryo production (IVP) in cattle; allowing to allocate oocytes and/or embryos per donor. As fresh embryo transfers on day 7 have higher pregnancy outcomes, the Corral® dish offers an added value for commercial OPU/IVP, since a higher blastocyst development at day 7 is obtained when the Corral® dish is used during IVM and IVC.

Keywords: Corral® dish, In vitro embryo production, Bovine, Donor

Background

Currently, many bovine embryos are being generated in vitro for commercial embryo transfer. In 2013, more than 500,000 embryos have been produced worldwide by ovum pick up (OPU) and in vitro embryo production (IVP) technologies, with South America taking the lead in OPU/IVP. However, during the last decade there has been an almost threefold rise in OPU/IVP embryos produced in Europe and North America, indicating an increasing interest in this application [1]. Since OPU/IVP has become an alternative and highly competitive technique for multiple ovulation and embryo transfer [2], much research has been done to optimize the OPU technique because numerous factors can influence the oocyte yield, such as hormone treatment prior to oocyte collection [3], OPU equipment [4] and interval between OPU sessions [5]. However, an average of only eight oocytes per Holstein–Friesian donor are obtained, a breed particularly used in Europe [6]. When these oocytes are being matured, they are grouped per individual donor, since the genetic identity of the OPU/IVP embryo needs

*Correspondence: Maaike.Catteeuw@Ugent.be
[1] Department of Reproduction, Obstetrics, and Herd Health, Faculty of Veterinary Medicine, Ghent University, Salisburylaan 133, 9820 Merelbeke, Belgium

to be preserved. This implies that during OPU/IVP, only small numbers of oocytes and embryos are cultured together. Moreover, quality of oocytes derived after OPU is very variable since some oocytes lack cumulus cells due to vacuum pressure [7]. The quality of the oocyte is however crucial and is predictive of the developmental potential of the resulting embryo [8]. It has been demonstrated that in vitro production starting from oocytes surrounded by few cumulus cells or denuded oocytes resulted in a lower blastocyst formation compared to IVP starting from oocytes surrounded by compact layers of cumulus cells [6, 9]. Due to the scarcity of the oocytes retrieved per donor, a strict selection including only the best cumulus oocyte complexes (COCs) prior to the in vitro process is not always possible. In commercial settings, where oocytes and embryos are cultured separately per donor, an average blastocyst rate of 16–18% is obtained [10, 11]. Besides the low blastocyst yield, there are also indications that grouping small numbers of embryos results in a lower total cell number and a higher rate of apoptosis compared with embryos cultured in large groups (77.16 cells versus 98.48 cells and 24.17% versus 12.14%, respectively) [12]. In mice [13, 14], cattle [15, 16] and humans [17], pooling oocytes and embryos in large groups increases blastocyst yield up to 40%. This beneficial effect of group culture has been related to a higher concentration of embryo secreted factors in the surrounding culture media, such as insulin-like growth factor-I [18] or platelet activating factor [19]. These secreted factors act potentially as a survival factor by preventing apoptosis of the embryonic cells or as a mitogenic factor [20]. In addition, during in vitro maturation cumulus cells and oocytes are also able to secrete signalling molecules. Oocyte secreted factors, such as bone morphogenetic protein 15 and growth differentiation factor 9, regulate a variety of cumulus cell functions associated with growth and differentiation, which in turn may regulate and stimulate the developmental competence of the oocyte [21]. These paracrine and autocrine factors require a close interaction between groups of COCs and subsequently embryos, thus creating a supporting microenvironment for development.

The Corral® dish, designed especially for human in vitro embryo production, consists of two central wells that are divided into four quadrants by a semi-permeable wall (Fig. 1a). In human IVP, a single embryo, having a larger diameter than the gaps between the wall, is placed per quadrant, with a maximum of two times four embryos of the same female patient per Corral® dish. This makes individual monitoring of embryo development possible while the medium and embryotrophic factors can flow through the quadrants (Fig. 1b) [17]. In human studies, single embryo culture has been applied

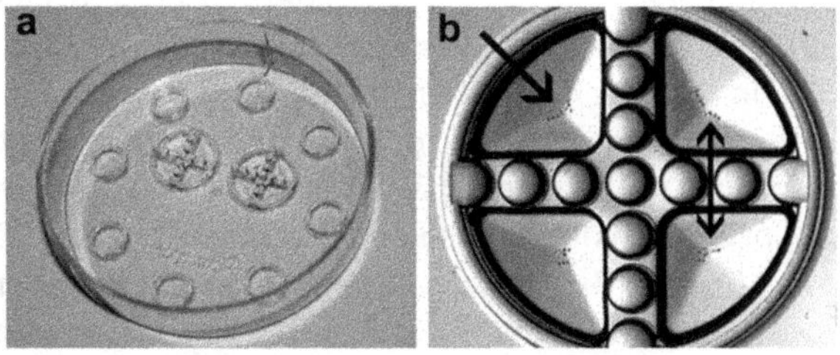

Fig. 1 Design of the Corral® dish. **a** The Corral® dish consists of two central wells. **b** These central well is divided into quadrants by a solid wall with numerous posts on top, allowing medium and embryotrophic factors to pass (*double arrow*) but oocytes or embryos remained per individual donor in a quadrant (*arrow*). Each quadrant of the Corral® dish contains the oocytes or embryos of one specific donor and is filled with 30 μL medium

in a Corral® dish setting [17], where only one embryo was placed in one quadrant, but in our study, we chose to allocate eight embryos belonging to the same donor in one quadrant, since embryo culture in small groups is routinely used in bovine OPU/IVP [15]. We hypothesized that the embryonic development would be stimulated in the common medium by the exchange of putative autocrine factors between the donor cows, while individual allocation of oocytes and subsequently embryos per donor cow still remained possible.

Methods

Media and reagents

Basic Eagle's Medium amino acids, Minimal Essential Medium (MEM) non-essential amino acids (100×), TCM-199-medium, kanamycin and gentamycin were purchased from Life Technologies Europe (Ghent, Belgium) and all other components were obtained from Sigma (Schnelldorf, Germany), unless otherwise stated. All the media were filter-sterilized using a 0.22 μm filter (Pall Corporation, Ann Arbor, MI, USA) before use.

In vitro embryo production protocol

Bovine embryos were produced by adapting previously described routine in vitro methods [22]. Briefly, ovaries were collected per slaughtered cow in separate plastic bags in a local slaughterhouse and processed within 2 h. Follicles between 2 and 8 mm diameter were punctured. Subsequently, COCs and embryos were strictly kept per donor cow during the complete procedure. From each donor, the first 8–10 COCs visible in the Petri dish were collected, without selection based on the quality of these COCs, only denuded oocytes were discarded. If fewer than eight COCs were available, the donor was excluded from the experiments. The COCs were transferred to maturation medium, which consisted of modified bicarbonate-buffered TCM-199 supplemented with 50 μg/

mL gentamycin and 20 ng/mL epidermal growth factor (EGF). Subsequently, COCs were matured for 22 h at 38.5 °C in 5% CO_2 in humidified air.

Fertilization occurred per donor with the semen of the same proven bull. Frozen-thawed spermatozoa were separated over a discontinuous Percoll gradient (45 and 90%; GE Healthcare Biosciences, Uppsala, Sweden). Sperm concentration was adjusted to 1×10^6 spermatozoa/mL using IVF-Tyrode's Albumin-Pyruvate-Lactate (TALP), which consisted of bicarbonate buffered Tyrode's solution, supplemented with BSA (Sigma A8806; 6 mg/mL) and heparin (25 μg/mL). The mature oocytes were incubated in 500 μL IVF-TALP with spermatozoa for 21 h at 38.5 °C in 5% CO_2 in humidified air.

After fertilization, excess spermatozoa and cumulus cells were removed by vortexing. Eight presumptive zygotes per donor were transferred to synthetic oviductal fluid (SOF) supplemented with essential and non-essential amino acids (SOFaa), 0.4% BSA (Sigma A9647) and ITS (5 μg/mL insulin, 5 μg/mL transferrin and 5 ng/mL selenium) and were incubated at 38.5 °C in 5% CO_2, 5% O_2 and 90% N_2 till 8 days post insemination (dpi). During this culture period, embryos were kept in the same culture dish and no renewal of SOF medium was performed.

Experiment 1: Embryo culture in the Corral® dish

For the first experiment, ovaries from individual donor cows were collected and processed separately. This experiment was conducted 4 times (4 replicates), for each replicate the ovaries of 16 different donor cows were collected. From each donor, 8–10 COCs were matured in 500 μL maturation medium in separate 4-well dishes. Subsequently, the oocytes were fertilized per donor in four-well dishes. After fertilization, the first eight presumptive zygotes were grouped, without prior selection and cultured per donor. Half of these donor groups were allocated to a droplet and the other half to a quadrant of the Corral® dish, this was chosen completely at random. Culture droplets consisted of 30 μL medium, eight droplets were made per culture dish (IVF Petri dish, Nunc®, Thermo Fisher, Denmark) and 8.5 mL mineral oil was covering these droplets (Drop IVC). In the Corral® dish, the two central wells were filled with 120 μL culture medium, each quadrant containing 30 μL (Corral® IVC). Mineral oil (8.5 mL) was used to cover the droplets of medium to prevent evaporation. Because of the typical structure of the Corral® dish, zygotes of eight different donors were grouped in those two central wells. An overview of COC and embryo distribution is shown in Fig. 2a.

Experiment 2: Oocyte maturation and embryo culture in the Corral® dish

Comparable to experiment 1, this experiment was conducted four times (4 replicates). For each replicate, ovaries from 16 different donors were collected separately. From each donor, ten COCs were matured in a quadrant of the Corral® dish. Each quadrant contains 30 μL maturation medium. In one central well, 40 COCs of four different donors were matured in 120 μL medium, each donor separated by the semi-permeable wall dividing the Corral® dish in quadrants. Both central wells were covered with 8.5 mL mineral oil. Routine fertilization occurred per donor in four-well dishes. As described in the first experiment, eight presumptive zygotes were cultured per donor either in a 30 μL drop of medium (Corral® IVM) or in a quadrant of the Corral® dish (Corral® IVM/IVC). In the latter, eight different donors were again grouped in the two central wells. An overview of COC and embryo distribution is shown in Fig. 2b.

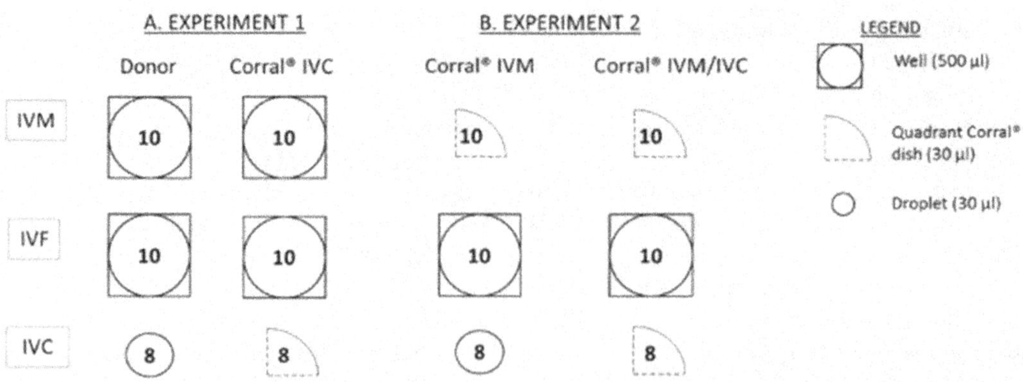

Fig. 2 Schematic illustration of the two experiments. As indicated in the legend, oocytes and embryos were grouped per donor in a four-well dish, a droplet or in a quadrant of the Corral® dish during the different phases of the in vitro embryo production (in vitro maturation-IVM, in vitro fertilization-IVF, in vitro culture-IVC). Furthermore, the number of oocytes and embryos grouped together is indicated in the icons. *(A)* In experiment 1, embryos were placed per donor in the Corral® dish or in a separate drop during IVC. *(B)* In experiment 2, oocytes and embryos were assigned per donor to the Corral® dish during IVM or during IVM and IVC

Evaluation of embryo development and embryo quality

To evaluate the embryo development, the cleavage rate was assessed at 45 h post insemination (hpi) as the percentage of presumed zygotes that cleaved. Blastocyst stages were evaluated according to the fourth edition IETS manual at 7 and 8 dpi. At 8 dpi, hatching rate was evaluated as the percentage of hatching or hatched blastocysts. Subsequently, total cell number (TCN) of the blastocysts was assessed by Hoechst 33342 staining. Briefly, day 8 blastocysts were fixed in 2% paraformaldehyde during 20 min and subsequently stained for 10 min with 0.1% Hoechst 33342. The stained blastocysts were evaluated using a 400× magnification fluorescence microscope (Leica DM 5500 B).

Statistical analysis

Statistical analyses were carried out with IBM SPSS Statistics 23. Differences at *P*-value <0.05 were considered statistically significant. Cleavage, blastocyst and hatching rates were analysed using a binary logistic regression model with treatment (Drop IVC vs Corral® IVC and Corral® IVM vs Corral® IVM/IVC) and replicate as fixed effects. The effect of replicates was assessed and excluded from the final model if it was not significant. Total cell numbers were analysed using a mixed model analysis of variance, with treatment (Drop IVC vs Corral® IVC and Corral® IVM vs Corral® IVM/IVC) as fixed effect and replicate as random effect and are expressed as mean ± standard error of the mean (SEM). If the effect of replicates was not significant, this was excluded from the final model.

Results

Experiment 1: Embryo culture in the Corral® dish

There was no significant difference noted in embryonic development between embryos cultured in individual donor droplets (Drop IVC) or embryos cultured in the Corral® dish (Corral® IVC) (Table 1). Both cleavage and blastocyst rate were similar in both groups. At day 8, a blastocyst rate was reached of 26.9% in Corral® IVC and 24.8% in Drop IVC. Furthermore, no differences were observed in TCN of day 8 blastocysts (Drop IVC: 188.1 ± 10.49; Corral® IVC: 194.2 ± 13.59).

Experiment 2: Oocyte maturation and embryo culture in the Corral® dish

Cleavage rate did not differ between two groups. Significantly more blastocysts were observed in the Corral® IVM/IVC compared to the Corral® IVM, at 7 dpi ($P < 0.05$), respectively 22.8 and 12.9%. This was however no longer the case for blastocyst rate at day 8, 26.7% was reached in the Corral® IVM and 30.1% in Corral® IVM/IVC (Table 1). Furthermore, TCN of day 8 blastocysts in these two groups did not differ (Corral® IVM: 125.0 ± 3.21; Corral® IVM/IVC: 133.9 ± 3.87).

Cleavage (45 hpi), blastocyst (7 and 8 dpi) and hatching rates of embryos produced per donor in droplets (Drop IVC) or in a quadrant of the Corral® dish (Corral® IVC) during in vitro culture (experiment 1) and embryos produced per donor in a quadrant of the Corral® dish during in vitro maturation (Corral® IVM) or during in vitro maturation and culture (Corral® IVM/IVC) (experiment 2). Asterisks (*) in the same column indicate a statistical difference between treatments within the same experiment ($P < 0.05$).

Discussion

The overall aim of this study was to evaluate the efficiency of Corral® dish for commercial purposes. The Corral® dish allows grouping of embryos from different donor groups without losing track of genetic identity by placing the embryos of each donor in a quadrant of the central wells. This allows secreted embryotrophic factors to reach a larger group of embryos (32 instead of 8) since all embryos are exposed to the same surrounding medium. These factors stimulate growth and development, which would result in a higher blastocyst yield. In this study, there was no difference found in embryonic development when applying the Corral® dish during culture in comparison with the allocation of embryos per donor in a separate droplet of medium. This was similar to the study of Ebner et al. [17] on human embryos, where one embryo was allocated to either a quadrant of the central wells or one embryo allocated to one of the other wells. However, when the Corral® dish was used both during maturation and culture, blastocyst yield was increased at 7 dpi compared to its use only during maturation, but this effect was no longer noticed at

Table 1 Embryonic development in the different treatment groups of experiments 1 and 2

	Treatment	Number of oocytes	Cleavage (%)	Blastocysts D7 (%)	Blastocysts D8 (%)	% Hatched
Exp 1	Drop IVC	219	158 (72.1)	41 (18.7)	59 (26.9)	22.0
	Corral® IVC	234	169 (72.2)	38 (16.2)	58 (24.8)	17.2
Exp 2	Corral® IVM	255	186 (72.9)	33 (12.9)*	68 (26.7)	22.1
	Corral® IVM/IVC	246	191 (77.6)	56 (22.8)*	74 (30.1)	28.4

8 dpi. Because more embryos reach the blastocyst stage on day 7 in the Corral® dish, when used during IVM and IVC, it offers the opportunity to transfer more fresh IVP embryos, which may subsequently give rise to more pregnancies and live born calves. It has been reported that pregnancy outcome is the highest when transferring fresh day 7 in vitro blastocysts, after transfers with in vivo derived embryos [23, 24].

On the other hand, the Corral® dish, has a specific design which implicates also three main disadvantages. First, the distance between donor groups is over 4 mm (Fig. 3). Gopichandran and Leese [16] reported that an optimal blastocyst formation occurred when a distance of 165 μm between the embryos was achieved. In the Corral® dish, the distance components in the medium have to cross between two donor groups is probably too large for optimal exchange of autocrine factors. A mathematical model constructed by Matsuura [25] calculated the concentration of secreted factors by embryos cultured in microwells and concluded that macromolecules (growth factors) are

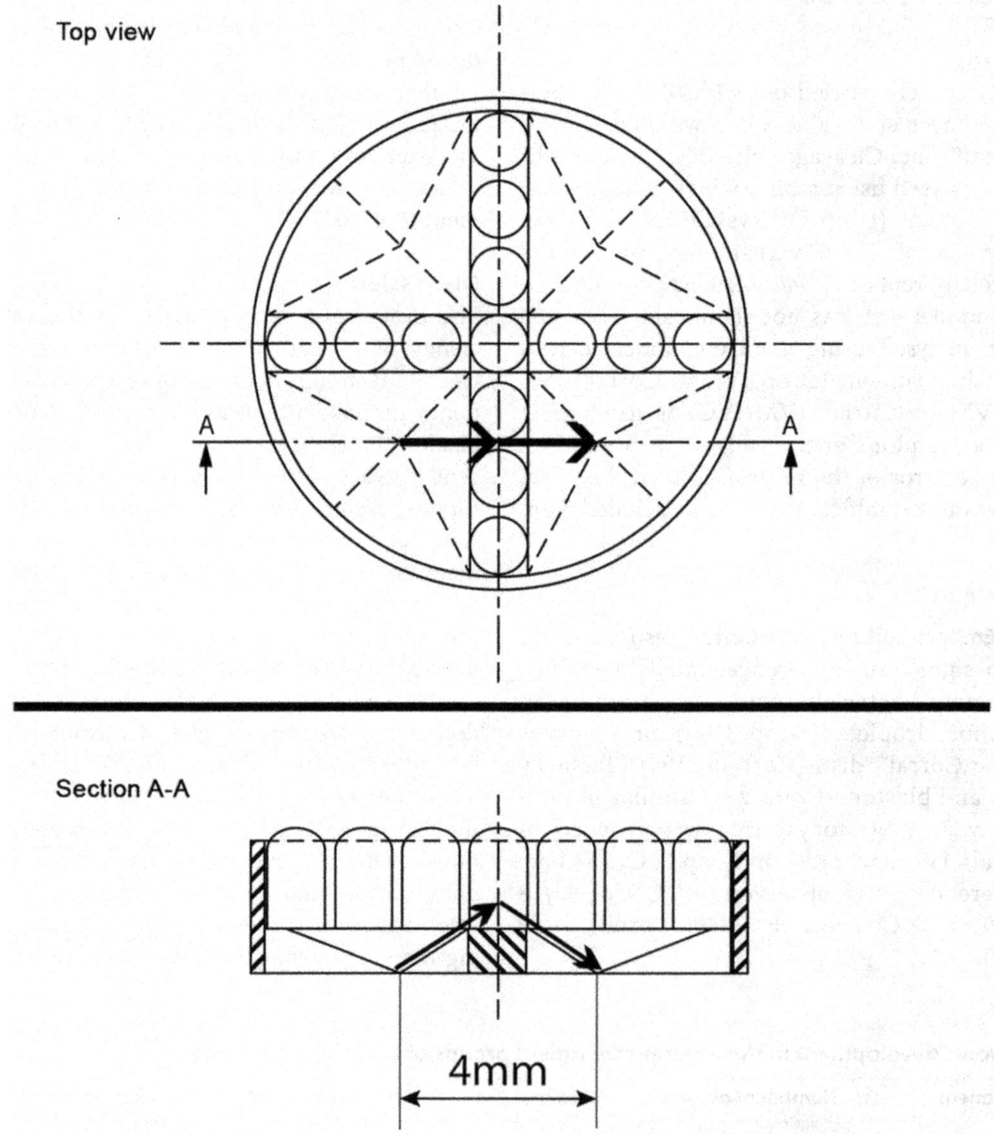

Fig. 3 Graphic design of the Corral® dish. This figure is pointing out a distance of 4 mm between the deepest sites of the quadrants. An even larger distance has to be covered by the embryotrophic factors, secreted by the allocated cumulus–oocyte complexes or embryos, to reach another quadrant. The diffusion of secreted factors can only appear in a vertical and oblique direction (*bold arrows*), due to the well-shaped quadrants and the in-between wall

slowly diluted and remain quite high in the neighbourhood of the embryo; while small molecules (waste materials) are rapidly diffusing away from the embryo. Due to the sloped sides of the quadrants (Fig. 3), diffusion of secreted factors could therefore be facilitated in a vertical and oblique direction, with growth factors remaining in the neighbourhood of the embryos located in the deepest point of the well. Second, each quadrant needs to be filled with 30 μL medium in order to connect the four quadrants. In this way, adjusting the incubation volume to the number of oocytes or embryos is impossible. This static design has therefore a major impact on oocyte/embryo density, which is referring to the number of embryos on a given amount in micro liter of medium and which is an important parameter during IVP [26–30]. Because of low embryo numbers in commercial practices, the medium volume cannot be decreased to achieve the ideal density of 1:1–1:3 [31–33]. The design of the Corral® dish could therefore be more suitable for donor cows having large numbers of COCs, since this is the only way to acquire a high embryo density in the Corral® dish. In Nelore cattle, a typical Brazilian breed, 30 or more oocytes can be collected per OPU session and this breed is therefore an excellent candidate for providing embryos for culture in the Corral dish [34]. Finally, from a sanitary point of view, possible transmission of pathogens can be considered as a risk factor between oocytes and embryos of different donors grouped in the Corral® dish. In theory, infection can be present as a consequence of intrafollicular infection or in vitro fertilization with infected semen. However, the risk of infection is rather small, since donor cows are carefully selected and tested for the absence of specific viral infections like bovine herpesvirus type 1 before entering an in vitro embryo program, and also every bull is tested for absence of infectious pathogens before he is allowed to enter an artificial insemination program. The zona pellucida plays a major role in protecting the embryo, and only very small viruses can form a risk for transzonal infection. Furthermore, before embryo transfer, washing embryos in combination with trypsin treatment is advised by sanitary procedures of the International Embryo Technology Society [35] to inactivate and remove possible viruses. In the end, it should still be advised to group oocytes and embryos of different donor cows in the Corral® dish only when the full health status is known.

Conclusions

A novel aspect of this study was that we used the Corral® dish for grouping small numbers of bovine oocytes and embryos per donor cow, whereas in other studies embryos have been cultured singly, thereby decreasing a possible beneficial effect of group culture. It is however doubtful whether the embryos can benefit from being grouped in the Corral® dish. Nonetheless, the Corral® dish is an easy applicable tool to produce in vitro embryos by grouping bovine oocytes and embryos per donor. Furthermore, the Corral dish® increases blastocyst development at 7 dpi, when used during IVM and IVC, and is therefore beneficial for commercial practice regarding embryo transfers as higher pregnancy rates are achieved with fresh day 7 blastocysts.

Abbreviations

COCs: cumulus oocyte complexes; dpi: days post insemination; IVC: in vitro culture; IVM: in vitro maturation; IVP: in vitro production; OPU: ovum pick up; TCN: total cell number.

Authors' contributions

MC conceived the study, collected the ovaries at the local slaughterhouse, evaluated the data, reviewed the literature and drafted the manuscript. AVS conceived, designed and coordinated the study, provided support and revised critically the manuscript. EW coordinated the study, performed statistical analysis, helped to draft and revised critically the manuscript. EM, HMK supported the study, provided advice and revised critically the manuscript. All authors read and approved the final manuscript.

Author details

[1] Department of Reproduction, Obstetrics, and Herd Health, Faculty of Veterinary Medicine, Ghent University, Salisburylaan 133, 9820 Merelbeke, Belgium. [2] CRV BV, Wassenaarweg 20, 6843 NW Arnhem, The Netherlands.

Competing interests

The authors declare that they have no competing interests.

Acknowledgements

The authors wish to thank Isabel Lemahieu and Petra Van Damme for their excellent technical assistance.

Funding

This research was supported by a doctoral grant funded by the Faculty of Veterinary Medicine, Ghent University, Belgium.

References

1. George P. Statistics of embryo collection and transfer in domestic farm animals. Embryo Transf Newsl. 2013;2014:14–26.
2. Boni R. Ovum pick-up in cattle: a 25 yr retrospective analysis. Anim Reprod. 2012;9:362–9.
3. De Roover R, Feugang JMN, Bols PEJ, Genicot G, Hanzen C. Effects of ovum pick-up frequency and FSH stimulation: a retrospective study on seven years of beef cattle in vitro embryo production. Reprod Domest Anim. 2008;43:239–45.
4. Bols PEJ, Ysebaert MT, Van Soom A, de Kruif A. Effects of needle tip bevel and aspiration procedure on the morphology and developmental capacity of bovine compact cumulus oocyte complexes. Theriogenology. 1997;47:1221–36.

5. Ding LJ, Tian HB, Wang JJ, Chen J, Sha HY, Chen JQ, Cheng GX. Different intervals of ovum pick-up affect the competence of oocytes to support the preimplantation development of cloned bovine embryos. Mol Reprod Dev. 2008;75:1710–5.
6. Merton J, de Roos APW, Mullaart E, de Ruigh L, Kaal L, Vos P, Dieleman SJ. Factors affecting oocyte quality and quantity in commercial application of embryo technologies in the cattle breeding industry. Theriogenology. 2003;59:651–74.
7. Bols PEJ, Van Soom A, Ysebaert MT, Vandenheede JMM, de Kruif A. Effects of aspiration vacuum and needle diameter on cumulus oocyte complex morphology and developmental capacity of bovine oocytes. Theriogenology. 1996;45:1001–14.
8. Goovaerts IGF, Leroy JLMR, Jorssen EPA, Bols PEJ. Noninvasive bovine oocyte quality assessment possibilities of a single oocyte culture. Theriogenology. 2010;74:1509–20.
9. Khurana NK, Niemann H. Effects of oocyte quality, oxygen tension, embryo density, cumulus cells and energy substrates on cleavage and morula/blastocyst formation of bovine embryos. Theriogenology. 2000;54:741–56.
10. Merton JS, de Roos APW, Koenen EPC, Roelen BAJ, Vos PLAM, Mullaart E, Knijn HM. Bovine OPU-derived oocytes can be matured in vitro for 16–28 h with similar developmental capacity. Reprod Domest Anim. 2012;47:1037–42.
11. Machado SA, Reichenbach HD, Weppert M, Wolf E, Goncalves PBD. The variability of ovum pick-up response and in vitro embryo production from monozygotic twin cows. Theriogenology. 2006;65:573–83.
12. Cebrian-Serrano A, Salvador I, Silvestre MA. Beneficial effect of two culture systems with small groups of embryos on the development and quality of in vitro-produced bovine embryos. Anat Histol Embryol. 2014;43:22–30.
13. Dai SJ, Xu CL, Wang J, Sun YP, Chian RC. Effect of culture medium volume and embryo density on early mouse embryonic development: tracking the development of the individual embryo. J Assist Reprod Gen. 2012;29:617–23.
14. Lane M, Gardner DK. Effect of incubation volume and embryo density on the development and viability of mouse embryos in vitro. Hum Reprod. 1992;7:558–62.
15. O'Doherty EM, Wade MG, Hill JL, Boland MP. Effects of culturing bovine oocytes either singly or in groups on development to blastocysts. Theriogenology. 1997;48:161–9.
16. Gopichandran N, Leese HJ. The effect of paracrine/autocrine interactions on the in vitro culture of bovine preimplantation embryos. Reproduction. 2006;131:269–77.
17. Ebner T, Shebl O, Moser M, Mayer RB, Arzt W, Tews G. Group culture of human zygotes is superior to individual culture in terms of blastulation, implantation and life birth. Reprod Biomed Online. 2010;21:762–8.
18. Spanos S, Becker DL, Winston RML, Hardy R. Anti-apoptotic action of insulin-like growth factor-I during human preimplantation embryo development. Biol Reprod. 2000;63:1413–20.
19. O'Neill C. The role of paf in embryo physiology. Hum Reprod Update. 2005;11:215–28.
20. O'Neill C. The potential roles for embryotrophic ligands in preimplantation embryo development. Hum Reprod Update. 2008;14:275–88.
21. Gilchrist RB, Thompson JG. Oocyte maturation: emerging concepts and technologies to improve developmental potential in vitro. Theriogenology. 2007;67:6–15.
22. Wydooghe E, Heras S, Dewulf J, Piepers S, Van den Abbeel E, De Sutter P, Vandaele L, Van Soom A. Replacing serum in culture medium with albumin and insulin, transferrin and selenium is the key to successful bovine embryo development in individual culture. Reprod Fert Develop. 2014;26:717–24.
23. Hasler JF. The current status of oocyte recovery, in vitro embryo production and embryo transfer in domestic animals, with an emphasis on the bovine. J Anim Sci. 1998;76:52–74.
24. Hasler JF, Henderson WB, Hurtgen PJ, Jin ZQ, McCauley AD, Mower SA, Neely B, Shuey LS, Stokes JE, Trimmer SA. Production, freezing and transfer of bovine IVF embryos and subsequent calving results. Theriogenology. 1995;43:141–52.
25. Matsuura K. Numerical calculations for diffusion effects in the well-of-the-well culture system for mammalian embryos. Reprod Fertil Develop. 2014;26:742–51.
26. Reed ML. Culture systems: embryo density. Methods Mol Biol. 2012;912:273–312.
27. Fujita T, Umeki H, Shimura H, Kugumiya K, Shiga K. Effect of group culture and embryo-culture conditioned medium on development of bovine embryos. J Reprod Develop. 2006;52:137–42.
28. Hoelker M, Rings F, Lund Q, Phatsara C, Schellander K, Tesfaye D. Effect of embryo density on in vitro developmental characteristics of bovine preimplantative embryos with respect to micro and macroenvironments. Reprod Domest Anim. 2010;45:E138–45.
29. Vajta G, Peura TT, Holm P, Paldi K, Greve T, Trounson AO, Callesen H. New method for culture of zona-included or zona-free embryos: the Well of the Well (WOW) system. Mol Reprod Develop. 2000;55:256–64.
30. Feng WG, Sui HS, Han ZB, Chang ZL, Zhou P, Liu DJ, Bao S, Tan JH. Effects of follicular atresia and size on the developmental competence of bovine oocytes: a study using the well-in-drop culture system. Theriogenology. 2007;67:1339–50.
31. Ferry L, Mermillod P, Massip A, Dessy F. Bovine embryos cultured in serum-poor oviduct-conditioned medium need cooperation to reach the blastocyst stage. Theriogenology. 1994;42:445–53.
32. Carolan C, Lonergan P, Van Langendonckt A, Mermillod P. Factors affecting bovine embryo development in synthetic oviduct fluid following oocyte maturation and fertilization in-vitro. Theriogenology. 1995;43:1115–28.
33. Donnay I, Van Langendonckt A, Auquier P, Grisart B, Vansteenbrugge A, Massip A, Dessy F. Effects of co-culture and embryo number on the in vitro development of bovine embryos. Theriogenology. 1997;47:1549–61.
34. Pontes JHF, Sterza FAM, Basso AC, Ferreira CR, Sanches BV, Rubin KCP, Seneda MM. Ovum pick up, in vitro embryo production, and pregnancy rates from a large-scale commercial program using Nelore cattle (*Bos indicus*) donors. Theriogenology. 2011;75:1640–6.
35. Stringfellow DA. Recommendation for the sanitary handling of in vivo-derived embryos. In: Stringfellow DA, Givens MD, editors. Manual of the International Embryo Transfer Society. Savoy: IETS. p. 79–84.

8

Twenty-four-hour ambulatory electrocardiography characterization of heart rhythm in *Vipera berus*-envenomed dogs

Anna Rave Vestberg[1*], Anna Tidholm[2,3] and Ingrid Ljungvall[3]

Abstract

Background: *Vipera berus* has a worldwide distribution and causes high morbidity in dogs annually. A complication to envenomation may be cardiac arrhythmias. The purpose of this study was to investigate the prevalence, types, and timing of arrhythmias, using 24-h ambulatory electrocardiography (24-AECG), in dogs bitten by *V. berus* in the first 24–32 h after envenomation. In addition, this study aimed to investigate if there were differences in selected clinical and hematological- and biochemical variables (including cardiac troponin I) at admission between *V. berus*-envenomed dogs with and without detected pathologic arrhythmias. Seventeen prospectively recruited client-owned dogs acutely envenomed by *V. berus*, were therefore examined clinically and echocardiographically, sampled for blood, hospitalized, and monitored by 24-AECG.

Results: Clinically significant pathologic arrhythmias in this study were of ventricular origin, such as frequent single ventricular premature contractions (VPCs) and couplets of VPCs, episodes of ventricular tachycardia and idioventricular rhythm, and "R-on-T phenomenon". Variations of these arrhythmias were detected by 24-AECG in eight (47%) of included dogs. No arrhythmias were detected by cardiac auscultation. Twenty-four hours following envenomation, four out of eight dogs experienced decreases (all $P < 0.039$), and three out of eight dogs experienced increases (all $P < 0.034$), in arrhythmic episodes. All four dogs bitten on a limb developed pathologic arrhythmias. Otherwise, no significant differences in clinical, hematological or biochemical variables were seen between dogs with pathologic arrhythmias and those without.

Conclusion: Forty-seven percent of dogs bitten by *V. berus* included in this study experienced pathologic arrhythmias of abnormal ventricular depolarization. During the first 24–32 h from the snakebite, some dogs experienced a decrease in arrhythmic episodes and others an increase in arrhythmic episodes. These findings indicate a potential value of repeated or prolonged electrocardiography monitoring of envenomed dogs for identification of which dogs that might benefit the most from prolonged hospitalization for optimal monitoring and treatment of cardiac abnormalities. In the present study, dogs that developed arrhythmias could not be differentiated from dogs that did not based on clinical findings or hematological or biochemical variables obtained at admission.

Keywords: *Vipera berus*, ECG, Ambulatory ECG, Dog, Arrhythmia, Snakebite

Background

Snakes of the Viperidae family, which has a worldwide distribution, yearly cause a significant number of envenomations in dogs [1–3]. *Vipera berus* is the only poisonous snake in Scandinavia and the United Kingdom [4]. The mortality rate of bitten dogs has been reported to vary from 0 to 7% [3, 5–8].

Most dogs are bitten on the nose or limbs and typical clinical signs include local swelling, edema and pain, as well as lethargy, depression, hyperthermia, salivation, and tachycardia [3, 5–7]. Various cardiac arrhythmias have been described as a complication to envenomation [9, 10]. Monitoring envenomed dogs for arrhythmias by auscultation is

*Correspondence: anna.vestberg@anicura.se
[1] Anicura Regional Animal Hospital, Ljusnevägen 17, 12848 Bagarmossen, Sweden
Full list of author information is available at the end of the article

challenging because sustained supraventricular-, idioventricular-, or ventricular tachycardia frequently present as a regular rhythm [11]. Electrocardiography (ECG) is therefore required to diagnose rhythm disturbances. Few studies have investigated arrhythmias secondary to *V. berus* and *Vipera palaestinae* envenomation [9, 10, 12]. In a prospective study of 24 dogs bitten by *V. berus* examined by standard (short-time) ECG, six dogs presented with arrhythmias at the initial clinical examination and ten dogs had arrhythmias 12–24 h after admission [10].

However, studies have shown that in-hospital ECGs of 2–5 min are insensitive for detecting arrhythmias [13, 14] which suggests that the arrhythmic incidence reported in earlier studies of snake bitten dogs might be underestimated.

A study describing ECG abnormalities using continuous 24-h ambulatory electrocardiography (24-AECG) in horses bitten by rattlesnakes has been published [15], but, to the authors' knowledge, 24-AECG studies investigating dogs bitten by viper snakes are lacking.

Abnormal hematological findings such as coagulopathy, neutrophilia, hemoconcentration, leukocytosis, and thrombocytopenia have been reported after envenomation by *V. berus* and *V. palaestinae* [1, 5–7, 12, 16, 17]. The reported biochemical abnormalities suggest mild multiple organ pathology, and elevated concentrations of muscle enzymes as a consequence of the envenomation [1, 5–7, 12, 16, 17].

Few studies have investigated circulating concentrations of cardiac specific troponin I (cTnI) in regards to envenomation by viper snakes. Concentrations of cTnI above reference ranges have been reported both at admission and 12–24 h after admission [9, 10, 12]. Increased cTnI concentrations do not seem to correlate with the presence of arrhythmias as some snake bitten dogs with arrhythmias have been shown to have normal concentrations of cTnI and vice versa [9, 10].

Increased knowledge of types of arrhythmias and when they potentially develop in relation to the envenomation episode would be beneficial to optimize monitoring and treatment strategies of dogs bitten by *V. berus*.

Therefore, the purpose of this study was to investigate the prevalence, types, and timing of arrhythmias, using 24-AECG, in dogs bitten by *V. berus* in the first 24–32 h after envenomation. In addition, we aimed to investigate the possible differences in selected clinical and hematological- and biochemical variables (including cTnI) at admission between *V. berus*-envenomed dogs with and without detected pathologic arrhythmias.

Methods

The study was approved by the Local Ethical Committee of Animal Experiments (S56-13) and the Swedish Board of Agriculture (5.2.18-10320/13). All owners signed a written consent form prior to inclusion in the study.

Dogs bitten between March 2014 and June 2015, presented to Anicura Regional Animal Hospital, Stockholm, Sweden, were prospectively recruited to the study. To be included in the study, dogs had to exhibit typical clinical signs of envenomation (sudden pain, swelling, and edema) and the snake had to have been observed by the owner, either as it bit the dog or in the near proximity of the dog.

Dogs with primary cardiac disease (other than trivial mitral- or tricuspid insufficiency with normal valvular morphology), systemic disease or that were treated with any type of medication prior to arrival at the hospital were excluded from the study. In addition, dogs that were bitten more than 8 h before presentation were also excluded.

Clinical evaluation and treatment strategy

Veterinary clinicians involved in the study had received oral instructions on how to examine the dogs and use the predesigned study protocol. Upon arrival at the animal hospital, dogs that met the inclusion criteria were examined by a veterinary clinician. The owners were interviewed about the time of the snake bite and the medical history of the dogs. Clinical findings with emphasis on the location of the snake bite, the appearance of the area of the bite (degree of swelling graded subjectively as no swelling or mild, moderate or severe swelling), and the dog's cardiovascular and mental status (graded subjectively as normal or mildly, moderately or severely depressed), were recorded in the study protocol and in the dog's medical record.

All dogs had a venous catheter placed in the distal cephalic vein and blood was sampled in EDTA, non-additive (serum), and heparin tubes, immediately after the clinical examination. The dogs were allowed short walks five times per 24 h. All dogs were treated according to the animal hospital's treatment strategies of viper bites, and administered constant rate infusion of intravenous crystalloids[1] and buprenorphine intravenously every eighth hour, at rates and doses at the discretion of the attending veterinary clinician. The morning after arrival, and every 24 h as long as the dogs were hospitalized, the clinical examination was repeated. The heart was auscultated every fourth hour by the attending veterinary clinician. It was the decision of the veterinary clinician in charge as to when the dog could be discharged. All dogs were recommended a revisit about 14 days after discharge from the animal hospital and the dogs were only permitted short leash walks until the revisit. At the time of the revisit, the owner was interviewed about any possible complications

[1] Ringer Acetat, Baxter Medical AB, Kista, Sweden.

to the snakebite, the dog's mental status and the appearance of the bite-area, and a clinical examination was performed. To investigate possible complications due to the snake bite, telephone interviews were conducted with the dog owners a minimum of 1 year after the snake bite.

Laboratory analysis

Blood was collected for hematologic analyses in EDTA tubes and analyzed by an automated laser-based hematology analyzer.[2] Blood smears were evaluated, and a manual differential count performed. Blood collected in serum tubes for biochemical analyses (C-reactive protein (CRP), glucose, urea, alanine amino transferase (ALAT), alkaline phosphatase (ALP), creatinine, albumin, total protein, total calcium, phosphate, bile acids, sodium, potassium, and chloride) was centrifuged (1500G, 5 min) 30 min after collection and analyzed by spectrophotometric methods.[3] All the mentioned analyses were performed immediately after centrifugation.

Blood collected in heparin tubes for plasma cTnI analysis was centrifuged (1500*g*, 5 min) immediately after sampling and thereafter transferred to cryotubes, and stored in −20 °C for a maximum time of 3 months after which time the samples were transported in frozen form to −80 °C and stored for a maximum time of 29 months. Batched-analysis was performed with a commercially available high-sensitivity, enzyme-linked immunosorbent assay[4], previously validated for use in dogs [18]. The lower detection limit of the assay was 0.01 ng/ml. All samples were analyzed in duplicate and the mean cTnI concentration for every dog was used for statistical analyses. The samples that contained a cTnI concentration lower than the detection limit of the assay was assigned a concentration of 0.005 ng/ml.

Echocardiography

To rule out primary cardiac disease, the dogs underwent a standard two-dimensional echocardiographic examination[5] immediately after the clinical examination. When this was impossible due to practical reasons, an echocardiographic examination was performed the following day or at the time of the revisit. The echocardiographic examinations were performed on unsedated and mildly restrained dogs in lateral recumbency. The left ventricular and right ventricular measurements were obtained from the right parasternal long and short axis views and the left atrial to aortic root ratio from the right parasternal short axis view, as previously described [19, 20]. Doppler examinations of all valves were performed and peak flow velocities were recorded.

Electrocardiographic evaluation

The dogs were shaved behind the elbows and on the chest, and the skin was cleaned with alcohol. The electrodes[6] were placed in a seven-lead precordial system and connected to a 24-AECG.[7] The system was covered by a monitoring vest and set to record for 24 h while the dogs were hospitalized.

Arrhythmia analyses

The recordings were analyzed by one of the authors (ARV) by a software[8] designed for humans. All recordings were manually checked and adjusted. Only examinations of a minimum of 18 h of recordings were included in the study. The time of the snake bite was set as hour zero for every dog and the number of hours from the time of the bite to the start of the 24-AECG recordings were calculated to ensure correct comparison of the hourly summaries of the recordings between the different dogs. The electrodes and recorder were removed after 25 h unless the electrodes had not detached prematurely.

The 24-AECG recordings were reviewed according to the definitions presented in Table 1. Dogs were divided into two groups as follows: dogs with pathologic arrhythmias and dogs without pathologic arrhythmias, and the criteria for the division was based upon findings in previous published studies of 24-AECG in dogs [13, 21–24]. Dogs that had less than 50 single and sporadic ventricular premature complexes (VPCs) per 24 h were considered normal, and dogs that had more than 50 single VPCs per 24 h (Fig. 1a), couplets of VPCs (Fig. 1b), ventricular tachycardia (VT) (Fig. 1c) or "R-on-T phenomenon" (Fig. 1d) were considered to have pathologic arrhythmias.

Statistical analysis

Statistical analyses were performed using a commercially available software program.[9] A value of $P < 0.05$ was considered significant for the analyses. Group data such as dog characteristics, clinical findings, and arrhythmia variables are presented as medians and interquartile range (IQR). A logarithmic transformation was performed to achieve a normal distribution for skewed variables.

[2] Sysmex-XT2000iV, Sysmex Corporation, Kobe, Japan.

[3] Roche Cobas C311, Roches Diagnostics GmBH, D-68298 Mannheim, Germany.

[4] Access Systems AccuTnI Assay, Beckman Coulter Inc, Fullerton, CA.

[5] GE Vivid E9/Logic E9, GE Medical, Milwaukee WI, USA.

[6] Ambu®Blue Sensor M REF: M-00-s/50, Ambu AS, Ballerup, Denmark.

[7] Trillium Platinum 5000 Forest Medical, East Syracuse, NY.

[8] Trillium Platinum version 4.32 software, Forest Medical, East Syracuse, NY.

[9] JMP, version 11.0.0, SAS Institute Inc. Cary, NC.

Table 1 List of variables derived from the 24-h ambulatory electrocardiography and the respective definitions

Maximum, minimum, and mean heart rate during 24 h and for every hour
Total number of episodes of bradycardia [minimum of four consecutive sinus beats at the rate of <45 beats per minute (BPM)] during 24 h and for every hour
Total number of episodes of tachycardia (minimum of four consecutive sinus beats at the rate of >150 BPM) during 24 h and for every hour
Total number of sinus pauses (defined as the absence of sinus P waves for more than 2 s) in 24 h and for every hour
Total number of single atrial premature complexes (APCs) (defined as a premature normally appearing QRS complex with an abnormal P wave morphology) in 24 h and for every hour
Total number of couplets (two consecutive) of APCs in 24 h and for every hour
Total number of episodes of supraventricular tachycardia (SVT) (defined as an episode of ≥3 normally appearing QRS complexes with a rate of >150 BPM that commence with a complex of abnormal P wave morphology and whose N–N interval is equal to or less than the previous N–N interval) in 24 h and for every hour
Total time of SVT during 24 h
Total number of single ventricular premature complexes (VPCs) (defined as a premature complex with a bizarre and abnormally wide morphology and large T wave of opposite polarity) in 24 h and for every hour
Total number of couplets of VPCs in 24 h and for every hour
Total number of episodes of ventricular tachycardia (VT) (defined as an episode of ≥3 VPCs with at the rate of >100 BPM) in 24 h and for every hour
Total number of VPCs in episodes of ventricular tachycardia in 24 h and for every hour
Total time of VT in 24 h
Total number of idioventricular episodes (defined as an episode of >3 VPCs at a rate of <100 BPM) in 24 h and for every hour
Total number of idioventricular complexes (defined as a VPC at a rate of <100 BPM) in 24 h and for every hour
Total number of ventricular depolarizations (defined as the sum of single and couplet VPCs, number of VPCs in episodes of VT, and number of complexes in episodes of IVR) in 24 h and for every hour
Total number of episodes of "R-on-T phenomenon" (defined as an episode where a VPC interrupts the T wave of the preceding beat) in 24 h and for every hour
Presence of second-degree AV block (defined as a P wave not conducting a QRS complex)

BPM beats per minute, *APC* atrial premature complex, *SVT* supraventricular tachycardia, *VPC* ventricular premature complex, *VT* ventricular tachycardia, *AV block* atrioventricular block

The non-parametric Mann–Whitney U test was used to compare continuous variables such as age, body weight, time from snake bite to admission and 24-AECG, duration of hospitalization, number of days from hospitalization to revisit, hematologic- and biochemical variables (including cTnI concentrations), and dose of buprenorphine, between dogs with pathologic arrhythmia and those without. The Chi square test was used for comparisons between categorical variables such as sex (female/male), area of bite (nose/limb), no/mild/moderate/severe swelling at admission and hospitalization, normal- and mildly/moderately/severely depressed mental status at admission, hospitalization, at home, and at revisit, and month of envenomation (subdivided into March–May and June–September) between dogs with pathologic arrhythmias and those without. To enable statistical analyses, no swelling and normal mental status were assigned 1, and mild(ly), moderate(ly), and severe(ly) swelling and depressed mental status were assigned 2, 3, and 4 respectively.

Univariate regression analyses were used to evaluate potential associations between hour after snakebite and the various ECG variables (listed in Table 1) and continuous and categorical variables described above for dogs with pathologic arrhythmias.

Results

Clinical findings

Breeds included Labrador retriever (n = 3), mixed breed (n = 3), German shepherd (n = 2), flat coated retriever (n = 1), Gonczy Polski (n = 1), Irish setter (n = 1), Jack Russel terrier (n = 1), Nova Scotia duck tolling retriever (n = 1), English pointer (n = 1), Rhodesian ridgeback (n = 1), Samoyed (n = 1), and Welsh springer spaniel (n = 1). Dog characteristics and clinical findings other than breed are summarized in Table 2.

Echocardiography

Four dogs (24%) underwent echocardiographic examinations at admission, five (29%) dogs the day after admission, and eight (47%) dogs at the revisit.

All dogs had unremarkable echocardiograms except one dog with trivial mitral insufficiency.

Electrocardiographic evaluation and arrhythmia analysis

All dogs had complete recordings of 24 h except three dogs that lacked 1, 2, and 6 h respectively. Clinically significant arrhythmias were of ventricular origin, and in the 24-AECG recordings, pathologic arrhythmias were found in eight of the 17 (47%) included dogs. Of the nine dogs with normal 24-AECG, none had more than seven

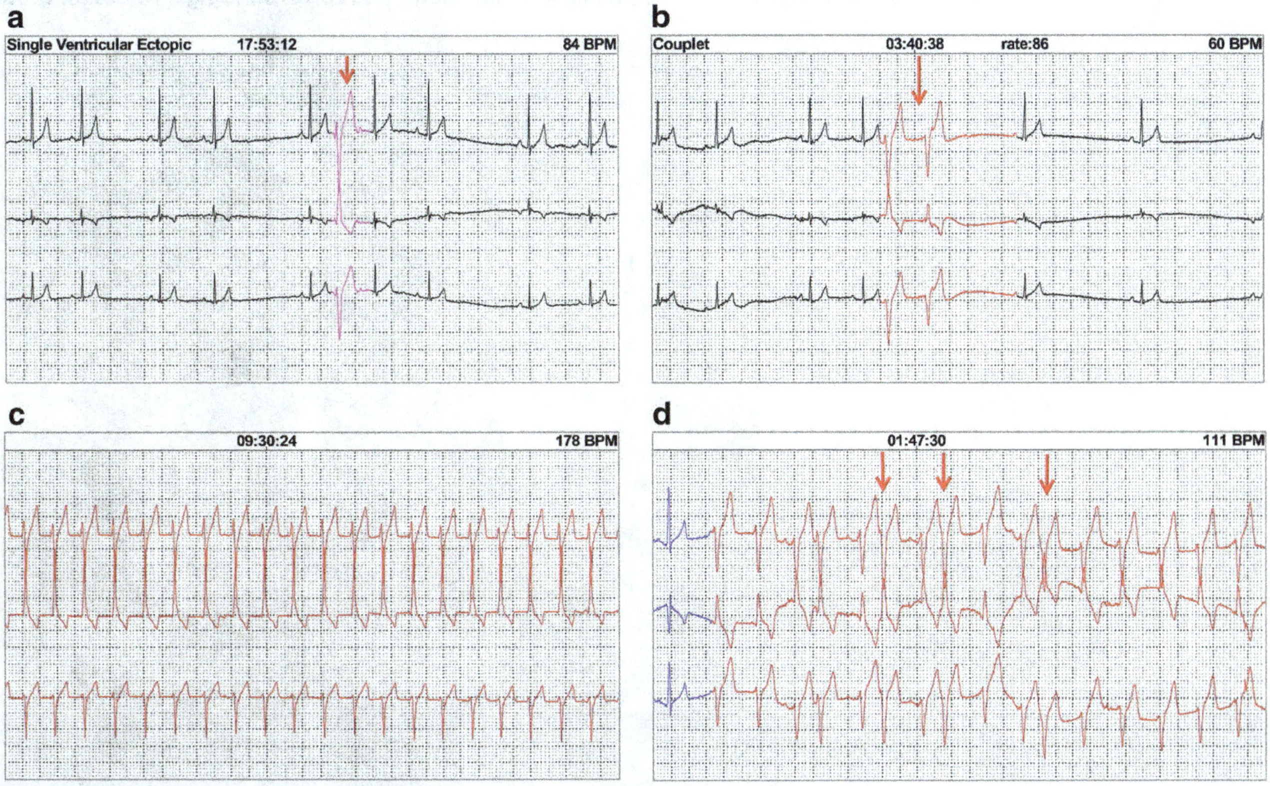

Fig. 1 24-h ambulatory electrocardiography strips recorded from selected dogs envenomed by *Vipera berus* to illustrate some abnormalities of ventricular depolarization used to separate dogs with and without pathologic arrhythmias. Dogs with the following abnormalities were considered to have pathologic arrhythmias. **a** More than 50 single ventricular premature complex (VPC) *(arrow)*. **b** Couplets of VPCs *(arrow)*. **c** Episodes of ventricular tachycardia. **d** "R-on-T phenomenon" *(arrow)*

ventricular depolarizations in total. None of the eight dogs with arrhythmias had less than 568 abnormal ventricular depolarizations. No dog had supraventricular arrhythmias other than single and sporadic atrial premature complexes (APCs). Sporadic events of second degree atrioventricular (AV) block was identified in four dogs in the group of dogs with pathologic arrhythmias and four dogs in the group of dogs without pathologic arrhythmias. A summary of dog characteristics and clinical findings in dogs with and without pathologic arrhythmias and *P* values obtained from the non-parametric Mann–Whitney U test and Chi square test are shown in Table 2.

Median and IQR for 12 selected 24-AECG variables of the eight dogs with pathologic arrhythmias are included in Table 3.

Characterization and timing of arrhythmias

Four of the eight dogs with pathologic arrhythmias experienced a decrease in episodes of arrhythmias in the 24 h following the snakebite. Two of these four dogs experienced a decrease (all $P < 0.039$) in each of the following categories: number of single VPCs, number of episodes of VT, total number of VPCs in episodes of VT, and total number of ventricular depolarizations (Fig. 2). One dog experienced a decrease in number of couplets of VPCs ($P = 0.005$, $R^2 = 0.47$). One dog experienced a decrease in the number of idioventricular episodes ($P = 0.001$, $R^2 = 0.53$), and one dogs had three episodes of "R-on-T phenomenon", one episode occurring 7 h and two episodes occurring 13 h after the snake bite.

Three dogs with pathologic arrhythmia experienced an increase in episodes of arrhythmias in the 24 h following the snake bite. All three dogs experienced increases in the total number of ventricular depolarizations during the recorded 24 h (all $P < 0.019$) (Fig. 2). One dog experienced an increase in each of the following categories: number of single VPCs ($P = 0.014$, $R^2 = 0.24$), number of episodes of VT ($P = 0.034$, $R^2 = 0.20$), and total number of VPCs in episodes of VT ($P = 0.0001$, $R^2 = 0.53$). Two of the dogs had 13 and 27 episodes of "R-on-T phenomenon" respectively. No correlation between time and episodes of "R-on-T phenomenon" was found for the former dog but for the latter dog, there was a decrease in the

Table 2 Dog characteristics and clinical findings for *Vipera berus*-envenomed dogs, and corresponding *P* values for group comparisons

Group	Dogs with pathologic arrhythmias	Dogs without pathologic arrhythmias	*P* value
Number	8/17	9/17	
Sex (female/male)	6/2	3/6	0.09
Age (years)	3.16 (IQR 1.62–4.34)	3.26 (IQR 1.02–5.45)	1.00
Weight (kg)	25.2 (IQR 20–29.9)	22 (IQR 17.6–36.4)	0.92
Month of bite (March–May/June–September)	4/4	5/4	0.82[a]
Area of bite (nose/limb)	4/4	9/0	0.02[b]
Time from bite to admission (hours)	1.85 (IQR 2.96–1.03)	2 (IQR 2–3)	0.89
Time from bite to 24-AECG (hours)	2 (IQR 1.25–3.75)	2 (IQR 2–3)	0.76
Mental status at admission (normal/mildly depressed/moderately depressed/severely depressed)	2/2/3/1 2.5 (IQR 1.25–3)	2/4/2/1 2 (IQR 1.5–3)	0.73
Degree of swelling of bite area at admission (normal/mildly/moderately/severely)	0/3/3/2 3 (IQR 2–3.75)	0/0/5/4 3 (IQR 3–4)	0.13
Mental status day after hospitalization (normal/mildly depressed/moderately depressed/severely depressed)	5/3/0/0 1 (IQR 1–2)	8/1/0/0 1 (IQR 1–1)	0.21
Degree of swelling of bite area day after hospitalization (normal/mildly/moderately/severely)	1/2/4/1 3 (IQR 2–3)	0/2/4/3 3 (IQR 2.5–4)	0.28
Mental status at home (normal/mildly depressed/moderately depressed/severely depressed)	8/0/0/0 I (IQR 1–1)	7/2/0/0 1 (IQR 1–1.75)	0.14
Mental status at revisit (normal/mildly depressed/moderately depressed/severely depressed)	7/0/0/0[b] 1 (IQR 1–1)	7/0/0/0[c] 1 (IQR 1–1)	1.00
Dose buprenorphine (mg/kg)	0.01 (IQR 0.006–0.012)	0.012 (IQR 0.011–0.013)	0.37
Arrhythmia or murmur detected with cardiac auscultation during hospitalization (yes/no)	0/9	0/9	
Additional clinical findings during hospitalization	Hematoma gingiva (n = 1) Edema limb (n = 1) Edema scrotum (n = 1) Diarrhea (n = 1)	Hematoma gingiva (n = 5)	
Additional medications during hospitalization	Maropitant (n = 1) Omeprazole (n = 1) Sucralfate (n = 2)	Maropitant (n = 1)	
Duration of hospitalization (days)	1.5 (IQR 1–2.75)	1 (IQR 1–2)	0.52
Time to revisit (days)	15 (IQR 11–17)	14 (IQR (13–16)	0.90
Concentration cTnI at admission	0.015 (IQR 0.006–0.039)[c]	0.01 (IQR (0.01–0.02)	1.00
Long-term complications to snake-bite (yes/no)[d]	0/8	0/5	

No swelling and normal mental status were assigned 1, and mild(ly), moderate(ly), and severe(ly) swelling and depressed mental status were assigned 2, 3, and 4 respectively. Dogs without pathologic arrhythmias had less than 50 single and sporadic VPCs per 24 h. Dogs with pathologic arrhythmias had more than 50 VPCs per 24 h, couplets of VPCs, VT or R-on-T. Group data is presented as medians and interquartile range (IQR)

[a] *P* value for testing March–May/June–September by pathologic arrhythmia yes/no

[b] *P* value for testing area of snakebite by pathologic arrhythmia yes/no

[c] seven dogs

[d] 13 dogs (four dog owners could not be contacted). 24-h ambulatory ECG (24-AECG). Cardiac troponin I (cTnI)

number of episodes of "R-on-T phenomenon" ($P = 0.017$, $R^2 = 0.53$) during the 24 h following the snakebite.

Laboratory analysis

Hematologic and serum biochemistry variables were within reference intervals for the majority of the dogs with a few exceptions. Three dogs had mild leukocytosis (15.1×10^6, 15.4×10^6, 16.2×10^6/l; reference interval 4.9–14.7 $\times 10^6$/l) and one dog had mild erythrocytosis (9.25×10^9/l; reference interval 6.2–8.9 $\times 10^9$/l). Two dogs had mild hyperglycemia (6.84, 7.2 mmol/l; reference interval 3.7–6.6 mmol/l) and elevated CRP (52, 57 mg/l; reference interval <20 mg/l). One dog had elevations in each of ALP (2.3 μkat/l; reference interval <1.4 μkat/l), creatinine (136 μmol/l; reference interval <135 μmol/l), phosphorus (2.9 mmol/l; reference interval 0.7–1.9 mmol/l), and bile acids (21 μmol/l; reference interval <20 μmol/l).

Table 3 Selected 24-h ambulatory electrocardiography variables derived from eight *Vipera berus*-envenomed dogs with pathologic arrhythmias

Variables 24-AECG	Median	IQR
Total number of QRS complexes	117,861	102,484–134,638
Maximum HR (BPM)	196	189–200
Minimum HR (BPM)	39.5	36–44.5
Average HR (BPM)	83.5	76.25–88.5
Single VPC	670	277–1626
Couplet VPC	155	55.5–416
Episodes of VT	200	33–331
Total number of VPCs in episodes of VT	3503	703–5720
Episodes of IVR	52	25.5–151
Total number of complexes in episodes of IVR	152	68–284
Total number of ventricular depolarizations	5241	1554–8059
Episodes of "R-on-T phenomenon"	0	0–4.8

Total number of ventricular depolarizations is defined as the sum of single and couplet VPCs, number of VPCs in episodes of VT, and number of complexes in episodes of IVR

24-AECG 24-h ambulatory ECG, *IQR* interquartile range, *HR* heart rate, *BPM* beats per minute, *VPC* ventricular premature complex, *VT* ventricular tachycardia, *IVR* idioventricular rhythm

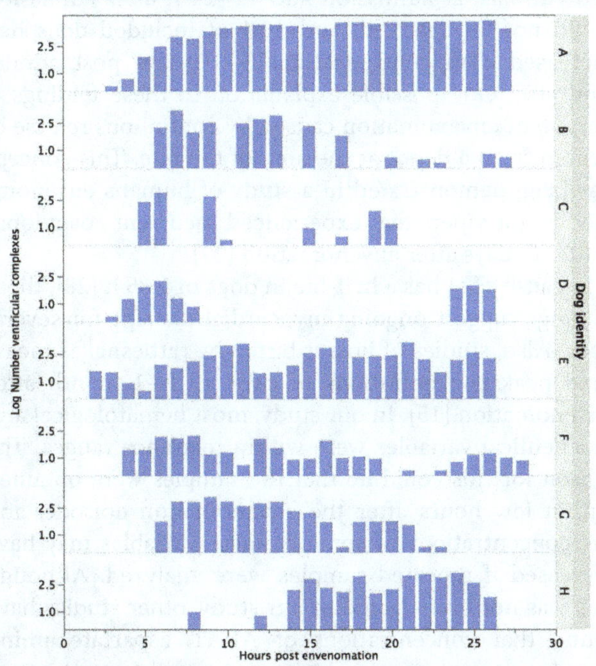

Fig. 2 Total number of ventricular depolarizations in the first 24 h (+ number of hours from envenomation episode until start of 24-h ambulatory ECG recordings) after *Vipera berus* envenomation in eight dogs with pathologic arrhythmias. Dogs with identities *B* and *F* experienced a decrease (all $P < 0.039$) in total number of ventricular depolarizations. Dogs with identities *A*, *E*, and *H* experienced an increase (all $P < 0.019$) in total number of ventricular depolarizations. A logarithmic transformation of the total number of ventricular depolarizations was performed to achieve a normal distribution. *P* values are from the univariate regression models

Plasma cTnI was analyzed in 15 dogs. The median cTnI value at admission was 0.01 ng/ml (IQR 0.01–0.02 ng/ml). All dogs had plasma cTnI concentrations <0.2 ng/ml.

No significant differences in hematologic and serum biochemistry variables were found between dogs with and without pathologic arrhythmias.

Discussion

The clinically significant arrhythmias detected in this study were of ventricular origin. Pathologic arrhythmias were detected in 47% of included dogs bitten by *V. berus*. Of these eight dogs, four dogs experienced a significant decrease and three a significant increase in arrhythmic episodes in the first 24–32 h following envenomation. All four dogs that were bit on a limb had pathologic arrhythmias. Otherwise, no significant clinical, hematological or biochemical differences between dogs with pathologic arrhythmias and dogs without were found in this study.

In our study, clinically significant arrhythmias were of ventricular origin, whereas other studies of viper envenomation also report of sinus tachycardia, APCs, ST-depression, and sinus arrest [9, 12]. There was a clear distinction between dogs with normal and pathologic 24-AECG recordings, and in no dog, were the findings equivocal. Of the eight dogs with pathologic arrhythmias, arrhythmic events decreased with time in four dogs. This indicates that the venom's cardiotoxic effects decreased during the 24 h following the snake bite, judged by the waning of ECG abnormalities. On the contrary, in three dogs with pathologic arrhythmias, arrhythmic events significantly increased with time; which implies myocardial damage worsening over time. In one study of *V. berus*-envenomed dogs examined with standard (short-time) ECGs, clinically relevant arrhythmias were detected at admission, between 6–7 h after the snakebite, but not at 12, 24, or 36 h after the bite in one dog [9]. In four of the dogs of this study, arrhythmias were detected either at 12, 24, or 36 h after the snakebite, but not at admission one to 6 h after the bite [9]. In a similar study of 24 dogs, six dogs had arrhythmias at admission and additionally four had arrhythmias 12–24 h post admission, the time lag from envenomation to admission was not reported [10]. Several factors, such as individual susceptibility, site of snake bite, season, and toxicity and volume of injected venom, might influence the presence or absence and timing of arrhythmias. By using a 24-AECG, in the present study, we were able to quantify all arrhythmic variables in the first 24–32 h, and follow possible variations in arrhythmic episodes after the snakebite, which would have been difficult if we had used multiple repeated short-time ECG examinations.

However, 24-AECG might not be an ideal method for use in clinical practice. Interpreting and analyzing the

24-AECG is made after completion of the recording, which would prevent immediate attention to and treatment of arising arrhythmias. Telemetric ECG equipment could be a valuable alternative clinical tool to monitor the individual snake bitten hospitalized dog.

Forty-seven percent of dogs bitten by *V. berus* included in this study experienced pathologic arrhythmias of abnormal ventricular depolarization. Other studies of viper envenomation report lower frequencies of arrhythmic events compared to our study [6, 7, 9, 10, 12, 17]. In publications of viper-bitten dogs where repeated ECG examinations were not performed, arrhythmias were detected by cardiac auscultation in 2–8% of included dogs [6, 7, 17]. Few studies of dogs bitten by vipers have included ECG examinations at predetermined time intervals of 8 or 12 h, to screen for ECG abnormalities, and in these the incidence of arrhythmias was 25, 29, and 42%, respectively [9, 10, 12]. Based on these findings, it appears likely that many arrhythmias remain undetected unless snake bitten dogs undergo repeated ECG examinations or 24-AECG. In fact, arrhythmic events were not detected by auscultation in any of the dogs in the present study. In cases of non-sustained VT, arrhythmias might have been missed if the heart was auscultated in periods of normal sinus rhythm. Furthermore, presence of idioventricular rhythms or VT, with heart rate within normal limits for normal sinus rhythm, might potentially explain the disagreement between auscultatory findings and ECG findings in the present study. Because the 24-AECG recordings were analyzed at the termination of the study, and no arrhythmias were detected by auscultation, none of the studied dogs were treated with any anti-arrhythmic medication.

All four dogs bitten on a limb developed pathologic arrhythmias. However, only four dogs were bitten on a limb, and such a potential association needs to be investigated further by studying a larger number of dogs. The prognosis for included dogs in this study was good regardless of area of bite. However, a study of *V. berus*-envenomated dogs suggested that there might be a correlation between limb envenomation and a poor prognosis [8]. Moreover, a study of *V. palaestinae* envenomation in dogs have found limb envenomation and a body weight less than 15 kg to be significantly associated with increased mortality [1]. This may suggest that the volume of venom injected by vipers in relation to the dog's size is of importance, and that this volume is inadequate to severely affect large dogs. In addition, dogs younger than 4 years had a lower risk of mortality than older dogs [1]. In the present study, all dogs recovered well from the snakebites. As most dogs were bitten on the nose, and the median age and weight 3 years and 22 and 25 kg respectively, their phenotype might have been favorable in regards to outcome. To further investigate a potential association between bite site and pathologic arrhythmias, studies including a greater number of dogs need to be conducted in the future.

In a study of 24 dogs bitten by *V. berus*, five dogs had elevated serum concentrations of cTnI in the absence of ECG abnormalities [9]. All dogs in the present study had low concentrations of plasma cTnI, analyzed using a high-sensitivity assay, at admission. The blood used for this analysis was sampled only a few hours after envenomation, which might have affected these results.

In humans, a rise in cTnI generally occurs 2–3 h after a myocardial injury [25], and release kinetics of cTnI in dogs appear similar [26]. The median time between snakebites and admission for all the included dogs in the present study was 1.8 h. This short time interval gave limited time for venom absorption from the bite site to the general circulation. As a result, there might have been insufficient time for the circulating venom to cause myocardial injury. This indicates that the peak concentrations of cTnI in our study might not have been detected. However, in a study of dogs envenomated by *V. berus*; differences in cTnI concentrations in dogs, with and without arrhythmias, at admission and 12–24 h after admission could not be detected, and 30% of included dogs had increased cTnI concentrations 5–10 days post admission [10]. One possible explanation to these findings is persistent envenomation caused by continuous release of venom from a depot at the area of the bite. This concept has been demonstrated in a study of humans envenomated by pit vipers that experienced recurrent coagulopathy 2–14 days after envenomation [27].

Because cTnI has a half-life in dogs of 1.85 h [28], these findings suggest ongoing myocardial damage for several days. Also, studies of horses bitten by rattlesnakes measured peak concentrations of cTnI 12 h–1 month after envenomation [15]. In our study, most hematological and biochemical variables were within reference ranges. The reason for this could be that the samples were obtained within few hours after the envenomation episode, and the concentrations of some of these variables may have increased if repeated samples were analyzed. Although this was not investigated in our study, other studies have found that concentrations of ALAT, aspartate amino transferase, and creatine kinase increased from the time of admission to 12–24 h after admission in dogs bitten by *V. palaestinae* and *V. berus* [7, 12].

The mode in which viper toxin causes myocardial damage is not entirely clear. Cardiotoxic components increase cellular membrane permeability to ions; resulting in altered fiber excitability damaging the myocardium and cardiac conduction [2]. This may explain the presence of arrhythmias in the absence of elevated cTnI concentrations seen in other studies [9]. In addition, studies suggest that the systemic inflammation caused by the snake bite, as measured by elevated concentrations of CRP, may injure the myocardium [10]. Also, CRP concentrations in snake bitten dogs have been shown to positively correlate with cTnI concentrations at admission, 12–14 h post-admission, and 5–10 days post-admission [6, 10]. In our study, only two dogs had elevated concentrations of CRP at admission, which made statistical analysis to investigate potential associations with cTnI and the presence of arrhythmias impossible.

There are some study limitations. Although 24-AECG analyses were made by the same person, the included dogs were otherwise examined and treated by different veterinary clinicians (using the same study protocol). This makes comparison of subjective variables between different dogs problematic. Because dogs were examined by 24-AECG in the hospital, they were mostly kept in cages. The results of this study might; therefore, not be directly applicable to dogs that are allowed unrestricted exercise. Another weakness of the study was the small number of included dogs. Included dogs were only examined for 24 h, and ECG findings after the first 24–32 h following a viper bite, could therefore not be evaluated in the present study. Only one blood sample for each dog for hematological and biochemical analyses was obtained at admission, and we were thus unable to investigate variations in concentrations of these variables with time after the snake bites. Moreover, three dogs did not have complete ambulatory ECG recordings of 24 h, and samples for cTnI analysis was lacking for two dogs, which may have affected the final analysis. The samples for cTnI analysis, awaiting transport for storage in −80 °C, were stored in −20 °C. Even though studies of cats have shown that storing samples at −20 °C for a maximum time of three, but not four, months is acceptable, this may have slightly altered the plasma concentrations of cTnI [29].

Conclusions

In this study of viper-envenomed dogs, the clinically significant arrhythmias were of ventricular origin. Forty-seven percent of included dogs suffered from abnormalities of ventricular depolarization based on findings on the 24-AECG. Dogs experienced a variation of patterns in arrhythmic episodes; some had a decrease and others an increase in abnormal ventricular depolarizations during 24–32 h following the snake bite. Based on findings from the present study, envenomed dogs should be monitored with repeated or continuous ECG-recordings, as differentiating dogs that will develop pathologic arrhythmias from those that will not, using clinical findings and hematologic or biochemical variables obtained at admission appears to be difficult. Dogs that have an increase in pathologic arrhythmic events in the first 24-h following envenomation might benefit from prolonged hospitalization to enable optimal monitoring and treatment of cardiac abnormalities.

Abbreviations

24-AECG: 24-h ambulatory electrocardiography; ALAT: alanine amino transferase; ALP: alkaline phosphatase; APC: atrial premature complex; AV block: atrioventricular block; BPM: beats per minute; CRP: C-reactive protein; cTnI: cardiac troponin I; ECG: electrocardiography; HR: heart rate; IQR: interquartile range; SVT: supraventricular tachycardia; *V. berus*: *Vipera berus*; *V. palaestinae*: *Vipera palaestinae*; VPC: ventricular premature complex; VT: ventricular tachycardia.

Authors' contributions

ARV participated in the design of the study, carried out the echocardiographic examinations, analyzed the 24-h ambulatory ECG recordings, interpretation of data, and drafted the manuscript. AT participated in the design of the study and helped to revise the manuscript. IL participated in the design of the study, performed the statistical analysis and interpretation of data, and helped to revise the manuscript. All authors read and approved the final manuscript.

Author details

[1] Anicura Regional Animal Hospital, Ljusnevägen 17, 12848 Bagarmossen, Sweden. [2] Anicura Albano Animal Hospital, Rinkebyvägen 21a, 18236 Danderyd, Sweden. [3] Department of Clinical Sciences, Faculty of Veterinary Medicine and Small Animal Sciences, Swedish University of Agricultural Sciences, P.O. Box 7084, 75007 Uppsala, Sweden.

Acknowledgements

The authors would like to acknowledge participating dogs, dog owners, veterinary clinicians, and veterinary technicians at Anicura Region Animal Hospital.

ARV would like to thank Suzanne Gundler for continued support and excellent mentorship.

Competing interests

The authors declare that they have no competing interests.

References

1. Segev G, Shipov A, Klement E, Harrus S, Kass P, Aroch I. *Vipera palaestinae* envenomation in 327 dogs: a retrospective cohort study and analysis of risk factors for mortality. Toxicon. 2004;43:691–9.
2. Goddard A, Schoeman JP, Leisewitz AL, Nagel SS, Aroch I. Clinicopathologic abnormalities associated with snake envenomation in domestic animals. Vet Clin Pathol. 2011;40:282–92.
3. Sutton NM, Bates N, Campbell A. Canine adder bites in the UK: a retrospective study of cases reported to the Veterinary Poisons Information Service. Vet Rec. 2011;169:607.
4. McDiarmid R, Campbell J, Toure T. Snake species of the world: a taxonomic and geographic reference. 1st ed. Washington: Herpetologist's League; 1999.
5. Turkovic V, Teichmann S, Dorfelt R. European adder bites in dogs in southern Germany. A retrospective study over a 6.5-year period. Tierarztl Prax K H. 2015;43:221–30.
6. Brandeker E, Hillström A, Hanås S, Hagman R, Holst BS. The effect of a single dose of prednisolone in dogs envenomated by *Vipera berus*—a randomized, double-blind, placebo-controlled clinical trial. BMC Vet Res. 2012. doi:10.1186/s12917-015-0352-6.

7. Lervik JB, Lilliehöök I, Frendin JHM. Clinical and biochemical changes in 53 Swedish dogs bitten by the European adder-*Vipera berus*. Acta Vet Scand. 2010. doi:10.1186/1751-0147-52-26.
8. Kängström L-E. Huggormsbett hos hund och katt. Svensk Veterinärtidning. 1989;41(Suppl 19):38–46.
9. Pelander L, Ljungvall I, Häggström J. Myocardial cell damage in 24 dogs bitten by the common European viper (*Vipera berus*). Vet Rec. 2010;166:687–90.
10. Langhorn R, Persson F, Åblad B, Goddard A, Schoeman JP, Willesen JL, et al. Myocardial injury in dogs with snake envenomation and its relation to systemic inflammation. J Vet Emerg Crit Care. 2014;24:174–81.
11. Kittleson MD, Kienle RD. Small animal cardiovascular medicine. 1st ed. St. Louis: Mosby Inc.; 1998.
12. Segev G, Ohad DG, Shipov A, Kass PH, Aroch I. Cardiac arrhythmias and serum cardiac troponins in *Vipera palaestinae* envenomation in dogs. J Vet Intern Med. 2008;22:106–13.
13. Wess G, Schulze A, Geraghty N, Hartmann K. Ability of a 5-min electrocardiography (ECG) for predicting arrhythmias in Doberman pinschers with cardiomyopathy in comparison with a 24-h ambulatory ECG. J Vet Intern Med. 2010;24:367–71.
14. Meurs KM, Spier AW, Wright NA, Hamlin RL. Comparison of in-hospital versus 24-h ambulatory electrocardiography for detection of ventricular premature complexes in mature boxers. J Am Vet Med Assoc. 2001;218:222–4.
15. Gilliam LL, Holbrook TC, Ownby CL, McFarlane D, Sleeper MM, Martin S, et al. Cardiotoxicity, inflammation, and immune response after rattlesnake envenomation in the horse. J Vet Intern Med. 2012;26:1457–63.
16. Aroch I, Yas-Natan E, Kuzi S, Segev G. Haemostatic abnormalities and clinical findings in *Vipera palaestinae*-envenomed dogs. Vet J. 2010;185:180–7.
17. Aroch I, Harrus S. Retrospective study of the epidemiological, clinical, haematological and biochemical findings in 109 dogs poisoned by *Vipera xanthina palestinae*. Vet Rec. 1999;144:532–5.
18. Oyama MA, Solter PF. Validation of an immunoassay for measurement of canine cardiac troponin I. J Vet Cardiol. 2004;6:17–24.
19. Thomas WP. Two-dimensional, real-time echocardiography in the dog Technique and anatomic validation. Vet Radiol. 1984;25:50–64.
20. Hansson K, Haggstrom J, Kvart C, Lord P. Left atrial to aortic root indices using two-dimensional and M-mode echocardiography in cavalier King Charles spaniels with and without left atrial enlargement. Vet Radiol Ultrasound. 2002;43:568–75.
21. Ulloa HM, Houston BJ, Altrogge DM. Arrhythmia prevalence during ambulatory electrocardiographic monitoring of beagles. Am J Vet Res. 1995;56:275–81.
22. Stern JA, Meurs KM, Spier AW, Koplitz SL, Baumwart RD. Ambulatory electrocardiographic evaluation of clinically normal adult boxers. J Am Vet Med Assoc. 2010;236:430–3.
23. Meurs KM, Spier AW, Lost D, Hamlin RL. Use of ambulatory electrocardiography for detection of ventricular premature complexes in healthy dogs. J Am Vet Med Assoc. 2001;218:1291–2.
24. Rasmussen CE, Vesterholm S, Ludvigsen TP, Häggström J, Pedersen HD, Moesgaard SG, et al. Holter monitoring in clinically healthy cavalier King Charles spaniels, wire-haired dachshunds, and Cairn terriers. J Vet Intern Med. 2011;25:460–8.
25. MacRae AR, Kavsak PA, Lustig V, Bhargava R, Vandersluis R, Palomaki GE, et al. Assessing the requirement for the 6-h interval between specimens in the American Heart Association classification of myocardial infarction in epidemiology and clinical research studies. Clin Chem. 2006;52:812–8.
26. Langhorn R, Willesen JL. Cardiac troponins in dogs and cats. J Vet Intern Med. 2016;30:36–50.
27. Boyer LV, Seifert SA, Clark RF, McNally JT, Williams SR, Nordt SP, et al. Recurrent and persistent coagulopathy following pit viper envenomation. Arch Intern Med. 1999;159:706–10.
28. Dunn ME, Coluccio D, Hirkaler G, Mikaelian I, Nicklaus R, Lipshultz SE, et al. The complete pharmacokinetic profile of serum cardiac troponin I in the rat and the dog. Toxicol Sci. 2011;123:368–73.
29. Langhorn R, Tarnow I, Willesen JL, Kjelgaard-Hansen M, Skovgaard IM, Koch J. Cardiac troponin I and T as prognostic markers in cats with hypertrophic cardiomyopathy. J Vet Intern Med. 2014;28:1485–91.

9

Psychometric evaluation of the canine brief pain inventory in a Swedish sample of dogs with pain related to osteoarthritis

Ann Essner[1,2*], Lena Zetterberg[1], Karin Hellström[1], Pia Gustås[3], Hans Högberg[4] and Rita Sjöström[5,6]

Abstract

Background: To evaluate intervention, implement evidence-based practice and enhance the welfare of dogs with naturally occurring osteoarthritis (OA), access to valid, reliable and clinically relevant outcome measures is crucial for researchers, veterinarians and rehabilitation practitioners. The objectives of the present study were to translate and evaluate psychometric properties, in terms of internal consistency and construct validity, of the owner-reported measure canine brief pain inventory (CBPI) in a Swedish sample of dogs with pain related to OA.

Results: Twenty-one owners of clinically sound dogs and 58 owners of dogs with pain related to OA were included in this observational and cross-sectional study. After being translated according to the guidelines for patient-reported outcome measures, the CBPI was completed by the canine owners. Construct validity was assessed by confirmatory factor analysis, by repeating the principal component analysis and by assessing for differences between clinically sound dogs and dogs with pain related to OA. Internal consistency was estimated by Cronbach's α. Confirmatory factor analysis was not able to confirm the factor-structure models tested in our sample. Principal component analysis showed a two-component structure, pain severity and pain interference of function. Two components accounted for 76.8% of the total variance, suggesting an acceptable fit of a two-component structure. The ratings from the clinically sound dogs differed from OA dogs and showed significantly lower CBPI total sum. Cronbach's α was 0.94 for the total CBPI, 0.91 for the pain severity and 0.91 for the pain interference of function.

Conclusions: The results indicate that the translated version of the CBPI is valid for use in the Swedish language. The findings suggest satisfying psychometric properties in terms of high internal consistencies and ability to discriminate clinically sound dogs from OA dogs. However, based on the confirmatory factor analysis, the original factor structure in the CBPI is not ideally suited to measure pain related to OA in our sample and the hypothesis of the presented two-factor structure was rejected. Further research needs to be conducted to determine whether the original psychometric results from CBPI can be replicated across different target groups and particularly with larger sample size.

Keywords: CBPI, Dogs, Measurement properties, Osteoarthritis, Pain, Physiotherapy, Rehabilitation

Background

To evaluate intervention, implement evidence-based practice and enhance the welfare of dogs with naturally occurring osteoarthritis (OA), access to valid, reliable and clinically relevant outcome measures is crucial for researchers, veterinarians and rehabilitation practitioners [1–3]. In human medicine, the use of patient-reported outcome measures in clinical practice is essential in patient-centered healthcare to follow the impact of interventions, choose the appropriate treatment and to capture the effect perceived by the patient [4]. Brief pain inventory is a well-known self-reported generic measure that originally was developed to capture pain intensity and pain interference with function in daily life in human cancer patients [5]. Over the years the human

*Correspondence: ann.essner@evidensia.se
[1] Department of Neuroscience, Faculty of Physiotherapy, Uppsala University, Husargatan, Biomedical Centre, Box 593, 751 24 Uppsala, Sweden
Full list of author information is available at the end of the article

brief pain inventory has been validated across languages and cultures and in different diseases [6–8]. Brown et al. [9, 10] adapted the instrument for use in dogs with OA related pain and pain in bone cancer. The canine brief pain inventory (CBPI) is a questionnaire intended to capture different dimensions of dog owners' perceptions of canine OA pain. To measure pain severity and how pain interferes with function in the daily life in dogs, the answers of the items in the questionnaire are given by a person living in the same household as the dog of interest, i.e. the owner of the dog [9]. Other owner-reported instruments have been used such as the Helsinki Chronic Pain Index [11], the Liverpool osteoarthritis in dogs [12] and the canine orthopedic index [13], besides the CBPI, in canine OA. Pain is a subjective unpleasant sensory and emotional experience in animals, as well as in humans, and their inability to communicate their experience in words makes it impossible to use self-reporting instruments to directly assess pain severity and pain interference with function [1]. Recognizing and assessing pain in a dog is challenging and even in humans, who are able to communicate their pain experience, it has been shown that there may be discrepancies in the agreement between the perceived intensity of pain assessed by the individual experiencing pain and the individual's pain as estimated by a parent [14]. Owner-reported pain instruments are based on canine behavioural changes affected by pain and the ability of the naïve observers, i.e. the owners, to recognize the behavioural signs in their dogs [15]. It has been shown by Hielm-Björkman et al. [16] that the ability of untrained owners to report the level of pain associated with OA on a visual analogue scale is limited, as they may not recognize the subtle signs of pain. Pain associated with OA may be manifested as changes in movement behaviour in the dog and gait evaluation during pain management is widely used in clinical settings. However, visual movement assessment and assigning levels and grades of lameness have shown poor intra- and inter-rater reliability among owners [17] and veterinarians [17, 18]. Hence, there is a challenge in constructing owner-reported instruments that prove adequate measurement properties.

Despite the challenges to owners to estimate pain experienced by their dogs, psychometric testing of the CBPI has shown adequate construct and criterion validity to assess owner-perceived pain. Psychometric testing refers to the construction and evaluation of an instrument developed to assess an unobservable concept, such as chronic pain [9, 11] and health related quality of life [19] in dogs. During the development of the CBPI, an exploratory factor analysis (EFA) was used to explore the relationships among the observed variables (items in a questionnaire), and to study the construct and subdomains. Brown et al. [9] extracted two subdomains in the CBPI; pain severity and pain interference with function in daily activities, in a group of dogs with pain related to OA, prior to treatment with anti-inflammatory drugs [9]. Later, Walton et al. [12] repeated an EFA in another sample of dogs with pain related to OA. In their sample, all CBPI items loaded heavily on one component, which they did not define [12]. Psychometric testing of the CBPI has also shown good internal consistency [9], moderate to strong test–retest reliability and a clinically significant responsiveness to change in the owners' perception of pain in dogs after anti-inflammatory treatment [9, 20, 21]. Nevertheless, when animal health-care professionals and researchers are selecting appropriate owner-reported outcome measures for pain associated to OA, considerations should be given to the purpose of the assessment and the context in which it is being used. The measurement properties, i.e. validity, reliability and responsiveness, should be established in the population of interest [4, 22, 23] and an instrument should be properly translated to the target language [24, 25]. The CBPI was originally validated in a group of untreated dogs with OA pain. To use the CBPI in a more diverse group of dogs with OA pain, e.g. dogs presented for physiotherapy, the instrument should to be psychometrically tested for its construct validity, and considered adequate. Construct validity concerns internal relationships, i.e. structural validity, and relationships to scores of other instruments or differences between known groups, i.e. hypothesis testing and cross-cultural validity [26]. The validity in a clinical target group, may differ from original psychometric testing. For instance, undergoing treatment, e.g. anti-inflammatory medication, may change the measurement properties of the CBPI, possibly threatening the validity of the CBPI as an outcome measure along the rehabilitation process. Dogs presented for physical rehabilitation in a veterinary primary care unit are a heterogeneous group of individuals and anti-inflammatory drugs are common treatment options in canine OA [1]. The psychometric properties of the CBPI has not yet been documented in such a diverse sample of dogs and our knowledge about whether the validity of the CBPI extends to a group including dogs that have ongoing anti-inflammatory treatment, i.e. are under pain management treatment, needs to be supplemented. In addition, the CBPI has not been translated from English to Swedish. Consequently, to assess the construct validity of the CBPI in a new target group, and to use the CBPI in the original target group, e.g. in a clinical protocol and for research, the CBPI questionnaire needs to be translated to the target language. In the present study, we hypothesized that the two-factor representation in the CBPI, pain severity and interference of pain with function, would be confirmed in a group of owners with dogs with OA pain presented for physical rehabilitation in a veterinary primary care unit. We also hypothesized that clinically sound dogs would show lower CBPI scores than OA dogs. Thus, the objectives of the present study were to translate the original CBPI and evaluate psychometric properties, in terms of internal consistency and construct validity, of the CBPI in a clinical sample of OA dogs referred for physiotherapy.

Methods

Study design

This study was an observational and cross-sectional study consisting of two groups of dogs that were consecutively recruited.

Study group and procedure

To determine the size of the sample we used a subject-to-item ratio 5:1 [27, 28]. The subject-to-item ratio was determined by the number of CBPI items rated by the owners; hence 10 items generated a sample size of 50 dogs. The sample size was overestimated by 10% to cover possible losses and altogether we aimed for 60 dogs with OA. We aimed for approximately 20 dogs in a control group and when the number was reached, it became clear that the respondents in the control group scored mainly zero in pain severity and pain interference with function items, yielding no more information from the owner-perceived answers.

Sixty-one dogs referred from primary care veterinarians for physical rehabilitation interventions due to naturally occurring OA were included in the OA group. A group of 21 clinically sound dogs participated as controls. Of these, 19 clinically sound dogs and their owners also participated as controls in another research study conducted by two of the authors (PG and AE) (unpublished data). All dogs, in both groups, were clinically examined by a veterinarian prior to enrolment in the study. The OA dogs were diagnosed before they were recruited to the study. None of the control dogs had a history or current clinical evidence of OA. At a visit to a registered animal physiotherapist (AE), the clinical history was collected and the owners, whose dogs fulfilled the inclusion criteria, answered the Swedish version of the CBPI. The CBPI questionnaire was administered to the owners at the veterinary clinic and the owners were instructed according to the user guide available for the CBPI (www.canineBPI.com). Collection of the questionnaire was performed on the same occasion. Nineteen of the owners of the clinically sound dogs received the questionnaire from a veterinarian (PG). The inclusion criteria were as follows: dog >1 year of age, dog >9 kg body weight, clinical evidence of OA of at least one synovial joint, radiographic evidence of osteoarthritis of at least one synovial joint. The following were exclusion criteria: the owner completing the questionnaire lacked an understanding of written Swedish, other concurrent disease interfering with the dogs' mobility, activity or health related quality of life. The dogs and the owners in the control group fulfilled the same inclusion and exclusion criteria as the OA group, except the clinical and radiographic evidence of OA. All dogs were client-owned and informed owner consent was obtained. The study protocols were approved by the Local Ethical Committee in Uppsala, Sweden (C81/12, C111/12, C17/2016).

Instruments

Canine brief pain inventory is a 10-item questionnaire. The first four items consist of eleven-point (0–10) rating scales asking the owners to rate the pain intensity in their dogs during the last seven days, addressing pain "at its worst", "at its least", "on average" and "right now". Zero indicates "no pain" and 10 represents "extreme pain". The remaining six items cover the degree to which the owners rate the pain interference with function for their dog. In the interference items, 0 indicates "does not interfere" and 10 indicates "interferes completely". CBPI scores are aggregated in two dimensions: (1) pain severity, using the four items (items 1–4) on pain intensity, and (2) pain interference, using the six items (items 5–10) on pain interference with function. The minimum sum of CBPI is 0 and the maximum sum in the pain severity items is 40 and in the pain interference 60. The sums of the two dimensions may be averaged to deliver a pain severity score and a pain interference score.

Body condition score was assessed by palpation and visual inspection by two of the investigators (AE and PG). A nine-point scale, reaching from one (severely underweight) to nine (obese), was used to assign the dogs to a body condition score, and in addition bodyweight was determined with digital scales [29]. Additional descriptive measures were collected on the same occasion that the owners answered the questionnaires (Table 1). The age (years) and body weight (kg) of the dogs were

Table 1 Demographic data of the cohort (n = 79)

	OA group (n = 58)	Control group (n = 21)
Age (years)	7 (1–12)	5 (1–10)*
Body weight (kg)	30.4 (9–56)	26 (9–53)
Body condition score	5.5 (3–8)	4 (4–5)*
Anti-inflammatory medication	46 (79%)	0 (0%)
Gender (female)	25 (43%)	13 (62%)

Values are presented in median (range) and frequencies (proportions)

OA osteoarthritis

* Significant difference estimated with Mann–Whitney's U test

documented together with data on treatment with anti-inflammatory medication.

Translation and back translation

Permission to translate the CBPI into Swedish was obtained in a written consent from the copyright holder Dr. Dorothy Cimino Brown. Standard procedure for translation of instruments designed for self-reported outcome was used [25]. The English versions of the CBPI instrument were translated into Swedish with a forward and backward procedure as follows: a translation from English to Swedish was done from the original language, i.e. English, by two independent native Swedish persons who were fluent in the target language and who had good understanding of the original language. Further, the Swedish version of CBPI was back translated into the original language by two independent native English persons who were fluent in the original language and had good understanding of the target language. The translation processes described by Wild et al. [24] and Terwee et al. [25] were used as guidelines and the questionnaire was pretested in a pilot study on the target sample. The translations were reviewed until a consensus about a translated version was reached. The pilot study was not included in this study.

Statistical analysis

Descriptive statistics comprised baseline data on age, bodyweight, body conditions score, on-going use of anti-inflammatory medication, presented as median (min–max) and frequencies (proportion). The pain severity sum, pain interference sum, total CBPI sum, pain severity score and pain interference with function score are presented as median (min–max). The internal consistency of the questionnaire was estimated to examine the extent to which items in the questionnaire correlated and measured the same concept. In accordance with Nunnelly and Bernstein [30] Cronbach's α >0.70 was considered acceptable.

Construct validity (structural validity) was assessed by confirmatory factor analysis (CFA) and EFA [22, 25]. When there already is an accepted theory or empirical knowledge about the relationships between the latent, e.g. pain severity and pain interference, and observed variables, e.g. the items in the CBPI questionnaire, a confirmatory factor analysis (CFA) can be used to establish and possibly confirm construct validity [6, 7]. The CFA was used to test a specification of a model with several factors, based on previous research focusing on the factor structure by means of goodness-of-fit. A CFA by maximum likelihood method was conducted to test the hypothesis that the two-factor representation in the CBPI would be confirmed (Fig. 1).

The following goodness-of-fit indices were assessed: model-Chi^2, degrees of freedom and Chi^2/df, comparative fit index (CFI), root mean square error of approximation (RMSEA) with 90% confidence intervals, normed fit index (NFI), and parsimony adjusted normed fit index (PNFI). These fit indices show the extent to which the proposed model fit the data and thus indicate whether the specified structure may be confirmed. According to the guidelines by Hu and Bentler [31] acceptable model fit values are RMSEA values close to 0.06 or less; and CFI values are close to 0.90 or higher; NFI >0.95. The PNFI should be used in conjunction with NFI and could have values as low as 0.5 when NFI is as high as 0.9. Model Chi^2 should lead to a high P value ($P > 0.05$) for a good model, and relative to its degrees of freedom, Chi^2/df <2.0. The CBPI has a theoretical foundation that indicates two domains; pain intensity and pain interference with function [9], although Walton et al. [12] presented only one dimension. Based on the EFA presented by Walton et al. [12] and Brown et al. [9] we also tested a one-factor model with all CBPI items. Because the ordered data from CBPI items are not normally distributed and not on a quantitative measurement scale, we also estimated the models by bootstrapping and by Bayesian methods [32]. These methods do not change the goodness-of-fit indices, but do reveal differences in estimated factor loadings and variances.

We repeated an EFA by principal component model with subsequent varimax rotation, to study the interitem relationship and to explore the factor structure in our target group. Factors were extracted according to Kaiser's rule; eigenvalues >1. Kaiser–Meyer–Olkin measure of sampling adequacy was calculated to assess whether our data was appropriate for factor analysis. Kaiser–Meyer–Olkin values between 0.5 and 0.7 was considered mediocre, 0.7–0.8 good, 0.8–0.9 high and above 0.9 excellent [33]. In addition, a significant Bartlett's test of sphericity was also required for our data to be suitable for factor analysis [34].

When a marked proportion of the respondents score their dogs at the minimum, a floor effect occurs. Due to the notable item level and total sum floor effect in the group of OA dogs, we created a subgroup in which the owners reported pain related to OA, CBPI total sum $\geq$1. The CFA and EFA were repeated in the subgroup of dogs ($n = 49$).

By assessing for differences between sound dogs and dogs diagnosed with OA, using Mann–Whitney U test, the construct validity (hypothesis testing) and the ability of the CBPI to discriminate dogs with OA was tested [22, 25]. The nonparametric Mann–Whitney U test was used due to the non-normality of the ordered scaled data received from the CBPI items.

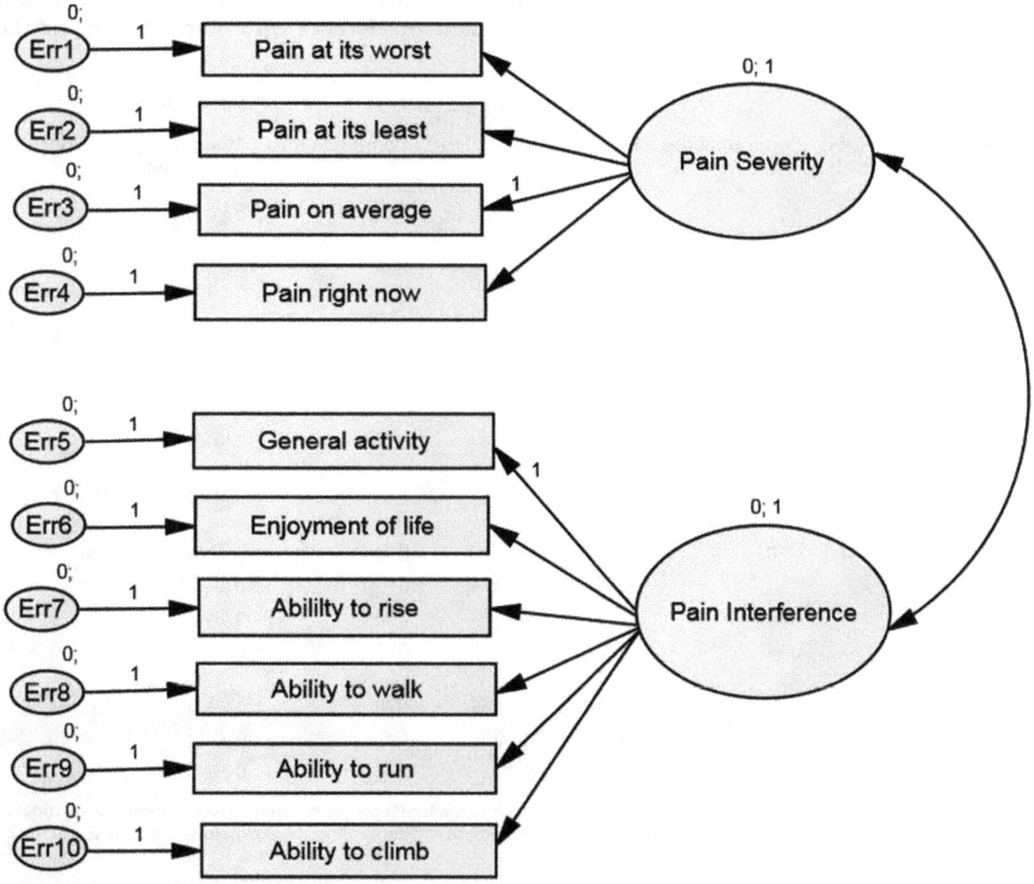

Fig. 1 Confirmatory factor model for the two-factor solution

Values of $P < 0.05$ were considered statistically significant and two-tailed assessments were used for all analyses. SPSS (Version 20, IBM Statistical Package for Social Science Statistics for Windows, Armonk, NY: IBM Corp) was used for descriptive statistics group comparisons, internal consistency and EFA. AMOS (IBM, SPSS, AMOS 22.0., AMOS Development Corporation, Spring House, PA) was used for CFA.

Results

Data from 79 adult dogs (38 females and 41 males) were included in this observational cross-sectional case–control study with the objective to translate the CBPI and validate the CBPI in a Swedish sample of OA dogs presented for physiotherapy. Inadequate completion of the CBPI questionnaire was present in three cases. Those were handled as internal missing values and the total completion rate was 97.5%. Translation of the CBPI showed that semantic equivalents were found in Swedish and that the conceptual meaning in the translated version of the questionnaire could be kept unchanged. There were significant demographic differences between control dogs and OA dogs in terms of age and body condition score. OA dogs were older and had higher body conditions scores. Most OA dogs (79%) had ongoing anti-inflammatory medication (Table 1). Descriptive information about the breeds included in the cohort can be found in Additional file 1.

Internal consistency and floor effect

Cronbach's α was 0.94 in the total CBPI, and 0.91 in the pain severity domain and 0.91 in the pain interference with function domain ($n = 58$). All items but "enjoyment of life" showed high levels of communality (>0.6) (Table 2). In the OA group ($n = 58$), more than 20% of the respondents rated floor value (score of 0) in all items, generating a floor effect. There was also a floor effect present in the pain severity sum and the pain interference with function sum (Table 2). In the group of owners rating presence of pain related to OA in their dogs ($n = 49$), the pain severity average (min–max) was 2.5 (0.0–5.8) and the pain interference with function average (min–max) was 2.3 (0.3–7.7). Including the owners that did not rate presence of pain related to OA ($n = 58$), the

Table 2 Pain severity (items 1–4) and pain interference with function (items 5–10) scores, percentage of minimum scoring and communalities for the CBPI items, pain severity sum, pain interference with function sum and the CBPI items totaled

All OA dogs (n = 58)				OA dogs with CBPI ≥1 (n = 49)			Control dogs (n = 21)		
CBPI item	Median (min–max)	% Floor[c]	Communalities	Median (min–max)	% Floor[c]	Communalities	Median (min–max)	% Floor[c]	Communalities
Pain at its worst[a]	3 (0–8)	24.6	0.76	4 (0–8)	12.2	0.74	0 (0–1)	95.2	NA
Pain at its least[a]	0 (0–5)	54.1	0.80	1 (0–5)	46.9	0.76	0 (0–0)	100	NA
Pain on average[a]	2 (0–6)	31.7	0.95	2 (0–6)	20.4	0.94	0 (0–0)	100	NA
Pain right now[a]	1 (0–6)	42.6	0.82	2 (0–6)	32.7	0.78	0 (0–0)	100	NA
General activity[b]	2 (0–10)	34.4	0.77	3 (0–10)	22.4	0.72	0 (0–0)	100	NA
Enjoyment of life[b]	1 (0–9)	44.1	0.57	1 (0–9)	34.7	0.53	0 (0–0)	100	NA
Ability to rise[b]	2 (0–9)	28.3	0.68	3 (0–9)	16.3	0.60	0 (0–0)	100	NA
Ability to walk[b]	1.5 (0–8)	31.7	0.84	2 (0–8)	20.4	0.82	0 (0–0)	100	NA
Ability to run[b]	2 (0–10)	31.7	0.81	2 (0–10)	20.4	0.78	0 (0–0)	100	NA
Ability to climb[2]	1 (0–10)	43.3	0.67	2 (0–10)	32.7	0.62	0 (0–0)	100	NA
PS sum	7.5 (0–23)	25.9	NA	10 (0–23)	12.2	NA	0 (0–1)	95.2	NA
PI sum	12.5 (0–46)	15.5	NA	14 (2–46)	0	NA	0 (0–0)	100	NA
CBPI total sum	19.5 (0–66)	15.5	NA	24 (2–66)	0	NA	0 (0–1)	95.2	NA

Values are presented as median (minimum–maximum). Proportion (%) of scoring minimum value (floor) value. Communalities showing proportions of variance for each item that can be explained by the two components, pain severity and pain interference with function, in the exploratory factor analysis by principal component analysis

CBPI canine brief pain inventory, *OA* osteoarthritis, *PS* pain severity (item 1–4), *PI* pain interference with function (item 5–10), *NA* not applicable

[a] Range 0–10 (no pain, extreme pain)

[b] Range 0–10 (does not interfere, interferes completely)

[c] % Scoring minimum value

pain severity average (min–max) was 1.9 (0.0–5.8) and the pain interference with function average (min–max) was 2.1 (0.0–7.7).

Construct validity; structural validity

In the CFA, both one- and two-factor models had similar CFI and RMSEA values. The CFI and NFI values were too low, the ratios Chi^2/df were small and the RMSEA were too high to be acceptable in all models. Altogether, this indicates that the proposed models could not be confirmed based on our data and we thereby do not show any estimated factor loadings and covariances. The fit indices for the confirmatory factor models by maximum likelihood estimation method are displayed in Table 3. Analysis by bootstrap modelling and by Bayesian estimations led to estimates of factor loadings, variances and covariances. These estimates differed somewhat from the maximum likelihood estimates. These results are shown in Additional file 2.

After a CFA we continued the analysis of the factor structure with an EFA (Table 4). Kaiser–Meyer–Olkin values of the CBPI were high, 0.88 in the whole group of dogs studied and 0.85 in the subgroup OA dogs with CBPI ≥1. Bartlett's test of sphericity was significant, altogether indicating our data were suitable for EFA. Exploratory factor analysis by principal component analysis showed a one-component structure with an eigenvalue of 6.7, in the total OA group (n = 58). One component showed an eigenvalue of 0.99 and was extracted together with the first component. Those two components accounted for 76.8% of the total variance (66.9 and 9.9% respectively), suggesting an acceptable fit of a two-component structure. Interitem correlations were good (overall > 0.35) and mean interitem correlation was 0.79 for severity items and 0.60 for interference items. In the group of OA dogs with CBPI total sum ≥1 (n = 49) two components with eigenvalues >1 were extracted. These components accounted for 60.9 and 11.9% of the total variance of the CBPI respectively. Together the

Table 3 Fit indices for the confirmatory factor models by maximum likelihood estimation method in all dogs with pain associated with osteoarthritis (n = 58) and dogs with osteoarthritis pain and CBPI ≥1 (n = 49)

Model	Chi²	Df	Chi²/df	CFI	NFI	PNFI	RMSEA	90% CI
1-factor (all OA)	156.81	36	4.36	0.775	0.730	0.584	0.243	0.204–0.282
1-factor(OA CBPI ≥1)	123.66	36	3.44	0.769	0.708	0.567	0.225	0.183–0.269
2-factor (all OA)	162.97	36	4.53	0.763	0.720	0.576	0.249	0.211–0.288
2-factor (OA CBPI ≥1)	126.55	36	3.52	0.761	0.702	0.561	0.229	0.186–0.273

Fit indices estimated were Chi²

df degrees of freedom, *Chi²/df* model *Chi²* related to its degrees of freedom, *CFI* comparative fit index, *NFI* normed fit index, *PNFI* parsimony adjusted normed fit index, *RMSEA* root mean squared error of approximation, *CBPI* Canine Brief Pain Inventory, *CI* confidence intervals, *OA* osteoarthritis

Table 4 Factor loadings in the exploratory factor analysis by principal component analysis with subsequent varimax rotation for the CBPI (two factors extracted) in all dogs with osteoarthritis (n = 58), and dogs with osteoarthritis and CBPI ≥1 (n = 49)

CBPI item	All OA dogs		OA dogs with CBPI ≥1	
	Factor 1	Factor 2	Factor 1	Factor 2
Pain at its worst	0.83	0.27	0.85	0.14
Pain at its least	0.87	0.22	0.85	0.21
Pain on average	0.90	0.38	0.91	0.34
Pain right now	0.82	0.38	0.80	0.37
General activity	0.66	0.58	0.66	0.53
Enjoyment of life	0.48	0.58	0.45	0.57
Ability to rise	0.59	0.57	0.57	0.52
Ability to walk	0.14	0.91	0.04	0.91
Ability to run	0.37	0.82	0.33	0.82
Ability to climb	0.45	0.69	0.42	0.66

CBPI canine brief pain inventory, *OA* osteoarthritis

components accounted for 72.8% of the total variance. Mean interitem correlations was in total 0.55. For severity items mean interitem correlation was 0.75 and for interference items 0.53.

Construct validity; hypothesis testing

Clinically sound dogs differed from OA dogs by showing significantly lower CBPI total sum, and significantly lower pain severity and pain interference with function sums.

Discussion

In this study, the CBPI was psychometrically tested in two groups of dogs to investigate internal consistency and construct validity in a Swedish context and in a heterogeneous group of dogs with pain associated with OA. The results from our study supplements the existing knowledge with the CBPI by confirming good to excellent internal consistency, the ability to discriminate OA dogs from clinically sound dogs and the number of components extracted in EFA. The number of components retained and the eigenvalues of each component were similar in the group of dogs with CBPI ≥1 and the group of dogs studied by Brown et al. [9] during the original development and psychometric testing of CBPI. The internal consistencies were also similar. In comparison, Cronbach's α for the total CBPI sum was 0.91 in the present study and 0.92 in the study conducted by Brown et al. [9]. Cronbach's α for severity of pain and pain interference with function were 0.91 and 0.91 respectively in our study, and 0.93 and 0.89 in the study by Brown et al. [9].

The demographic data showed statistical differences in age and body condition score between OA dogs and controls. Control dogs were slightly younger and had lower body condition score compared to OA dogs. In contrast to previous studies on the measurement properties of the CBPI the majority of dogs had ongoing treatment with anti-inflammatory medications, which is common in an applied clinical setting. Our more diverse study sample contributes to knowledge about the differences among individuals (Tables 1, 2). The median, minimum and maximum values of each CBPI item indicate that a considerable number of dogs are still reported with major OA symptoms, i.e. pain and functional impairments in: general activity, enjoyment of life, ability to rise, ability to run, and ability to climb. Our results are consistent with previous reports on the efficacy of anti-inflammatory drugs in dogs with OA, showing that pain control is not complete with one modality only [21, 35]. Although 79% of the OA dogs had ongoing on anti-inflammatory medication the canine owners still report presence of pain symptoms and that pain interferes with daily activities and mobility. The present study is not designed for the assessment of cross-cultural differences among dog owners in Sweden compared to dog owners in the US, since our sample is based on a new target group. However, the pain severity score, the pain interference with function score and the CBPI total sum (Table 2) in the present study allow for comparisons with the CBPI scores reported in several drug intervention studies for canine osteoarthritis [21, 35]. The pain severity score, pain interference score and the CBPI total sum in owners rating presence of pain related to OA in their dogs in our study are similar to those previously reported after two weeks of treatment with anti-inflammatory drugs [21, 35]. When the dog owners who did not rate presence of pain in their dogs were included, the CBPI scores and the present study were lower compared to the values reported to Brown et al. [21], but in the total CBPI sum was in consistence with the value reported by Wernham et al. [35]. The findings in the present study consist of a systematic examination of the CBPI in a new diverse target group, revealing an item level, as well as a total score, floor effect in dogs with pain related to OA. The proportion of respondents scoring zero in the pain severity sum was 12.2% in the group with CBPI ≥1. Floor effects of about 15–20% indicate that the true level of owner-perceived symptoms of pain would not be adequately represented by the CBPI in our sample [36]. Hence, there may be more variance in the concept, i.e. chronic pain, that may not be measured by the CBPI. It should be mentioned that the owner-reported ratings in the present study may be attributed to a response shift in the internal standards of the owners of the OA dogs undergoing pain management. And, as with the owners rating pain intensity in their dogs using a visual analogue scale [16], they may have a lack of recognition of subtle behavioural signs related to persistent OA pain in their dogs. The later may explain the higher proportion of floor effects in the pain severity items. Consequently, the changes in scores may be limited by the floor effect, and the responsiveness of the CBPI may be reduced because many dogs would not be able to change their item score despite the likelihood of clinical improvement. However, the sum of pain interference with six daily activities, i.e. general activity, enjoyment of life, rising to standing, walking, running, and climbing, showed no floor effect in the group of dogs rated CBPI >1 (Table 2), suggesting the pain interference items may be more sensitive to change in dogs undergoing multimodal OA management. However, it was not within the scope of this study to assess the responsiveness of the instrument.

The fit indices achieved in the CFA were not acceptable according to the guidelines by Hu and Bentler [31]. Because neither of our proposed CFA models could be confirmed, the hypothesis of the presented two-factor representation in the CBPI, was rejected as causal structure underlying the construct. The subsequent principal component analysis performed in our study showed that three of the CBPI items loaded equally on the two extracted factors, i.e. general activity, enjoyment of life and ability to rise, indicating that the items are influenced by both the pain severity and the pain interference factor. Since the factor loading is the correlation between the factor and the item, it seems like three of the pain interference items also may assess the pain severity factor in our sample. All the CBPI items are still important in the instrument because they show heavy positive loadings (>0.4), but the factor structure seems to differ from the original. In the original psychometric testing, Brown et al. [9] presented that item 1–4 in the CBPI questionnaire loaded heavy on pain severity, and item 5–10 loaded heavy on the pain interference factor. As indicated in Table 4 the factor loadings were rather equal in several items, and the one-factor and two-factor model analyzed in our CFA did not allow for the dual loading.

Since we performed a comprehensive linguistic translation process with high quality, according to guidelines for translation and cross-cultural adaption [24, 25], we do not relate the failure of the one-factor and the two-factor model in the CFA to the translation process. Instead we consider several other possible reasons why the original two-factor factor model in the CFA did not fit our Swedish sample. We know that our samples vary in comparison with the study that performed the original psychometric testing of CBPI because we also enrolled dogs with ongoing anti-inflammatory medication. Moreover, the proportion of the floor effect of the CBPI in our study group, in combination with a small sample size and equal factor loading in three of the interference items, may also have contributed to skewness in data leading to computational difficulties in the CFA. Analyzing ordinally scaled items as they were on a continuous scale may also have consequences for the results. The difference in estimates we found in the Bayesian estimation support this.

Our results highlight the importance of validated instruments to increase the certainty with which they accurately reflect what they are supposed to measure. The concepts within an instrument may differ with context, culture and/or time, which in turn may bias a study if the equality is not ensured across different target groups. The cohort included in this study consisted of canine owners who rated the severity of pain and the pain interference with function in dogs undergoing medical pain management, as well as dogs not undergoing medical treatment, which is highly applicable in clinical settings at veterinary primary care units and canine rehabilitation facilities. Indeed, it has been shown that ratings of the perceived level of pain in another individual is difficult and may differ in humans e.g. between parental caregivers and children experiencing pain [14]. Pain in dogs is hence not an easy phenomenon to quantify. The clinical picture of a dog with persistent OA pain or chronic pain behaviour associated with OA, includes changes in several dimensions and may be evaluated by deconstruction of the pain behaviour. In contrast to the CBPI, the Helsinki Chronic Pain Index is a chronic pain questionnaire that allows the canine owners to describe the behaviour of the dog rather than to rate the level of pain or the level of interference of pain on function [37, 38]. A description of each canine chronic pain behaviour under investigation may contribute to make the ratings more defined, which may overcome part of the subjectivity in rating a sensory and emotional pain experience of an animals [39, 40].

Our data showed a high level of communalities (all but one >0.6) in the EFA which we considered to be good enough to consistently reproduce the factor loadings even in a small sample. A limitation of our study was that although communalities were high in the EFA the sample size was small, but still fair, for factor analysis. However, according to the COSMIN checklist manual, our assessment of the structural validity of the CBPI in a diverse group of dogs with pain related to OA was excellent in all other aspects [22, 25].

Conclusions

The quality of our comprehensive Swedish translation of the CBPI was high and the translated version is valid for use in the Swedish language. The findings of this study suggest satisfying psychometric properties in terms of high internal consistencies and ability to discriminate clinically sound dogs from OA dogs, of the CBPI in a heterogenous Swedish sample of dogs with pain related to OA. Although, animal health-care professionals should be aware of the potential floor effect in a sample similar to ours and that the interpretability of the results from the CBPI may be affected. As the pain interference with function items showed no floor effect in owners reporting pain ≥ 1 in their dogs, we suggest that part of the CBPI can be used separately. With regard to the EFA, three of the pain interference items, i.e. general activity, enjoyment of life and ability to rise, were also correlated with pain severity. Furthermore, based on the CFA the original factor structure in CBPI is not ideally suited to measure owner-perceived pain related to OA in our diverse sample of dogs, and the hypothesis of the presented two-factor structure was rejected. Further research needs to be conducted to determine whether the original psychometric results from CBPI can be replicated across different target groups and particularly with larger sample size.

Authors' contributions

All authors contributed to the article. The idea for the article was conceived by AE. AE and RS made substantial contributions to conception and design of the article. AE and PG were responsible for the data acquisition. Data were processed by AE and HH. In addition, AE was the main author and RS, PG, HH, LZ, and KH contributed in drafting the article and revising it critically. All authors analyzed, interpreted and discussed the results, commented on the manuscript and gave final approval of the version to be submitted for publishing. All authors read and approved the final manuscript.

Author details

[1] Department of Neuroscience, Faculty of Physiotherapy, Uppsala University, Husargatan, Biomedical Centre, Box 593, 751 24 Uppsala, Sweden. [2] Evidensia Djurkliniken Gefle, Norra Gatan 1, 803 21 Gävle, Sweden. [3] Department of Clinical Sciences, Faculty of Veterinary Medicine and Animal Husbandry, Swedish University of Agricultural Sciences, Box 7054, 750 07 Uppsala, Sweden. [4] Department of Health and Caring Sciences, Faculty of Health and Occupational Studies, University of Gävle, 801 76 Gävle, Sweden. [5] Unit of Research Education and Development, Region Jämtland Härjedalen, Box 654, 831 27 Östersund, Sweden. [6] Department of Community Medicine and Rehabilitation, Faculty of Physiotherapy, Umeå University, 901 87 Umeå, Sweden.

Acknowledgements

We are grateful to the dogs and their owners who participated in this study. We also want to thank the translators for their contribution to our manuscript during the translation process of the Canine Brief Pain Inventory.

Competing interests

The authors declare that they have no competing interests.

Funding

The study was supported by Grants from Jan Skogsborg Foundation, and Agria Animal Insurance and the Swedish Kennel Club joint research fund.

References

1. Mathews K, Kronen PW, Lascelles D, Nolan A, Robertson S, Steagall PV, et al. Guidelines for recognition, assessment and treatment of pain. J Small Anim Pract. 2014;55:E10–68.
2. Lascelles BDX, Knazovicky D, Case B, Freire M, Innes JF, Drew AC, et al. A canine-specific anti-nerve growth factor antibody alleviates pain and improves mobility and function in dogs with degenerative joint disease-associated pain. BMC Vet Res. 2015;11:101.
3. Knazovicky D, Helgeson ES, Case B, Gruen ME, Maixner W, Lascelles BDX. Widespread somatosensory sensitivity in naturally occurring canine model of osteoarthritis. Pain. 2016;157:1325–32.
4. Kyte DG, Calvert M, van der Wees PJ, ten Hove R, Tolan S, Hill JC. An introduction to patient-reported outcome measures (PROMs) in physiotherapy. Physiotherapy. 2015;101:119–25.
5. Cleeland CS, Ryan KM. Pain assessment: global use of the brief pain inventory. Ann Acad Med Singap. 1994;23:129–38.
6. Lapane KL, Quilliam BJ, Benson C, Chow W, Kim M. One, two, or three? constructs of the brief pain inventory among patients with non-cancer pain in the outpatient setting. J Pain Symptom Manag. 2014;47:325–33.
7. Atkinson TM, Rosenfeld BD, Sit L, Mendoza TR, Fruscione M, Lavene D, et al. Using confirmatory factor analysis to evaluate construct validity of the brief pain inventory (BPI). J Pain Symptom Manag. 2011;41:558–65.
8. Williams VSL, Smith MY, Fehnel SE. The validity and utility of the BPI interference measures for evaluating the impact of osteoarthritic pain. J Pain Symptom Manag. 2006;31:48–57.
9. Brown DC, Boston RC, Coyne JC, Farrar JT. Development and psychometric testing of an instrument designed to measure chronic pain in dogs with osteoarthritis. Am J Vet Res. 2007;68:631–7.

10. Brown DC, Boston R, Coyne JC, Farrar JT. A novel approach to the use of animals in studies of pain: validation of the canine brief pain inventory in canine bone cancer. Pain Med Malden Mass. 2009;10:133–42.
11. Hielm-Björkman AK, Rita H, Tulamo R-M. Psychometric testing of the Helsinki chronic pain index by completion of a questionnaire in Finnish by owners of dogs with chronic signs of pain caused by osteoarthritis. Am J Vet Res. 2009;70:727–34.
12. Walton MB, Cowderoy E, Lascelles D, Innes JF. Evaluation of construct and criterion validity for the "Liverpool Osteoarthritis in Dogs" (LOAD) clinical metrology instrument and comparison to two other instruments. PLoS ONE. 2013;8:e58125.
13. Brown DC. The canine orthopedic index. Step 2: psychometric testing. Vet Surg. 2014;43:241–6.
14. Berntson L, Svensson E. Pain assessment in children with juvenile chronic arthritis: a matter of scaling and rater. Acta Paediatr. 2001;90:1131–6.
15. Egger CM, Love L, Doherty T. Pain management in veterinary practice. 1st ed. Chichester: Wiley-Blackwell; 2013.
16. Hielm-Björkman AK, Kapatkin AS, Rita HJ. Reliability and validity of a visual analogue scale used by owners to measure chronic pain attributable to osteoarthritis in their dogs. Am J Vet Res. 2011;72:601–7.
17. Burton NJ, Owen MR, Colborne GR, Toscano MJ. Can owners and clinicians assess outcome in dogs with fragmented medial coronoid process? Vet Comp Orthop Traumatol. 2009;22:183–9.
18. Quinn MM, Keuler NS, Lu Y, Faria MLE, Muir P, Markel MD. Evaluation of agreement between numerical rating scales, visual analogue scoring scales, and force plate gait analysis in dogs. Vet Surg. 2007;36:360–7.
19. Reid J, Wiseman-Orr ML, Scott EM, Nolan AM. Development, validation and reliability of a web-based questionnaire to measure health-related quality of life in dogs. J Small Anim Pract. 2013;54:227–33.
20. Brown DC, Bell M, Rhodes L. Power of treatment success definitions when the Canine Brief Pain Inventory is used to evaluate carprofen treatment for the control of pain and inflammation in dogs with osteoarthritis. Am J Vet Res. 2013;74:1467–73.
21. Brown DC, Boston RC, Coyne JC, Farrar JT. Ability of the canine brief pain inventory to detect response to treatment in dogs with osteoarthritis. J Am Vet Med Assoc. 2008;233:1278–83.
22. Mokkink LB, Terwee CB, Patrick DL, Alonso J, Stratford PW, Knol DL, et al. The COSMIN study reached international consensus on taxonomy, terminology, and definitions of measurement properties for health-related patient-reported outcomes. J Clin Epidemiol. 2010;63:737–45.
23. Mokkink LB, Prinsen CAC, Bouter LM, de Vet HCW, Terwee CB. The consensus-based standards for the selection of health measurement instruments (COSMIN) and how to select an outcome measurement instrument. Braz J Phys Ther. 2016;20:105–13.
24. Wild D, Grove A, Martin M, Eremenco S, McElroy S, Verjee-Lorenz A, et al. Principles of good practice for the translation and cultural adaptation process for patient-reported outcomes (PRO) measures: report of the ISPOR task force for translation and cultural adaptation. Value Health. 2005;8:94–104.
25. Terwee CB, Mokkink LB, Knol DL, Ostelo RWJG, Bouter LM, de Vet HCW. Rating the methodological quality in systematic reviews of studies on measurement properties: a scoring system for the COSMIN checklist. J Qual Life Res. 2012;21:651–7.
26. Mokkink LB, Terwee CB, Knol DL, Stratford PW, Alonso J, Patrick DL, et al. The COSMIN checklist for evaluating the methodological quality of studies on measurement properties: a clarification of its content. BMC Med Res Methodol. 2010;10:22.
27. O'Rourke N, Hatcher L. A step-by-step approach to using SAS for factor analysis and structural equation modeling. 2nd ed. Cary: SAS Institute Inc; 2013.
28. Russell DW. In search of underlying dimensions: the use (and abuse) of factor analysis in personality and social psychology bulletin. Personal Soc Psychol Bull. 2002;28:1629–46.
29. German AJ, Holden SL, Moxham GL, Holmes KL, Hackett RM, Rawlings JM. A simple, reliable tool for owners to assess the body condition of their dog or cat. J Nutr. 2006;136:2031S–3S.
30. Nunnally JC, Bernstein IH. Psychometric theory. 3rd ed. New York: McGraw-Hill; 1994.
31. Hu L, Bentler PM. Cutoff criteria for fit indexes in covariance structure analysis: conventional criteria versus new alternatives. Struct Equ Model Multidiscip J. 1999;6:1–55.
32. Byrne BM. Structural equation modeling with AMOS: Basic concepts, applications, and programming. 2nd ed. New York: Routledge; 2009.
33. Hutcheson G, Sofroniou N. The multivariate social scientist: introductory statistics using generalized linear models. 2nd ed. London: Sage Publications; 2009.
34. Bartlett MS. Tests of significance in factor analysis. Br J Stat Psychol. 1950;3:77–85.
35. Wernham BGJ, Trumpatori B, Hash J, Lipsett J, Davidson G, Wackerow P, et al. Dose reduction of meloxicam in dogs with osteoarthritis-associated pain and impaired mobility. J Vet Intern Med. 2011;25:1298–305.
36. Terwee CB, Bot SDM, de Boer MR, van der Windt DAWM, Knol DL, Dekker J, et al. Quality criteria were proposed for measurement properties of health status questionnaires. J Clin Epidemiol. 2007;60:34–42.
37. Hielm-Björkman AK, Kuusela E, Liman A, Markkola A, Saarto E, Huttunen P, et al. Evaluation of methods for assessment of pain associated with chronic osteoarthritis in dogs. J Am Vet Med Assoc. 2003;222:1552–8.
38. Mölsä SH, Hielm-Björkman AK, Laitinen-Vapaavuori OM. Use of an owner questionnaire to evaluate long-term surgical outcome and chronic pain after cranial cruciate ligament repair in dogs: 253 cases (2004–2006). J Am Vet Med Assoc. 2013;243:689–95.
39. Lindegaard C, Thomsen MH, Larsen S, Andersen PH. Analgesic efficacy of intra-articular morphine in experimentally induced radiocarpal synovitis in horses. Vet Anaesth Analg. 2010;37:171–85.
40. Holton L, Reid J, Scott EM, Pawson P, Nolan A. Development of a behaviour-based scale to measure acute pain in dogs. Vet Rec. 2001;148:525–31.

10

In vivo assessment of subcutaneous fat in dogs by real-time ultrasonography and image analysis

Rita Payan-Carreira[1*†], Luis Martins[2†], Sónia Miranda[1,2,3], Pedro Olivério[2] and Severiano R. Silva[1]

Abstract

Background: Systems for estimating body condition score (BCS) are currently used in canine practice to monitor fatness levels. These tools are cheap and easy to use but lack the necessary precision to monitor small changes in body fat, particularly during weight control treatments or in research. The present work aims to study the application of real-time ultrasonography (RTU) together with image analysis in the assessment of subcutaneous fat depots in dogs. Ultrasound images were collected from five anatomical locations (chest, flank, abdomen, thigh and lumbar) from 28 healthy dogs of different breeds and with a body weight (BW) ranging from 5.2 to 33.0 kg. BCS was collected by visual appraisal using a 5-point scale. Subcutaneous fat thickness (SFT) was estimated from RTU images, using the average of three measurements taken in fat deposits located above the muscles represented in each image. Correlations were established between SFT and BW or BCS as well as a classification of BCS-based fatness [*overweight* (BCS = 4), *ideal* (BCS = 3) and *lean* (BCS = 2)].

Results: SFT was found to differ between the five regions considered ($P < 0.001$). Abdomen and thigh were the areas displaying the widest variation for the different dogs included in the study and also those correlating most with BW, in contrast to the chest, which showed the least variation. Overall, a strong correlation was found between BCS and SFT. The highest correlations were established for the flank, abdomen and lumbar areas. In every anatomical area, a decrease in SFT was observed across all three BCS classes, ranging from 48 to 65 % among *overweight* and *ideal* dogs, and from 46 to 83 % among *ideal* and *lean* dogs.

Conclusions: Preliminary data showed that within this population there was a strong correlation between BCS and SFT estimated from RTU images. It was also observed that RTU measurements for fat thickness differed among the anatomical points surveyed suggesting differences in their sensitivity to a change in BCS. The images displaying the best prediction value for fatness variations were those collected at the lumbar and abdomen areas.

Keywords: Dog, Body condition score, Ultrasound, Subcutaneous fat thickness

*Correspondence: rtpayan@gmail.com
†Rita Payan-Carreira and Luis Martins contributed equally to this work
[1] Zootecnia Department, CECAV-Centro de Ciência Animal e Veterinária, Universidade de Trás-os-Montes e Alto Douro, Quinta de Prados, 5000-801 Vila Real, Portugal
Full list of author information is available at the end of the article

Background

Obesity is the most common nutritional disorder in dogs and is becoming a common health and welfare problem worldwide [1, 2]; it results from the intake of excessive dietary energy combined with poor lifestyle habits, particularly inactivity. According to different surveys, the prevalence of dog obesity ranges from 22 to 44 % [3]. In dogs, obesity is linked to both a shortened lifespan [4] and increased incidence of secondary diseases, including metabolic diseases, respiratory distress, hypertension, cardiac disease, neoplasia as well as orthopaedic and skin diseases [3, 5].

Surveying a dog's condition is a key aspect of routine clinical examination. Estimating body condition score (BCS) is the most commonly used method to estimate fatness in dogs [6] and to monitor the response to weight loss programs in daily practice. Knowledge of body composition, in particular the percentage of body fat, provides useful information about the physical and metabolic status of animals [7], allowing proper advice to be given on feeding and weight reduction programs [2, 8].

Over the years, several methods have been developed to accurately measure and estimate the percentage of body fat, and also to facilitate understanding of the causes and effects of obesity. These include dual-energy X-ray absorptiometry [7, 9], bioelectrical impedance [9], computed tomography [10] and magnetic resonance imaging [11]. Nevertheless, implementing such methods in clinical practice is difficult or expensive. Practitioners need simple, semi-quantitative methods to support their work, which may explain why body condition scoring remains the tool mostly used on a routine daily basis. While this procedure is cheap, easy to use and reproducible among operators [6], it is a subjective technique and lacks sharp sensitivity, being unable to detect minor variations in body composition over time and correlating poorly with body weight [6].

Several BCS charts for dogs are available, which use 5-, 7- or 9-point scores to estimate the degree of fatness. Charts which give a higher score correlate better to the amount of body fat percentage obtained from more accurate methods [2]. Although the accuracy of the 5-point scale may be increased by adding half-scores between the whole scores, the fact is that in Portugal, as in Japan [2], most veterinarians use the whole score 5-point scale in routine daily practice. However, BCS's sensitivity regarding a dog's overall fatness is generally considered lower than more expensive methods, mainly due to the particular pattern of fat distribution in this species [2]. Notably, it is hard to quantify fatness levels in borderline cases between two consecutive scores.

A growing number of clinics now use alternative and more precise methods to assess body fat distribution in animals, such as computer tomography or magnetic resonance imaging [7, 10, 11]. However, such techniques are generally not applied to BCS since the initial price, operating costs and the equipment's lack of mobility severely limit its use on a routine daily basis.

Over the last two decades, real-time ultrasonography (RTU) has become an increasingly important tool for the measurement of body fatness. RTU is used today in several domestic species to predict in vivo body fat covering [12–14]. It is widespread both in animal science and in clinical research, because of its relatively low cost, portability, robustness and easiness of use as well as its ability to obtain precise and highly reproducible images; moreover, it is well tolerated by animals and is well accepted by the public. Nevertheless, little information is available on the use of RTU to assess body fatness in dogs [15]. As the 5-point BCS system is not dependent on animals' weight and essentially displays the thickness of their fatness covering [15], we hypothesised that SFT estimated through RTU images would reflect the level of fatness covering, and would thus also be relatively independent of the size of the dog.

Therefore, the present study intends to assess body fat depots from five different anatomical sites in dogs using RTU and image analysis, seeking to validate RTU as a predictor of body fatness by establishing a relationship between BCS and subcutaneous fat measurements obtained by RTU.

Methods

Animals

Data were collected from 28 privately-owned mature dogs randomly recruited according to their BCS from among the patients at a private veterinary hospital. All the animals were indoor pet dogs or guide dogs for the blind that were assessed on routine veterinary visits, for treatments such as neutering, vaccination or deworming. All the animals were submitted to a physical examination and considered free of underlying pathologies. A positive pregnancy diagnosis was the sole additional excluding criterion imposed for the study.

Body size, weight and body condition score

The animals in the study were representative of both genders (14 males and 14 females) and also of different sizes (miniature-4; small-10; medium-14), weight (5.2–33.0 kg) and BCS (2–4, on a 5-point scale).

Two trained operators independently assigned the dogs' BCS, using visual appraisal and palpation, according to Hill's 5-point scale [16]. In the present study, BCS in dogs ranged from 2 (*lean* or *underweight*) to 4 (*overweight*). Additionally, dogs weight was assessed using an electronic scale displaying a sensitivity of 1 g.

Three morphometric variables were used to estimate the size of the dog, namely, height at withers, thoracic girth and the rump width. These were measured with the animal in standing position, looking straight ahead with the head in normal carriage position, using a measuring stick, callipers or a tape as appropriate. In the case of crossbred dogs, the height at withers and thoracic girth were used to establish the size of the dogs, following similarities with the body frame of breeds recognised by FCI (Fédération Cynologique Internationale) whose standards were used to define purebred size. In short, the height at withers and thoracic girth were used to distinguish between miniature and small sized dogs, while the height at withers was used to distinguish between small and medium sized dogs.

Ultrasound image acquisition

To obtain RTU images, a General Electric ultrasound scanner (GE logic book XP, General Electrics, Buckinghamshire, UK) was used which was equipped with a 39 mm-long multifrequency linear transducer (8LRS, 6–11 MHz; General Electrics, Buckinghamshire, UK), set to 10 MHz. RTU image acquisition was performed in right lateral recumbency, without the need for sedation or anaesthesia. There was no need for hair clipping at the image collection spots; ethanol and ultrasound gel served as a coupling medium.

Ultrasound image acquisition was performed from five anatomical sites (Fig. 1), selected according to their suitability from previous research on dogs [15] (flank, abdomen, thigh and lumbar) and also from the authors' perception of changes in subcutaneous fat deposits in obese dogs (chest). The locations used were:

1. Chest—at the entry of the chest, from the midline to the left, the transducer transversal to the *manubrium sterni*, over the *cleidocephalicus* muscle;
2. Flank—on the dog's left side, over the ninth intercostal space, just above the costochondral junction, the transducer transversal to the ribs over the *obliquus externus abdominis* muscle;
3. Abdomen—on the left lateral wall of the abdomen, midway on the perpendicular line between the *linea alba* and the tip of the *processus transversus* of the lumbar vertebrae, the transducer in vertical position over the *obliquus externus abdominis* muscle;
4. Thigh—on the inner face of the right thigh, midway on a diagonal line traced from the *tuber ischiaticum* to the *tuberositas tibiae*, the transducer placed transversal to the femur, between the *gracilis* and *semimembranosus* muscles;
5. Lumbar—between the third and the fifth lumbar vertebrae, over the *M. longissimus lumborum* covered by the thoracolumbar fascia, 2–3 cm to the left of the midline, the transducer parallel to the *processus spinosus* of the lumbar vertebrae.

All the RTU images were saved in 640 × 480 JPEG format for subsequent analysis.

Ultrasound image analysis and subcutaneous fat measurements

To eliminate subjective inter-operator bias, a single experienced operator analysed all the RTU images using ImageJ software (version 1.38x, NIH, USA; http://rsb.info.nih.gov/ij/download.html). Measures of subcutaneous fat thickness were estimated from the thickness of fat deposits located above the muscles displayed in the images, at all five anatomical sites. The skin was included in all thickness measurements. For each image, the average of the measurements taken at the three different locations was considered, so as to eliminate possible fluctuations that might exist in the thickness of subcutaneous fat. The first measurement was taken at the midline of the ultrasound image and the others were obtained equidistantly, 1.5 cm to each side.

Statistical analyses

Data were analysed using the JMP statistical analysis software (SAS Institute, Cary, NC, USA). A descriptive data analysis for body weight, BCS and subcutaneous fat thickness (SFT) at each point of collection was carried out by mean, standard deviation (SD), range and coefficient of variation (CV). The relationships between the BCS and SFT measurements obtained by RTU image analyses were computed using the correlation analysis procedure. The general linear model (GLM) procedure was used to fit two models showing the associations between BCS and SFT. The first model was developed to evaluate the effect of BCS on SFT at the five anatomical sites considered. In this model, three categories were used, based on BCS [*overweight* (BCS 4), *ideal* (BCS 3) and *lean* (BCS 2)], with the animal's body size being used as a covariate. The second model included the anatomical region as a factor of influence over SFT. This model used BCS and rump width as co-variables. For both models, least square (LS) means were determined and compared using an F-test protected LSD (least significant difference). A *P* value $\leq$0.05 was regarded as statistically significant.

Results

Overall values for body weight, BCS and subcutaneous fat thickness collected from the five selected anatomical sites used in the current study are presented in Table 1.

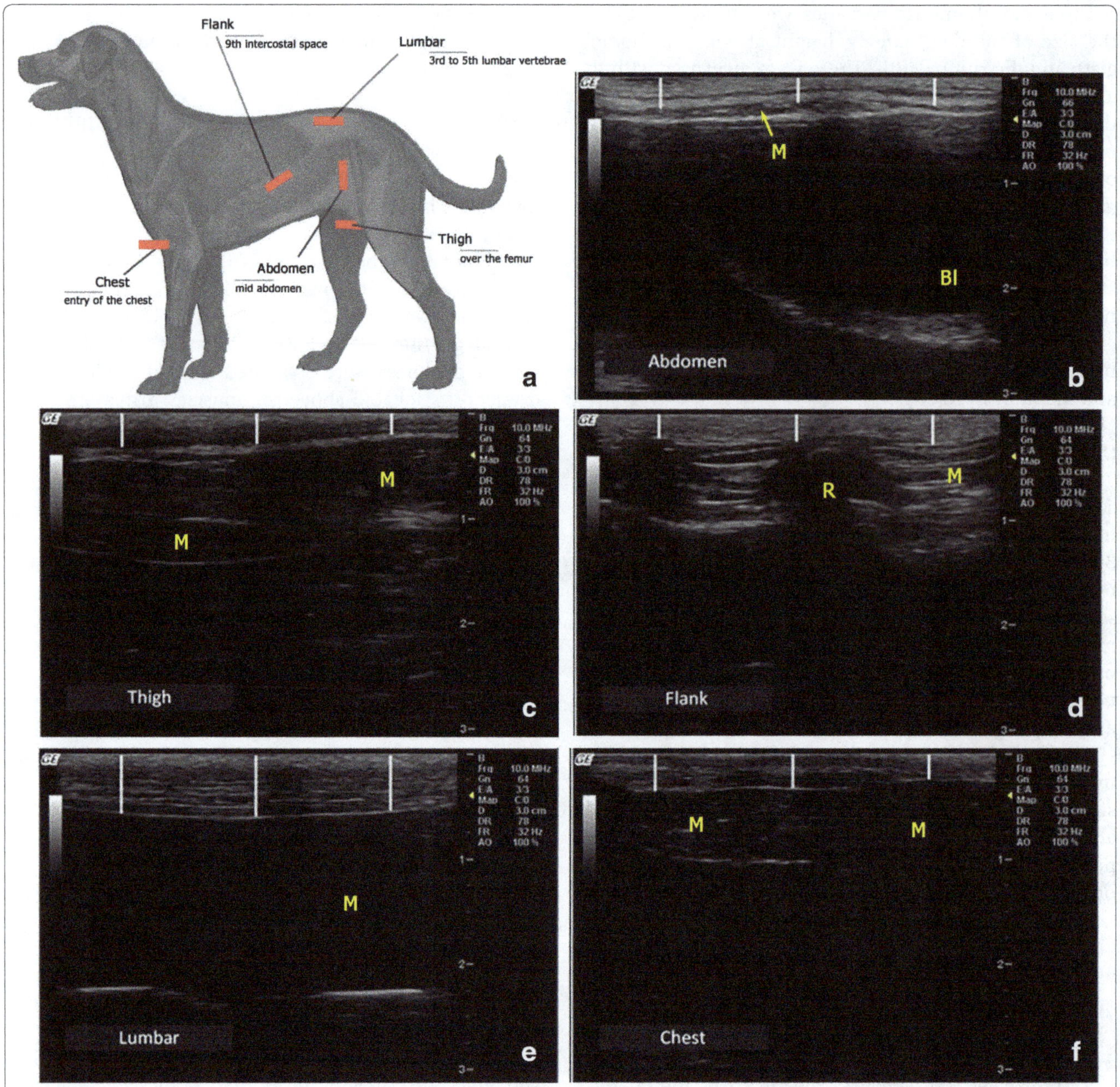

Fig. 1 Real-time ultrasonography (RTU) assessment of subcutaneous fat thickness (SFT) in dogs. **a** Schematic representation of the anatomical sites used in the study to assess SFT in dogs. The *red* box illustrates the transducer location in each of the five areas used in the study. **b–f** Representative RTU images from the five anatomical areas sampled. In each image, measurements of subcutaneous fat thickness (SFT) were taken at three different locations (*white vertical lines*) to estimate a mean SFT value. *M* muscle plan, *B* bladder, *R* ribs' acoustic shadow

Dogs in this study displayed a mean body weight of 17.5 kg, with values ranging from 5 to 33 kg. Median BCS in these 28 dogs was 3, ranging from 2 to 4 points (n = 4, n = 18 and n = 6, for BCS levels 2, 3 and 4, respectively). Animals displayed different body size, namely miniature (n = 4), small (n = 10) and medium-sized dogs (n = 14). Body weight varied noticeably among the dogs, presenting a coefficient of variation of 55.4 %, in contrast with the lower variation observed for BCS (CV = 19.7 %).

Subcutaneous fat thickness varied among different animals and anatomical sites (Table 1). Overall SFT levels obtained with RTU ranged from 1.02 to 7.88 mm with a coefficient of variation between 33.2 and 51.2 %. The highest variations were found in the abdomen (51.2 %),

Table 1 Body weight, BCS and subcutaneous fat thickness (SFT) in dogs (n = 28)

Traits	Mean	SD	Minimum	Maximum	CV (%)
Body weight (kg)	17.52	9.71	5.15	33.00	55.41
BCS (scores 1–5)	3.07	0.60	2.00	4.00	19.67
Subcutaneous fat thickness (mm)					
Abdomen	3.15	1.62	1.02	7.88	51.20
Thigh	2.63	1.27	1.11	5.95	48.31
Flank	2.28	0.93	0.98	4.21	40.83
Lumbar	2.89	1.15	1.14	6.31	39.56
Chest	2.39	0.79	1.22	4.02	33.19

Mean, standard deviation (SD), minimum, maximum and coefficient of variation (CV)

and the lowest in the chest (33.2 %). The coefficient of variation for SFT measurements in the different anatomical sites showed a pattern allowing them to be divided into three groups (Table 1): the abdomen and thigh with the highest variations (CV = 51.2 and 48.3 %, respectively); the flank and lumbar area with intermediate variations (CV = 40.8 and 39.6 %, respectively), and the chest, the area with least variation (CV = 33.2 %). Overall SFT variation was considerably higher than the variation observed for BCS; even when considering only the chest, variation was about 40 % higher in SFT measurements compared to BCS.

Data concerning the correlations between BCS, BW and SFT from the five anatomical sites analysed are presented in Table 2. The correlation between BW and BCS was low (r = 0.230, P > 0.05). In general, the correlations between BW and SFT measurements were also low (r between 0.214, P > 0.05 and 0.598, P < 0.01). The highest correlations between BW and SFT were obtained from the abdomen (r = 0.415, P < 0.05) and thigh (r = 0.598, P < 0.01). However, the correlation between BCS and SFT measurements proved to be high (r between 0.708 and 0.815, P < 0.01). A strong correlation was also obtained between SFT measurements collected from different anatomical sites (r > 0.654, P < 0.01) with emphasis on the correlation between SFT from the abdomen and the lumbar region (r = 0.873, P < 0.01) or the flank (r = 0.847, P < 0.01).

Subcutaneous fat thickness was significantly affected (P < 0.001) by the anatomical region used to collect RTU images (Table 3). The abdomen displayed the highest SFT (SFT = 3.15 mm), whereas the lumbar and thigh displayed similar SFT (2.89 and 2.63 mm, respectively), and the flank and chest showed the lowest SFT (2.28 and 2.39 mm, respectively; P < 0.05). No differences were found between SFT from lumbar and thigh regions or between SFT from flank and chest. Taking the difference between the largest and the smallest SFT value, a difference of 0.87 mm was observed, corresponding to a 28 % variation.

BCS categories (*lean, ideal* and *overweight*) significantly affect SFT measurements (P < 0.001) (Table 4). In general, a decrease in SFT levels at all the five anatomic sites sampled was observed between the *overweight* and *ideal* classes of dogs (P < 0.05) and between the *ideal* and *lean* (P < 0.05) classes. The only exception was the thigh, where measurements remained similar in animals classified as *ideal* and *lean* (P < 0.05). To sum up, differences in SFT measurements between *overweight* and *ideal* animals ranged between 1.21 and 2.63 mm (in the chest and abdomen, respectively), which represented a variation of 48–65 % in SFT levels among these two classes of fatness. Similarly, the variation in SFT between animals classified as *ideal* and *lean* ranged between 0.36 and 1.50 mm (in the thigh and abdomen, respectively), representing a variation of 46–83 % between those two BCS classes. In general, STF values increased between two to fourfold in *overweight* dogs, compared to *lean* dogs.

Discussion

The main purpose of the present study was to establish the association between BCS and subcutaneous fat thickness in five selected anatomic sites in dogs. Previous studies have confirmed the association between BCS and subcutaneous fat thickness estimated from thoracic

Table 2 Correlations between body weight, BCS and subcutaneous fat thickness (in mm) in the five anatomical sites studied (n = 28)

	BCS	Abdomen	Thigh	Flank	Lumbar	Chest
Body weight	0.230 ns	0.415*	0.598**	0.214 ns	0.361 ns	0.268 ns
BCS		0.799**	0.708**	0.815**	0.781**	0.776**
Abdomen			0.807**	0.847**	0.873**	0.799**
Thigh				0.697**	0.744**	0.654**
Flank					0.818**	0.812**
Lumbar						0.839**

Correlation coefficient values connected with ns P > 0.05; * P < 0.05; ** P < 0.01

Table 3 Least squares means of subcutaneous fat thickness (in mm) from the five anatomical sites studied

	Subcutaneous fat thickness (mm)
Body region	
Abdomen	3.15[a]
Thigh	2.63[b]
Flank	2.28[c]
Lumbar	2.89[b]
Chest	2.39[c]
Probability	0.001
SEM	0.13

BCS and rump width were used as co-variables

SEM standard error of means

a,b,c Within a column, least squares means followed by a common letter are not significantly different (P > 0.05)

Table 4 Least squares means for subcutaneous fat thickness (in mm) from five anatomical points according to body condition classes

	Abdomen	Thigh	Flank	Lumbar	Chest
Fat classification					
Overweight	5.43[a]	4.54[a]	3.61[a]	4.48[a]	3.45[a]
Ideal	2.80[b]	2.17[b]	2.08[b]	2.65[b]	2.24[b]
Lean	1.30[c]	1.81[b]	1.19[c]	1.61[c]	1.49[c]
Probability	0.001	0.001	0.001	0.001	0.001
SEM	0.38	0.29	0.21	0.28	0.20

Body size was used as co-variable

SEM standard error of means

a,b,c Least squares means within a column that are followed by a common letter are not significantly different (P > 0.05)

radiographs [17] or two-dimensional ultrasound images [18], suggesting that both methods would be suitable for use in routine practice, for prediction of body fatness in dogs, besides that they are easily performed at clinics.

The coefficient of variation was higher for BW than BCS. The differences in the size of dogs used in the present study could explain the coefficient of variation observed for BW. As expected the coefficient of variation was lower for BCS since the scores in BCS charts are independent of animals' weight and essentially refer to the distribution of fatness covering [15]. On this basis, we hypothesised that SFT estimated in RTU images would likewise reflect fat covering and would, therefore, be relatively independent of the size of the dog, though perhaps being dependent on the pattern of fat distribution in a breed. This hypothesis seems to be supported by the weak correlations between BW and BCS observed in the current work, which other studies have also shown [6], as well as those between BW and SFT. These weak correlations could be explained by the size differences among the dogs enrolled in the present study though it cannot be ruled out that breed specificities may also be involved in the distribution of body fat [9]. Dorsteen and Cooper [6] recognised that BCS is not sensitive enough to be used for research, although it may be useful as a tool for routine evaluation of adiposity in management practices.

In this study, the areas used to generate the RTU images included certain areas described as being of predictive value (flank, abdomen, tight and lumbar) [15], as well as what the authors perceived to be the peripheral morphological changes associated with increased overweight status and obesity (chest). Overall, the coefficient of variation differed among the anatomical sites assessed, in particular in the abdominal and thigh areas. These results agree with previous studies on body composition determined by dual-energy x-ray absorptiometry [7] and on subcutaneous fat thickness showing that diverse body regions yield different correlations with BCS [15]. This could result from existing species-specific differences in the pattern of fat deposition among dogs with increased BCS scores. This issue raises an additional concern which should be addressed in future research, namely, to ascertain which anatomical area can best predict fat content across all BCS scores.

The study by Wilkinson and McEwan [15] used A-mode (one-dimensional) ultrasonography, coupled with a high frequency (20 MHz) probe, enhancing the ability to discriminate small variations in SFT in different regions. However, in the present study, the use of a 10 MHz transducer set for small surface areas and in B-mode, was sufficient to detect SFT changes in lean dogs. In their study, Wilkinson and McEwan [15] determined the thickness of subcutaneous fat located between the *panniculus carnosus* (cutaneous muscle) and skin, which was not included in measurements, whereas in the current study SFT measurements included the skin. Also, in that study euthanized animals from a shelter were used, with an increased representation of young animals (below 3 years old), in contrast to our study, which included only clinically healthy privately-owned mature dogs. These major differences could explain the divergence in the results obtained in the present study regarding SFT in the four common anatomical sites assessed, which were particularly notable for maximum and mean SFT values. It is also worth mentioning that mean SFT values obtained in the present study are closer to the values obtained from histological measurements of subcutaneous fatness by Wilkinson and McEwan [15].

Data gathered herein also highlight the need to identify the most suitable anatomical sites to use in RTU prediction of body fat deposits in routine daily practice or research. Seeking the best anatomical site to measure subcutaneous fat has been a concern of other authors [18]. Morooka et al. [18], examining several points along the vertebral column, state that the lumbar region is the most suitable for sampling subcutaneous fat deposits with RTU.

This study revealed that strong associations exist between each of the five anatomical sites assessed; the highest associations were obtained for the abdominal and lumbar regions. Previous studies reported that the thickness of fat deposits in the lumbar area was closely related to the degree of adiposity in dogs [15, 18].

In the present study, dogs were grouped into three main BCS classes; *overweight*, *ideal* and *lean*. According to previous studies, assigning a BCS score may be challenging when animals approach the extremes between two consecutive scores [2, 19]. SFT data gathered in the present study showed that, on average, the difference in fat thickness between *overweight* or *lean* animals compared with *ideal* animals was higher than that reported to occur in body weight when BCS level changes, in accordance with studies using the same scoring scale as the one used here [6]. An overall reduction of 48–65 % was observed in the thickness of subcutaneous fat between *overweight* and *ideal* weighing animals, while the differences between *lean* and *ideal* animals ranged from 46 to 83 %. These results suggest that RTU is sensitive enough to detect smaller variations in subcutaneous fat than those perceived when using BCS in dogs.

All five anatomical regions used to collect RTU images were similarly sensitive to assess differences between categories. Nevertheless, the fat covering was thicker in the abdomen and the lumbar area, and thinner in the flank. Also, these two regions reveal strong correlations with BCS levels, suggesting that they may be the most suitable areas to collect information on SFT. Nevertheless, additional anatomical areas need to be identified, particularly considering that the interest of a site may change according to the pattern of fat deposition throughout different dogs' developmental stages (young, mature and old). Additionally, to strengthen the results obtained here, further studies should include the extremes of BCS levels.

Conclusions

In this preliminary study, it was demonstrated that RTU and image analysis can measure subcutaneous fat thickness and detect its changes with higher sensitivity than results obtained with the 5-point scale used for BCS. Additionally, in spite of the high correlations between SFT and BCS in all five anatomic sites analysed, the abdomen and lumbar areas were those where the greatest differences were observed within each category of fatness (*overweight*, *ideal* and *lean*) and will thus be the most useful to distinguish differences in the adiposity of dogs.

Abbreviations

BCS: body condition scoring; BW: body weight; CV: coefficient of variation; FCI: Fédération Cynologique Internationale; LS: least square; LSD: least significant difference; RTU: real-time ultrasonography; SD: standard deviation; SFT: subcutaneous fat thickness.

Authors' contributions

RP-C and SRS conceived and designed the study. LM, SM and PO contributed to data collection from dogs. LM and SRS performed image analysis and extracted the corresponding data. SRS, LM and RP-C contributed to writing the manuscript and reviewing the literature. SRS and RP-C contributed to the revision and final approval of the manuscript. All authors read and approved the final manuscript.

Author details

[1] Zootecnia Department, CECAV-Centro de Ciência Animal e Veterinária, Universidade de Trás-os-Montes e Alto Douro, Quinta de Prados, 5000-801 Vila Real, Portugal. [2] EUVG-Escola Universitária Vasco da Gama, Campus Universitário, Bloco B, Lordemão, 3020-210 Coimbra, Portugal. [3] HVBV-Hospital Veterinário do Baixo Vouga, Segadães, 3750-742 Águeda, Portugal.

Acknowledgements

This work was supported by the Portuguese Science and Technology Foundation (FCT) under Project PEst-OE/AGR/UI0772/2014.

Competing interests

The authors declare that they have no competing interests.

Declaration

Publication charges for this article were funded by the research platform Future Animal Health and Welfare at the Swedish University of Agricultural Sciences.

About this supplement

This article has been published as part of *Acta Veterinaria Scandinavica* Volume 58 Supplement 1, 2016: Animal Obesity—causes, consequences and comparative aspects: current research. The full contents of the supplement are available online at http://actavetscand.biomedcentral.com/articles/supplements/volume-58-supplement-1.

References

1. White G, Hobson-West P, Cobb K, Craigon J, Hammond R, Millar KM. Canine obesity: is there a difference between veterinarian and owner perception? J Small Anim Pract. 2011;52:622–6.
2. Li G, Lee P, Mori N, Yamamoto I, Kawasumi K, Tanabe H, Arai T. Supplementing five-point body condition score with body fat percentage increases the sensitivity for assessing overweight status of small to medium sized dogs. Vet Med Res Rep. 2012;3:71–8.
3. Gosselin J, Wren JA, Sunderland SJ. Canine obesity—an overview. J Vet Pharmacol Ther. 2007;30:1–10.
4. Laflamme DP. Obesity in dogs and cats: what is wrong with being fat? J Anim Sci. 2012;90:1653–62.

5. German AJ. The growing problem of obesity in dogs and cats. J Nutr. 2006;136:1940–6.
6. Dorsten CM, Cooper DM. Use of body condition scoring to manage body weight. Contemp Top Lab Anim Sci. 2004;43:34–7.
7. Speakman JR, Booles D, Butterwick R. Validation of dual energy X-ray absorptiometry (DXA) by comparison with chemical analysis of dogs and cats. Int J Obes Relat Metab Disord. 2001;25:439–47.
8. Elliott DA. Techniques to assess body composition in dogs and cats. Waltham Focus. 2006;16:16–20.
9. Jeusette I, Greco D, Aquino F, Detilleux J, Peterson M, Romano V, Torre C. Effect of breed on body composition and comparison between various methods to estimate body composition in dogs. Res Vet Sci. 2010;88:227–32.
10. Purushothaman D, Vanselow B, Wu S, Butler S, Brown WY. Whole body computed tomography with advanced imaging techniques: a research tool for measuring body composition in dogs. J Vet Med. 2013. doi: 10.1155/2013/610654.
11. Gifford A, Kullberg J, Berglund J, Malmberg F, Coate KC, Williams PE, Cherrington AD, Avison MJ, Welch EB. Canine body composition quantification using 3 tesla fat-water MRI. J Magn Reson Imaging. 2014;39:485–91.
12. Silva SR, Gomes MJ, Dias-da-Silva A, Gil LF, Azevedo JMT. Estimation in vivo of the body and carcass chemical composition of growing lambs by real-time ultrasonography. J Anim Sci. 2005;83:350–7.
13. Quaresma M, Payan-Carreira R, Silva SR. Relationship between ultrasound measurements of body fat reserves and body condition score in female donkeys. Vet J. 2013;197:329–34.
14. Scholz M, Bünger L, Kongsro J, Baulain U, Mitchell D. Non-invasive methods for the determination of body and carcass composition in livestock: dual-energy X-ray absorptiometry, computed tomography, magnetic resonance imaging and ultrasound: invited review. Animal. 2015;9:1250–64.
15. Wilkinson MJA, McEwan NA. Use of ultrasound in the measurement of subcutaneous fat and prediction of total body fat in dogs. J Nutr. 1991;121:4–7.
16. Alexander L, Buckley C, Merill R, Morris PJ, Stevenson A. WALTHAM® pocket book of healthy weight maintenance for cats and dogs. 2nd ed. In: German AJ, Butterwick R, editors. London: Beyond Design Solutions Ltd; 2010. p. 7. https://www.waltham.com/dyn/_assets/_pdfs/waltham-booklets/WALTHAMPocketBookOfHealthyWeightMaintenanceForCatsAndDogs.pdf. Accessed 15 June 2015.
17. Linder DE, Freeman LM, Sutherland-Smith J. Association between subcutaneous fat thickness measured on thoracic radiographs and body condition score in dogs. Am J Vet Res. 2013;74:1400–3.
18. Morooka T, Niiyama M, Saito M. Measurement of the back fat layer in beagles for estimation of obesity using two dimensional ultrasonography. J Small Anim Pract. 2001;42:56–9.
19. Burkholder WJ. Use of body condition scores in clinical assessment of the provision of optimal nutrition. JAVMA. 2000;217:650–4.

11

Serum concentration of gastrin, cortisol and C-reactive protein in a group of Norwegian sled dogs during training and after endurance racing

Marte Ekeland Fergestad[1,4†], Tuva Holt Jahr[2*†], Randi I. Krontveit[3] and Ellen Skancke[1]

Abstract

Background: High incidences of gastritis and gastric ulceration are observed in sled dogs participating in endurance races. Exercise-induced increases in hormones like gastrin and cortisol have been suggested as possible contributing factors. An increase in C-reactive protein (CRP) has also been observed in canines during physical exercise. The aim of this study was to evaluate the effect of long distance racing on the serum concentration of gastrin, cortisol and CRP in a group of sled dogs, by comparing the results achieved early in the training season and after participating in a long distance race; "Femundløpet". Dogs that only trained to the race, but did not compete in the race, were used as control dogs. Sixty-five sled dogs participated in the study; 46 competing dogs (25 completing and 21 non-completing the race) and 19 non-racing dogs (control dogs). The blood samples were collected in October 2012 and February 2013.

Results: The post-race serum concentration of gastrin, cortisol and CRP was significantly elevated in sled dogs participating in the race (both completing and non-completing dogs) when compared to the results from training. However, no significant differences were observed between the two sampling dates in the control dogs. Post-race results for completing and non-completing dogs were also compared. This demonstrated a significant elevation in gastrin in non-completing versus completing dogs, and a significant elevation in cortisol in completing compared to non-completing dogs.

Conclusions: Participation in a long distance race was associated with a significant increase in serum gastrin, cortisol and CRP in sled dogs.

Keywords: Sled dog, Canine, Long distance race, Gastrin, Cortisol, C-reactive protein, Gastritis, Gastric ulceration

Background

Physical activity can be associated with gastrointestinal dysfunction in both humans and dogs, although the pathophysiology is complex and not completely understood [1–5].

Sled dogs competing in endurance races have a high risk of gastric erosion, ulceration and bleeding [3, 4]. The prevalence of gastric lesions in dogs competing in the Iditarod race has been reported to be 48.5–61 % [3, 5]. By assessing necropsy findings of dogs deceased during or soon after competing in an endurance race, the two most common causes of death were found to be aspiration of gastric contents with subsequent aspiration pneumonia and acute blood loss due to gastric ulceration. Gastritis and gastric ulceration were common autopsy findings [4].

It has been suggested that gastritis and gastric ulcers in sled dogs, independent of the severity, often are

*Correspondence: tuva.holt.jahr@nmbu.no
†Marte Ekeland Fergestad and Tuva Holt Jahr contributed equally to this work
[2] Present Address: Department of Companion Animal Clinical Sciences, Faculty of Veterinary Medicine and Biosciences, Norwegian University of Life Sciences, PO Box 8146 Dep, 0033 Oslo, Norway

asymptomatic, and that gastric lesions do not necessarily affect the performance of racing dogs [6]. However, in humans these conditions are related to pain and discomfort [7]. As such, their high prevalence in sled dogs has significant animal welfare implications. This highlights the importance of understanding the pathophysiology and identifying the potential causes of exercise-related gastritis and gastric ulcers.

Release of gastrointestinal and stress-related hormones, like gastrin and cortisol, has been proposed as potential contributors to exercise-induced gastritis and gastric ulcers in sled dogs [1, 6].

In humans, participation in long distance races leads to an increase in serum gastrin [8–10]. The major effect of gastrin is stimulation of gastric acid release, and gastrin is therefore assumed to play a role in all gastric inflammatory processes [11]. If a similar rise in gastrin also exists in racing sled dogs, a possible gastrin-initiated increase in gastric acid may contribute to exercise-induced gastritis and gastric ulcers.

Physical exercise promotes release of cortisol in both humans [8, 9] and dogs [1, 12, 13]. An association between gastric lesions and an increase in endogenous cortisol has been demonstrated in racing sled dogs. It has been suggested that a rise in cortisol during training may be involved in the development of gastritis and gastric ulcers seen in racing sled dogs [1].

A rise in serum concentration of C-reactive protein (CRP) generally is related to trauma, inflammation or infection. Several studies have demonstrated an increase in CRP related to physical exercise [14–16], mostly due to muscle damage [16]. However, an exercise-induced increase in CRP together with other markers of gastric lesions may also indicate gastric inflammation during physical activity.

The aim of this study was to evaluate the effect of racing on the serum concentration of gastrin, cortisol and CRP in a group of sled dogs by comparing the results achieved early in the training season and after participating in a long distance race; "Femundløpet". Dogs only trained and not competing in the race, were used as control dogs.

Methods

Study design: clinical prospective cohort study.

"Femundløpet" is a long distance race of 600 km, arranged in Røros, Norway. Four mushers registered for participation in "Femundløpet" in February 2013, were contacted in October 2012. All agreed to let their dogs participate, and later signed a consent regarding the study.

Included dogs

In this study, a group of sixty-five sled dogs (n = 65) were observed during a training season from 2012 leading up the race in February 2013. The dogs were divided into three cohorts based on participation and outcome of the race: race completing (group 1) (n = 25), race non-completing (group 2) (n = 21) and non-competing/control dogs (group 3) (n = 19). Non-completing dogs were defined as dogs withdrawn from the race without considering the reason for the withdrawal, such as illness or other causes.

The dogs were classified by breed (Alaskan or Siberian husky), sex (male/female) and age (in years). Information regarding health, training and feeding routines during the training season was collected via questionnaires.

Blood sample collection

Blood samples were collected early in the training season (October 2012); samples A, and at the end of the observation period, shortly after the race (February 2013); samples B. Samples from the three groups were further subdivided into A1 and B1 (race completing), A2 and B2 (race non-completing) and A3 and B3 (non-competing/control dogs). The training data of the determined parameters served as control for the post-race values.

Prior to collection of samples A, the dogs had been rested and fasted for a minimum of 12 h. These samples were collected at the mushers' homes.

B1 samples were collected as soon as possible and within 1.5 h after the dogs crossed the finish line. The completing dogs were not fed prior to blood sampling at the finish line. B2 samples were collected at the checkpoints as soon as possible and within 8 h after the dogs were withdrawn from the race. Feeding prior to sampling in non-completing dogs was recorded at the checkpoints. Dogs that had not been fed prior to sample collection were categorized as unfed. There was no recording of feeding along the track. B3 Samples were collected at the mushers' homes 2 weeks after the race. The dogs had been resting and not fed for a minimum of 12 h prior to sampling.

Blood sampling and storage

Blood samples were obtained from the cephalic vein, and approximately 6 ml of whole blood were collected from each dog. Within 1 h the samples were centrifuged for 10 min, and serum was transferred to labelled serum tubes. Serum isolated after one centrifugation was reserved for gastrin analysis. Serum isolated after two centrifugations was reserved for CRP and cortisol analysis. The sampling procedure was the same for all blood samples.

Samples A1, A2, A3 and B3 were immediately transported in a cooler and frozen at −70 °C. Samples B1 were relocated to −20 °C within 1 h after sampling. Samples B2 were kept in a cooler, outdoors at approximately

−5 °C, and transferred to −20 °C within 2 days after collection. After the race, samples B1 and B2 were kept frozen during transport back to the Norwegian School of Veterinary Science and transferred to −70 °C. All samples were stored at −70 °C prior to analysing in March 2013.

Analysis of gastrin, cortisol and CRP

Analysis of serum gastrin was performed at Rikshospitalet University Hospital, Oslo. Measurement of serum gastrin was performed via GASTRIN (^{125} I) Radioimmunoassay Kit (MP Biomedicals, USA). This analysis is designed for human gastrin measurement, but is currently also applied for measurement of canine gastrin. The reference range for gastrin (10–40 pg/ml) used in this study is obtained from another laboratory, which uses the same method (Helen Evans, BSc Hons, Veterinary Services Operations Manager, Cambridge Specialist Laboratory Services, UK, personal communication).

Analysis of serum cortisol and CRP were performed at The Central Laboratory at the Norwegian University of Life Sciences. Serum cortisol was analysed using IMMULITE 2000 from Simens, both instruments and reagents. The cortisol analysis is a solid-phase, competitive chemiluminescent enzyme immunoassay (polyclonal rabbit anti-cortisol). Serum CRP was analysed by ADVIA 1800 from Siemens, Immunoturbidimetric assay (anti-human CRP antibody), reagents from Randox (RANDOX Laboratories Ltd., UK), and calibrator from Life Diagnostics, Inc USA: dog C-Reactive Protein (2250 mg/L). The laboratory's own reference values were employed (cortisol 20–250 nmol/L and CRP 0–15 mg/L).

Statistical analysis

Data was compiled in Microsoft® Excel (Microsoft Corporation, 1 Microsoft Way, Redmond, WA 98052-7329, USA) and subsequently imported in Stata 12 (Stata Corporation, 4905 Lakeway Drive, College Station, TX 778445, USA), which was used for all statistical analyses.

Distribution of gastrin, cortisol and CRP was assessed by histograms. Formal tests for normality (Shapiro-Wilks) were also applied. One-way ANOVA or Wilcoxon–Mann–Whitney tests were applied to test for differences in serum gastrin, CRP and cortisol between the variables breed, sex, age and fasting status. Wilcoxon–Mann–Whitney tests were used to compare median values of gastrin, cortisol and CRP in sample A1 with sample B1, A2 with B2, and A3 with B3. In addition, sample A1 was compared to A2 and A3 for possible differences before the race applying Wilcoxon–Mann–Whitney tests. Boxplots for gastrin, cortisol and CRP by the subgroups completing, non-completing and controls were generated.

For CRP, Wilcoxon signed rank test was used to test whether the median CRP values of A samples as well as A1, A2 and A3 were significantly different from and higher than the upper reference limit for CRP (15 mg/L). Because a few dogs in the B2 group (non-completing) were fed prior to blood sampling, the B2 group were divided in sub-groups fed and not-fed and compared to the respective A2 Samples applying Wilcoxon–Mann–Whitney tests. P values <0.05 were considered statistically significant.

To confirm results of the non-parametric testing, quantile regression with sample (A1, A2, A3, B1, B2, B3) as variable were performed for the three outcome variables gastrin, cortisol and CRP. Overall significance of the variable was tested using multiple Wald test. P values <0.05 were considered statistically significant. The Stata command lincom was used to generate contrasts among the different categories.

As sensitivity-analyses, statistical analyses excluding the whole team that withdrew during the race, were also performed.

Results

A total of 65 dogs, 18 Siberian huskies (28 %) and 47 Alaskan huskies (72 %), were included in the study. There were 32 females (49 %) and 33 males (51 %) with a mean age of 3.9 years, ranging from 1 to 9 years. There were no significant age or sex differences in the serum concentrations of gastrin, cortisol and CRP. However, there was a significant breed difference in the serum concentration of CRP ($P = 0.017$) (Table 1).

Summary statistics for the variables serum gastrin, cortisol and C-reactive protein (CRP) according to breed, age and sex in a group of Norwegian sled dogs, *Wilcoxon–Mann–Whitney test, **ANOVA.

Forty-six dogs (71 %) participated in "Femundløpet" 2013, while 19 dogs (29 %) were included as post-race controls. Twenty-five dogs (54 %) completed the 600 km race in 3–4 days, while 21 dogs (46 %), including a complete team of 12 dogs, were dropped at different times during the race. The team that withdrew completed 500 km of the race.

Information regarding health, training and feeding routines during the training season was considered approximately equal for all dogs. At the time of blood sampling in October 2012 (A1, A2 and A3), all dogs were considered healthy based on physical examination by the authors, and none had clinical signs of gastrointestinal dysfunction according to the owners' observations. This was also the case for the control dogs post-race in February 2013 (sample B3). Among the completing dogs (B1) no recording of possible illness, including signs of gastrointestinal dysfunction, was done by the authors. Non-completing

Table 1 Summary statistics for the variables gastrin, cortisol and CRP according to breed, age and sex

Variable	N (%)/mean (range)	Gastrin (pg/ml)		Cortisol (nmol/L)		CRP (mg/L)	
		Mean (sd)/median	*P* value	Mean (sd)/median	*P* value	Mean (sd)/median	*P* value
Breed			0.173*		0.20*		0.017*
Alaska husky	47 (72 %)	18.9 (11.7)/15.8		61.2 (24.4)/58.0		27.9 (16.7)/24.8	
Siberian husky	18 (28 %)	15.6 (6.8)/12.9		64.7 (23.4)/59.5		15.6 (18.2)/10.9	
Age	3.9 (1–9)	18.0 (10.7)/15.0	0.71**	62.3 (24.0)/58	0.67**	24.4 (17.9)/18.8	0.85**
Sex			0.13*		0.99*		0.23*
Male	33 (1 %)	15.2 (4.9)/14.3		63.0 (27.5)/58.0		27.1 (19.1)/21.8	
Female	32 (49 %)	21.1 (14.0)/15.0		61.3 (20.1)/57		21.5 (16.3)/17.8	

dogs (B2) were withdrawn due to various reasons, like lameness, depression, anorexia and/or dehydration. However, some of them did not have any signs of illness, which was the case with several of the dogs in the team withdrawn at 500 km.

Neither dogs during training (A1, A2, A3) nor the controls post-race (B3) were fed prior to blood sampling. Except for seven (15 %) non-completing dogs none of the competing dogs (85 %) were fed.

Sample A1 was compared to A2 and A3 for possible differences in gastrin, cortisol and CRP. No significant differences were found between A1 and A2, nor between A1 and A3. Summary statistics for these samples are outlined in Table 2.

Boxplot of the different subgroups are shown in Fig. 1. The following sections present the detailed results for gastrin, cortisol and CRP.

Summary statistics for the variables serum gastrin, cortisol and C-reactive protein (CRP) in a group of Norwegian sled dogs. Samples were taken early in the training season, after completing a long distance race, in dogs not completing the race and in non-competing control dogs. Reference values: gastrin 10–40 pg/ml, cortisol 20–250 nmol/L and CRP 0–15 mg/L. *Wilcoxon–Mann–Whitney test.

Gastrin

The serum concentration of gastrin was significantly increased ($P < 0.001$) when comparing samples B1–A1 (race-completing dogs) (Table 2). This was also the case when comparing samples B2–A2 (race non-completing dogs) ($P < 0.001$). There was no significant difference in gastrin serum concentration between samples B3 and A3 (control dogs). Serum concentration of gastrin was significantly elevated in samples B2 (non-completing dogs) when compared to samples B1 (completing dogs), ($P < 0.001$).

When comparing the post-race results in the fed and not-fed dogs among the non-completing dogs, no significant difference in median serum gastrin concentrations was detected. In the fed non-completing dogs there was significantly higher median gastrin in the post-race samples compared to their respective A samples ($P = 0.013$) (Table 2). In the not-fed non-completing dogs, the post-race samples were also compared to their respective samples A. Also in these dogs the median gastrin was significantly higher post-race ($P < 0.001$) (Table 2). Sensitivity-analyses excluding the entire team that withdrew had negligible influence on the results (data not shown, available upon request).

Quantile regression analysis confirmed the results; all categories except from B2 (race non-completing) had significantly lower median serum gastrin compared to the baseline category which was the race completing group (B1) (Table 3), and group B2 had significantly higher gastrin than A2 (race non-completing dogs) ($P < 0.001$) while the difference between B3 and A3 (control dogs) was not significant.

The sensitivity-analyses excluding the entire team that withdrew from the race decreased the difference between group B2 compared to B1 ($P = 0.094$), but had negligible influence on the other results (data not shown, available upon request).

Cortisol

The serum concentration of cortisol was significantly increased ($P < 0.001$) when comparing samples B1–A1 (race-completing dogs) (Table 2). This was also the case when comparing Samples B2–A2 (race non-completing dogs) ($P = 0.001$). There was no significant difference in cortisol serum concentration between Samples B3 and A3 (control dogs). Serum concentration of cortisol in post-race results was significantly higher ($P = 0.0039$) in completing dogs when compared to non-completing dogs. Sensitivity-analyses excluding the entire team that withdrew had negligible influence on the results (data not shown).

Quantile regression analysis confirmed the results; all categories had significantly lower median serum cortisol

Table 2 Summary statistics for the variables serum gastrin, cortisol and CRP

Sample category	N	Mean (sd)	Median (range)	P value*
Gastrin (10–40 pg/ml)				
A1 completing dogs	25	18.1 (11.2)	15.0 (8.3–62.4)	$P < 0.001$
B1 completing dogs	25	41.6 (17.8)	36.6 (13.5–71.1)	
A2 non-completing dogs	21	17 (12.2)	15.2 (9.1–64.7)	$P < 0.001$
B2 non-completing dogs	21	68.7 (28.3)	69.8 (16.4–120.8)	
Fed A2 non-completing dogs	7	21.9 (19.2)	15.9 (9.1–64.7)	$P = 0.013$
Fed B2 non-completing dogs	7	63.1 (28.9)	75.3 (17.1–95.5)	
Not-fed A2 non-completing dogs	14	15.9 (6.6)	14.35 (9.3–30)	$P < 0.001$
Not-fed B2 non-completing dogs	14	71.5 (28.6)	69.8 (16.4–120.8)	
A3 control dogs	19	18.1 (8.5)	14.7 (8.8–40.4)	$P = 0.7703$
B3 control dogs	19	20.5 (12.6)	18.2 (8.3–57.9)	
Cortisol (20–250 nmol/L)				
A1 completing dogs	25	60.8 (26.9)	57.0 (27–141)	$P < 0.001$
B1 completing dogs	25	153.2 (60.9)	147.0 (74–323)	
A2 non-completing dogs	21	58.1 (18.2)	57 (33–94)	$P = 0.001$
B2 non-completing dogs	21	103.7 (54.2)	80.0 (46–224)	
A3 control dogs	19	68.8 (25.7)	63.5 (41–135)	$P = 0.0752$
B3 control dogs	19	57.6 (23.3)	52 (34–125)	
C-reactive protein (0–15 mg/L)				
A1 completing dogs	25	25.8 (15.9)	22.1 (1.2–55.3)	$P < 0.001$
B1 completing dogs	25	90.6 (49.9)	75.1 (26.9–191.7)	
A2 non-completing dogs	21	20.4 (20.4)	13.5 (1.8–78.9)	$P < 0.001$
B2 non-completing dogs	21	104.5 (52.2)	89.7 (22.3–220.2)	
A3 control dogs	19	27.2 (17.5)	23.4 (5.3–63.3)	$P < 0.001$
B3 control dogs	19	15.3 (35.2)	3.2 (0–156.9)	

compared to the baseline category which was the race completing group (B1) (Table 3), while the differences between B2 and A2 (race non-completing dogs), and between B3 and A3 (control dogs) were not significant. The sensitivity-analyses excluding the entire team that withdrew increased the difference between B2 and A2 (race non-completing dogs) ($P = 0.002$), but had negligible influence on the other results (data not shown, available upon request).

Crp

Median CRP for samples A was significantly higher than the upper reference value for CRP ($P < 0.001$). For sample A1 and A3, median CRP was also significantly higher than the upper reference limit, $P = 0.004$ and 0.02, respectively. For samples A2 the median CRP appeared to be only numerically higher than the upper reference limit.

The serum concentration of CRP was significantly increased ($P < 0.001$) when comparing samples B1–A1 (race completing dogs) (Table 2). This was also the case when comparing samples B2–A2 (race non-completing dogs) ($P < 0.001$). There was a significant increase in serum CRP concentration in samples A3 compared to B3 (control dogs) ($P < 0.001$). Serum concentration of CRP in post-race results was elevated in non-completing dogs when compared to completing dogs, although this was not significant. Sensitivity-analyses excluding the entire team that withdrew had negligible influence on the results (data not shown, available upon request).

Quantile regression analysis confirmed the results; all categories except B2 (race non-completing dogs) had significantly lower median CRP compared to the baseline category, which was the race-completing group (B1) (Table 3). Group B2 had significantly higher CRP than A2 (race non-completing dogs), ($P < 0.001$), while the difference between B3 and A3 (control dogs) was not significant. The sensitivity-analyses excluding the entire team that withdrew had negligible influence on the results (data not shown, available upon request).

Quality control of gastrin, cortisol and CRP

MP Biomedicals inter-assay precision and intra-assay precision GASTRIN (^{125}I) Radioimmunoassay Kit is outlined in Table 4.

Discussion

Gastrin, cortisol and CRP are involved in different physiological mechanisms including secretion of gastric acid, stress response and inflammatory reactions. The main findings in this study were that dogs participating in this long distance race had an increase in serum concentration of gastrin, cortisol and CRP. It can be hypothesized that an increase in these parameters to some extent may indicate the general level of stress and inflammation arising during extreme physical exercise, but they may also be markers of gastrointestinal dysfunction.

Gastrin

Sled dogs that participated in a long distance race experienced a significant increase in serum gastrin. Previous human studies, which focused on gastrointestinal dysfunction during long distance races, also concluded that there is an exercise-induced increase in serum concentration of gastrin [8–10, 17].

Exercise-induced elevation in serum gastrin can be a result of several factors or mechanisms. Repetitive blows

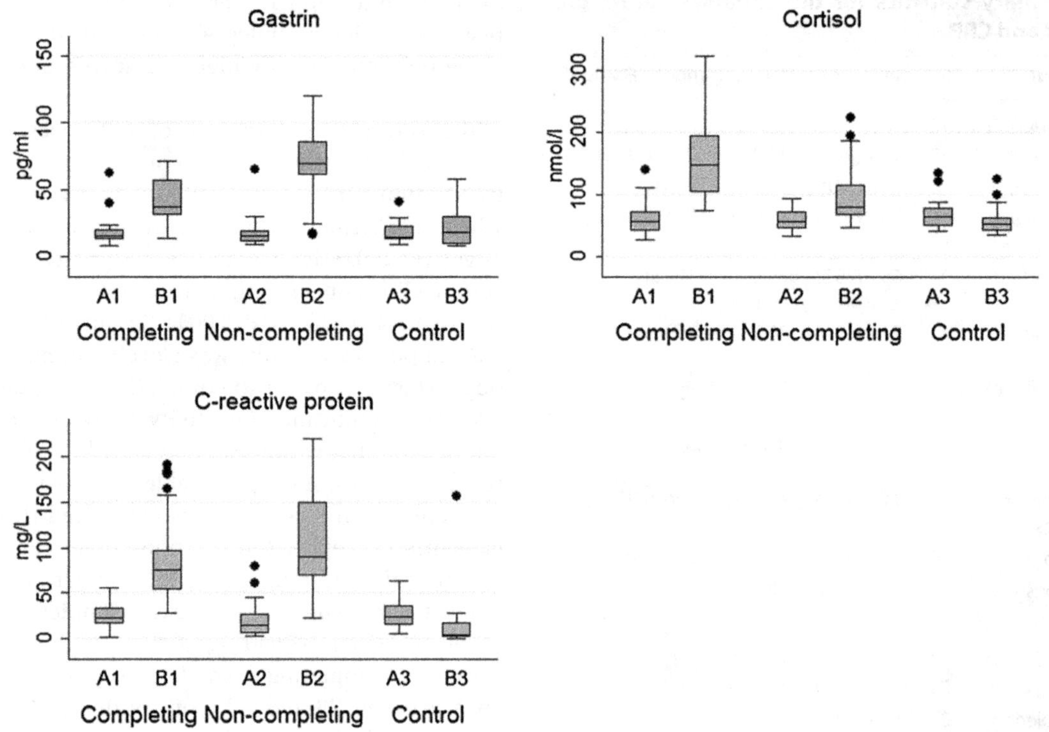

Fig. 1 Boxplots for gastrin, cortisol and C-reactive protein. Boxplots for gastrin, cortisol and C-reactive protein [CRP] by the subgroups completing, non-completing and control dogs in a group of sled dogs participating in a Norwegian long distance race

against visceral organs during running are in bipeds thought to trigger the release of gastrointestinal hormones, including gastrin [8], although this has not been documented in quadrupeds. In addition, renal inactivation of gastrin might be reduced during physical exercise, due to redistribution of blood supply from visceral organs to skeletal muscles [8]. However, a study concluded that renal hypoperfusion was less likely in exercising sled dogs [18]. Release of catecholamines due to physical activity [17] may stimulate the release of gastrin, although a study regarding exercising sled dogs showed minimal systemic release of catecholamines, making this mechanism of gastrin increase less likely [12].

Food intake, along with the expectation and smell of food, stimulates secretion of gastrin [19]. In humans and horses, food intake after physical exercise gives a significantly higher increase in serum gastrin compared to what is registered in fasted individuals [17, 20]. Sled dogs are snacked during racing, and this may give a higher exercise-induced increase of gastrin, similar to the rise seen in humans and horses. In this study, all dogs were supposed to be fasted prior to blood sampling, however the competing dogs might have received food along the trail, and seven non-completing dogs were fed prior to blood sampling. It is also possible that competing dogs were expecting food when approaching the checkpoints and finish line. These factors may contribute to the increase in serum gastrin detected in the competing dogs. Serum gastrin was significantly elevated in non-completing dogs when compared to completing dogs. If this is a result of different feeding patterns or may be associated with illness in non-completing dogs is not known and merits further investigation.

The major pathophysiologic factor causing gastritis and gastric ulceration is currently considered to be breakdown of the mucosal barrier, and not hyperacidity as earlier proposed [21]. Some studies have concluded that there is no decrease in gastric pH in humans or dogs during physical activity [8, 9, 22–24], which emphasizes that hyperacidity is not the causation of exercise-related gastritis and gastric ulceration. Release of various inhibitors, such as somatostatin, has been assumed to limit the release of gastric acid during physical exercise [8, 9].

On the other hand, several studies regarding sled dogs demonstrate a significant reduction in the severity of exercise-induced gastritis and gastric ulceration by preventive use of gastric acid reducing agents, like omeprazole and famotidine [25–27]. This would suggest that gastric acid is a contributing factor to exercise-induced gastritis and gastric ulceration in dogs. Further

Table 3 Quantile regression of serum gastrin, cortisol and C-reactive protein values

Variable and level	Coefficient (SE)	P value	95 % confidence interval
Gastrin			
Racing status		<0.001[a]	
A1 completing dogs	−21.6 (4.83)	<0.001[a]	−31.17; −12.03
B1 completing dogs	Baseline	–	–
A2 non-completing dogs	−21.4 (5.06)	<0.001[a]	−31.42; −11.38
B2 non-completing dogs	33.2 (5.06)	<0.001[a]	23.18; 43.22
A3 control dogs	−21.9 (5.20)	<0.001[a]	−32.20; −11.60
B3 control dogs	−18.40 (5.20)	<0.001[a]	−28.70; −8.10
Intercept	36.6 (3.42)	<0.001[a]	29.83; 43.37
Cortisol			
Racing status		<0.001[a]	
A1 completing dogs	−21.6 (4.83)	<0.001[a]	−31.17; −12.03
B1 completing dogs	Baseline	–	–
A2 non-completing dogs	−21.4 (5.06)	<0.001[a]	−31.42; −11.38
B2 non-completing dogs	33.2 (5.06)	<0.001[a]	23.18; 43.22
A3 control dogs	−21.9 (5.20)	<0.001[a]	−32.20; −11.60
B3 control dogs	−18.40 (5.20)	<0.001[a]	−28.70; −8.10
Intercept	36.6 (3.42)	<0.001[a]	29.83; 43.37
C-reactive protein (CRP)			
Racing status		<0.001[a]	
A1 completing dogs	−21.6 (4.83)	<0.001[a]	−31.17; −12.03
B1 completing dogs	Baseline	–	–
A2 non-completing dogs	−21.4 (5.06)	<0.001[a]	−31.42; −11.38
B2 non-completing dogs	33.2 (5.06)	<0.001[a]	23.18; 43.22
A3 control dogs	−21.9 (5.20)	<0.001[a]	−32.20; −11.60
B3 control dogs	−18.40 (5.20)	<0.001[a]	−28.70; −8.10
Intercept	36.6 (3.42)	<0.001[a]	29.83; 43.37

Results from quantile regression of the effect of racing status and time of blood sampling on serum gastrin, cortisol and C-reactive protein (CRP) in a group of sled dogs participating in a Norwegian long distance race

[a] Multiple wald test

investigation regarding exercise-induced increase in gastrin related to gastric pH should be done. Use of antacid medication, like omeprazole and famotidine, leads to an increase in serum gastrin concentration in dogs [28]. However, at the time of this study, use of such medications prior to and during race was not allowed in Norway. According to the mushers, none of the dogs were medicated prior to blood sampling during training. Therefore, use of antacids did not influence the gastrin results in this study.

Table 4 MP biomedicals inter-assay precision and intra-assay precision GASTRIN (^{125}I) radioimmunoassay kit

Sample	Control 1	Control 2	Control 3	Serum
Inter-assay precision, gastrin				
n	20	20	20	20
Mean, pg/mL	56.7	232	465	49.4
S.D.	2.59	9.56	26.1	2.91
% CV	4.6	4.1	5.6	5.9
Intra-assay precision, gastrin				
n	22	22	22	
Mean, pg/mL	56.0	225	474	
S.D.	5.91	16.8	37.2	
% CV	10.6	7.5	7.8	

Regarding cortisol quality control, the inter-assay CV was 10 % at 80 nmol/L and 8 % at 550 nmol/L

Regarding CRP Quality Control, for homemade dog serum pool, the inter-assay CV was 6 % at 27.4 mg/L

Cortisol

There was a significant increase in serum cortisol in the competing dogs after racing. These findings are in accordance with previous human, horse and canine studies [1, 8, 9, 13, 17, 29]. Also, anticipation of exercise before racing can cause increase in cortisol in sled dogs [30].

A negative energy balance during physical activity may trigger the release of cortisol [1, 12]. Racing sled dogs have high-energy requirements, and may not be capable of sufficiently increasing their food intake to meet these requirements. Racing sled dogs are also exposed to cold, which further increases energy demands [31].

Dogs that completed the race had significantly higher serum cortisol levels compared to dogs that did not complete. This may reflect the sustained strain that the dogs experience with greater distance, and the prolonged requirement for energy in completing dogs.

It has been proposed that exercise-induced increase in endogenous cortisol may contribute to development of gastritis and gastric ulceration in sled dogs. A study regarding sled dogs competing in the Iditarod race showed that dogs with abnormal gastroscopic findings after racing also had a significantly higher serum cortisol level, compared to dogs with normal gastroscopic findings. However, the association between endogenous cortisol and gastrointestinal ulceration was not possible to establish [1].

Crp

There was a significant increase in serum CRP in competing dogs. An increase in serum CRP after long distance racing has previously been reported in humans and canines [14–16, 32]. Muscle degradation with subsequent inflammation is assumed to be a contributing factor in humans and dogs [16, 33].

Serum CRP concentration was slightly higher in non-completing dogs compared to completing dogs, although the difference was not significant. It could be speculated that this may be due to injuries or illness causing an inflammatory response in the majority of the non-completing dogs. Studies with larger case numbers and appropriate statistical power are necessary to reveal a true difference and support the proposed hypothesis.

The control dogs had a significantly higher serum concentration of CRP during training compared to the results post-race. It is likely that they underwent less physical activity in the post-race period compared to the training season. Also, median CRP for Samples A was significantly higher than the upper reference value for CRP, implicating either an inflammatory state of all dogs or a methodical problem in the laboratory analysis of CRP bringing higher results than previously described for healthy dogs when using the same assay. The serum concentration of CRP was significantly higher in Alaska huskies compared to Siberian huskies. The Siberian huskies in the present study represented a single team and one musher, and the finding might be spurious and possibly not reflect true breed differences.

In a study with experimentally induced damage to the gastric mucosa in dogs, it was concluded that CRP could be a useful indicator for gastric lesions [34]. However, as serum CRP also increases as a result of exercise or general illness in sleds dogs, the use of serum CRP as a general diagnostic tool for gastritis or gastric ulceration may be limited in racing sled dogs.

Strengths and limitations

A strength of this study is the prospective design. The use of a control group for the post-race results and a genuine endurance race setting increase the external validity of this study. However, there were also limitations that need to be kept in mind.

Standardization of blood sampling during the race was difficult and not optimal. Appropriate storage of the blood samples was difficult to standardize completely, especially regarding the time passed before freezing at −70 °C. Although temperatures in February in this part of Norway are generally well below 0 °C, storage procedures could have influenced the results. It is known that serum gastrin concentration can decrease significantly if stored in room temperature for a few hours [35]. Likewise, the cortisol concentration can decrease if serum is stored at temperatures above 0 °C over several days [36]. CRP on the other hand is considered to be far more stable in different storage conditions, and it is likely that the serum concentration of CRP were not affected to the same extent as gastrin and cortisol, by transport and temperatures [37, 38]. It is therefore possible that an even greater rise in both serum gastrin and cortisol levels would have been measured, if the samples had been stored in optimal conditions.

Some samples from dogs that did not complete the race were collected after the dogs had been rested for up to 8 h. This could influence the values of the measured parameters. The impact of this resting period is probably a decrease in serum concentrations of gastrin, cortisol and CRP. It is possible that the measured values would have been even higher if the samples had been collected straight after racing.

Because the dogs were from different mushers, confounding factors in the dogs' home environment might influence the results and interpretation of the statistical analysis.

One musher and his team of dogs withdrew from the race after 500 km. All dogs belonging to this team were recorded as non-completing. Having a whole team of dogs not completing the race was not preplanned during the design of the study, but merely a result of the study being performed in a genuine race setting. Sensitivity-analyses excluding this team had negligible influence on the results and conclusions.

During a race non-completing dogs mostly withdraw due to clinical signs of disease. However, the presumption that they are clinically ill and that completing dogs are healthy, is not always correct. In the authors' experience, reasons for dropping may vary from observed clinical disease to consideration of a dog's fitness. Withdrawal of entire teams, including sick and healthy individuals, also happens. There may be different opinions regarding when it is unjustifiable to let a dog continue a race, making the definition sick relative and subjective. Completing dogs have additionally been observed with signs compatible with lethargy and diarrhea. Consequently, the dogs' health status should not be defined as healthy just because they have completed a race. These challenges need to be addressed in future studies.

No age or sex related differences in the serum concentrations of gastrin, cortisol or CRP could be detected in this study. This might be due to the sample size, and therefore could have appeared if the number of dogs included had been higher. However, it seems unlikely that there should be age or sex differences in either of these parameters. It can be speculated that a rise in CRP may appear with increasing age due to processes linked to ageing, or that a rise in cortisol may be observed in younger, inexperienced dogs due to a higher degree of psychological stress.

In the analysis of gastrin, both inter- and intra assay variation were available (Table 4), which strengthens the results of this study. CV was low and relatively similar for both inter- and intra-assay variation. In the analysis of cortisol and CRP, only inter-assay variation was measured. How this could have affected the results in this study is unknown.

Future research

Further investigation is needed to evaluate if an exercise-induced increase in serum gastrin and cortisol may contribute to gastritis and gastric ulceration in racing sled dogs. In future studies it would be interesting to focus on the association between distinct signs of illness and different biomarkers in completing and non-completing racing dogs. However, the clinical evaluation of the participating sled dogs needs to be done by the same person in a standardized matter, and clinical suspicion of gastrointestinal disease needs to be confirmed by diagnostic procedures. Because sled dogs with gastritis and gastric ulcers often are asymptomatic [7], gastroscopy together with measurement of biomarkers should be performed during training season, and immediately before and after participation in a race. This could increase our knowledge concerning exercise-induced metabolic changes in sled dogs during racing and enlighten possible causalities to gastritis and gastric ulceration in racing sled dogs.

Conclusions

This study indicated an exercise-induced increase in serum gastrin, cortisol and CRP in sled dogs participating in a long distance race. The results of this study have generated new knowledge on exercise-induced metabolic changes and can guide future research in this field (Additional file 1).

Authors' contributions

MRF and THJ participated in the design and coordination of the study, carried out the sample collection and drafted the manuscript. This was done as their final year research project at the Norwegian School of Veterinary Science. ES initiated the study as supervisor for the final year research project, participated in the design and coordination of the study and helped to draft the manuscript. RIK performed statistical analysis and helped to draft the manuscript. All authors read and approved the final manuscript.

Author details

[1] Department of Companion Animal Clinical Sciences, Faculty of Veterinary Medicine and Biosciences, Norwegian University of Life Sciences, PO Box 8146 Dep, 0033 Oslo, Norway. [2] Present Address: Department of Companion Animal Clinical Sciences, Faculty of Veterinary Medicine and Biosciences, Norwegian University of Life Sciences, PO Box 8146 Dep, 0033 Oslo, Norway. [3] Department for Pharmacoeconomics, Norwegian Medicines Agency, PO Box 63, Kalbakken, 0901 Oslo, Norway. [4] Present Address: Department of Food Safety and Infection Biology, Faculty of Veterinary Medicine and Biosciences, Norwegian University of Life Sciences, PO Box 8146 Dep, 0033 Oslo, Norway.

Acknowledgements

The authors would like to thank the participating mushers, all involved staff at Femundløpet 2013, participating vet nurse Dagrun Hansen Lia at Norwegian University of Life Sciences and the employees at The Central Laboratory at Norwegian University of Life Sciences, especially Stein Istre Thoresen for helpful feedback.

Competing interests

The authors declare that they have no competing interests.

Funding

"Smådyrpraktiserende veterinærers forenings faglige og vitenskapelige fond" and "Dyrlege Smiths legat" contributed with economic funding to this project.

References

1. Royer CM, Willard M, Williamson K, Steiner JM, Williams DA, David M. Exercise stress, intestinal permeability and gastric ulceration in racing Alaskan sled dogs. Equine Comp Exerc Physiol. 2005;2:53–9. doi:10.1079/ECP200446.
2. Moses FM. Gastrointestinal bleeding and the athlete. Am J Gastroenterol. 1993;88:1157–9.
3. Davis MS, Willard MD, Nelson SL, Mandsager RE, McKiernan BS, Mansell JK, et al. Prevalence of gastric lesions in racing Alaskan sled dogs. J Vet Intern Med. 2003;17:311–4.
4. Dennis MM, Nelson SN, Cantor GH, Mosier DA, Blake JE, Basaraba RJ. Assessment of necropsy findings in sled dogs that died during Iditarod Trail sled dog races: 23 cases (1994-2006). J Am Vet Med Assoc. 2008;232:564–73. doi:10.2460/javma.232.4.564.
5. Davis MS, Willard MD, Williamson KK, Steiner JM, Williams DA. Sustained strenuous exercise increases intestinal permeability in racing Alaskan sled dogs. J Vet Intern Med. 2005;19:34–9.
6. Ritchey JW, Davis MS, Breshears MA, Willard MD, Williamson KK, Royer CM, et al. Gastritis in Alaskan racing sled dogs. J Comp Pathol. 2011;145:68–76. doi:10.1016/j.jcpa.2010.11.008.
7. de Oliveira EP, Burini RC. The impact of physical exercise on the gastrointestinal tract. Curr Opin Clin Nutr Metab Care. 2009;12:533–8. doi:10.1097/MCO.0b013e32832e6776.
8. O'Connor AM, Johnston CF, Buchanan KD, Boreham C, Trinick TR, Riddoch CJ. Circulating gastrointestinal hormone changes in marathon running. Int J Sports Med. 1995;16:283–7. doi:10.1055/s-2007-973006.
9. Philipp E, Wilckens T, Friess E, Platte P, Pirke KM. Cholecystokinin, gastrin and stress hormone responses in marathon runners. Peptides. 1992;13:125–8.
10. Banfi G, Marinelli M, Bonini P, Gritti I, Roi GS. Pepsinogens and gastrointestinal symptoms in mountain marathon runners. Int J Sports Med. 1996;17:554–8. doi:10.1055/s-2007-972894.
11. Garcia-Sancho M, Rodriguez-Franco F, Sainz A, Rodriguez A, Silvan G, Illera JC. Serum gastrin in canine chronic lymphocytic-plasmacytic enteritis. Can Vet J. 2005;46:630–4.
12. Durocher LL, Hinchcliff KW, Williamson KK, McKenzie EC, Holbrook TC, Willard M, et al. Effect of strenuous exercise on urine concentrations of homovanillic acid, cortisol, and vanillylmandelic acid in sled dogs. Am J Vet Res. 2007;68:107–11. doi:10.2460/ajvr.68.1.107.
13. Huntingford JL, Levine CB, Mustacich DJ, Corrigan D, Downey RL, Wakshlag JJ. The effects of low intensity endurance activity on various physiological parameters and exercise induced oxidative stress in dogs. Open J Vet Med. 2014;4:11. doi:10.4236/ojvm.2014.47016.
14. Wakshlag JJ, Stokol T, Geske SM, Greger CE, Angle CT, Gillette RL. Evaluation of exercise-induced changes in concentrations of C-reactive protein and serum biochemical values in sled dogs completing a long-distance endurance race. Am J Vet Res. 2010;71:1207–13. doi:10.2460/ajvr.71.10.1207.
15. Kenyon CL, Basaraba RJ, Bohn AA. Influence of endurance exercise on serum concentrations of iron and acute phase proteins in racing sled dogs. J Am Vet Med Assoc. 2011;239:1201–10. doi:10.2460/javma.239.9.1201.

16. Fallon KE. The acute phase response and exercise: the ultramarathon as prototype exercise. Clin J Sport Med. 2001;11:38–43.
17. Sliwowski Z, Lorens K, Konturek SJ, Bielanski W, Zoladz JA. Leptin, gastrointestinal and stress hormones in response to exercise in fasted or fed subjects and before or after blood donation. J Physiol Pharmacol. 2001;52:53–70.
18. McKenzie EC, Jose-Cunilleras E, Hinchcliff KW, Holbrook TC, Royer C, Payton ME, et al. Serum chemistry alterations in Alaskan sled dogs during five successive days of prolonged endurance exercise. J Am Vet Med Assoc. 2007;230:1486–92. doi:10.2460/javma.230.10.1486.
19. James FE, Mansfield CS, Steiner JM, Williams DA, Robertson ID. Pancreatic response in healthy dogs fed diets of various fat compositions. Am J Vet Res. 2009;70:614–8. doi:10.2460/ajvr.70.5.614.
20. Furr M, Taylor L, Kronfeld D. The effects of exercise training on serum gastrin responses in the horse. Cornell Vet. 1994;84:41–5.
21. Wallace JL, Granger DN. The cellular and molecular basis of gastric mucosal defense. FASEB J. 1996;10:731–40.
22. Markiewicz K, Cholewa M, Lukin M. Gastric basal secretion during exercise and restitution in patients with chronic duodenal ulcer. Acta Hepatogastroenterol (Stuttg). 1979;26:160–5.
23. Feldman M, Nixon JV. Effect of exercise on postprandial gastric secretion and emptying in humans. J Appl Physiol Respir Environ Exerc Physiol. 1982;53:851–4.
24. Kondo T, Naruse S, Hayakawa T, Shibata T. Effect of exercise on gastroduodenal functions in untrained dogs. Int J Sports Med. 1994;15:186–91. doi: 10.1055/s-2007-1021045.
25. Williamson KK, Willard MD, McKenzie EC, Royer CM, Payton ME, Davis MS. Efficacy of famotidine for the prevention of exercise-induced gastritis in racing Alaskan sled dogs. J Vet Intern Med. 2007;21:924–7.
26. Williamson KK, Willard MD, Payton ME, Davis MS. Efficacy of omeprazole versus high-dose famotidine for prevention of exercise-induced gastritis in racing Alaskan sled dogs. J Vet Intern Med. 2010;24:285–8. doi:10.1111/j.1939-1676.2009.0454.x.
27. Davis MS, Willard MD, Nelson SL, McCullough SM, Mandsager RE, Roberts J, et al. Efficacy of omeprazole for the prevention of exercise-induced gastritis in racing Alaskan sled dogs. J Vet Intern Med. 2003;17:163–6.
28. Parente NL. Bari Olivier N, Refsal KR, Johnson CA. Serum concentrations of gastrin after famotidine and omeprazole administration to dogs. J Vet Intern Med. 2014;28:1465–70. doi:10.1111/jvim.12408.
29. Snow DH, Rose RJ. Hormonal changes associated with long distance exercise. Equine Vet J. 1981;13:195–7.
30. Angle CT, Wakshlag JJ, Gillette RL, Stokol T, Geske S, Adkins TO, et al. Hematologic, serum biochemical, and cortisol changes associated with anticipation of exercise and short duration high-intensity exercise in sled dogs. Vet Clin Pathol. 2009;38:370–4. doi:10.1111/j.1939-165X.2009.00122.x.
31. Hinchcliff KW, Reinhart GA, Burr JR, Schreier CJ, Swenson RA. Metabolizable energy intake and sustained energy expenditure of Alaskan sled dogs during heavy exertion in the cold. Am J Vet Res. 1997;58:1457–62.
32. McConkey B. C reactive protein concentrations during long distance running. Br Med J (Clin Res Ed). 1984;289:1696.
33. Burr JR, Reinhart GA, Swenson RA, Swaim SE, Vaughn DM, Bradley DM. Serum biochemical values in sled dogs before and after competing in long-distance races. J Am Vet Med Assoc. 1997;211:175–9.
34. Otabe K, Ito T, Sugimoto T, Yamamoto S. C-reactive protein (CRP) measurement in canine serum following experimentally-induced acute gastric mucosal injury. Lab Anim. 2000;34:434–8.
35. Mordecai A, Sellon RK, Mealey KL. Normal dogs treated with famotidine for 14 days have only transient increases in serum gastrin concentrations. J Vet Intern Med. 2011;25:1248–52. doi:10.1111/j.1939-1676.2011.00826.x.
36. Behrend EN, Kemppainen RJ, Young DW. Effect of storage conditions on cortisol, total thyroxine, and free thyroxine concentrations in serum and plasma of dogs. J Am Vet Med Assoc. 1998;212:1564–8.
37. Doumatey AP, Zhou J, Adeyemo A, Rotimi C. High sensitivity C-reactive protein (Hs-CRP) remains highly stable in long-term archived human serum. Clin Biochem. 2014;47:315–8. doi:10.1016/j.clinbiochem.2013.12.014.
38. Li Q, Kang T, Tian X, Ma Y, Li M, Richards J, et al. Multimeric stability of human C-reactive protein in archived specimens. PLoS One. 2013;8:e58094. doi:10.1371/journal.pone.0058094.

12

Risk factors associated with diarrhea in Danish commercial mink (*Neovison vison*) during the pre-weaning period

Julie Melsted Birch[1*], Jens Frederik Agger[1], Christina Dahlin[1], Vibeke Frøkjær Jensen[2], Anne Sofie Hammer[1], Tina Struve[3] and Henrik Elvang Jensen[1]

Abstract

Background: Pre-weaning diarrhea in mink, also known as "sticky kits", is a syndrome and outbreaks occur every year on commercial mink farms in all mink producing countries. Morbidity and mortality can be considerable on a farm with huge economic consequences for the farmer as well as compromised welfare for the mink kits. Although efforts have been taken to identify etiologic agents involved in outbreaks, the syndrome is still regarded as multifactorial and recurring problems on the same farms draw attention to management and environmental risk factors. In the pre-weaning period from May to June 2015, a case control study was carried out on 30 Danish mink farms. Data concerning management, biosecurity, hygiene, feed consumption, antibacterial prescription and production efficiency were analyzed.

Results: The proportion of 1-year old females, farm size (total number of females), energy supply per female in the late gestation period, and dogs accessing the farm area were significantly associated with being a case farm. Case farms were prescribed almost twice the amount of antibacterials per gestational unit (female and litter) as in control farms. Farmers on case farms spent significantly more time nursing and treating the animals and experienced more females with mastitis compared to farmers on control farms. No significant differences in cleaning practices or hygienic measures between case and control farms were found and there were no differences in drinking water quality, bedding material, composition neither of color types nor in management regarding litter equalization.

Conclusions: Results from this study showed an association between the occurrence of pre-weaning diarrhea on mink farms and parity profile, farm size and feeding intensity in the gestational period. The access of dogs to the farm area was a significant risk factor, but needs further clarification.

Keywords: "Sticky kits", "Wet kits", Wet kit syndrome, "Greasy kits", Risk factors, Farm level

Background

Diarrhea in the pre-weaning period of mink also known as "sticky kits", "wet kits" or "greasy kits" is a syndrome, which has been known in Denmark for more than 60 years [1]. Clinical signs are characterized by diarrhea and the appearance of a sticky exudate starting in the neck region, which to a variable extend may spread over the trunk and legs. Greasy, black claws maybe an early sign of the syndrome (Fig. 1). In fulminant, prolonged cases the perineal region becomes edematous and dehydration may develop together with a distressed vocalizing behavior [2].

Whole mink litters are affected and the morbidity rate vary from zero to more than 30% of the litters with a mortality of typically one or two kits per litter [3]. The syndrome is rather common in all mink producing countries although the number of farms and the severity of outbreaks vary from year to year [3]. The economic consequences for the mink farmers can

*Correspondence: jubi@sund.ku.dk
[1] Department of Veterinary and Animal Sciences, Faculty of Health and Medical Sciences, University of Copenhagen, Ridebanevej 3, 1870 Frederiksberg C, Denmark
Full list of author information is available at the end of the article

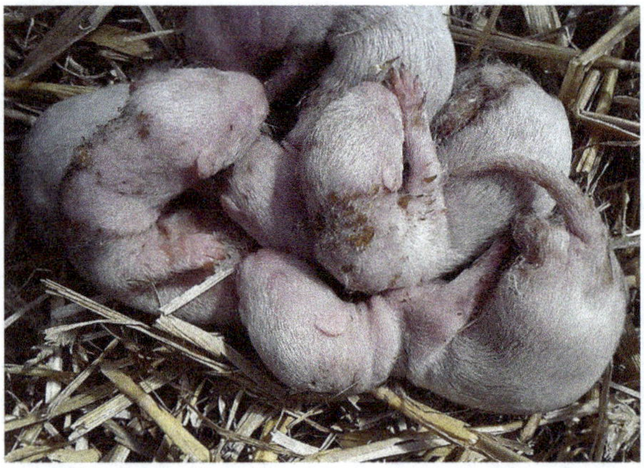

Fig. 1 A mink kit litter affected by pre-weaning diarrhea and a greasy/sticky appearance

be considerable due to cost for treatment and increased mortality. Efforts have been taken to identify etiologic microorganisms from outbreaks of pre-weaning diarrhea. *Staphylococcus delphini* and *Escherichia coli* have among other bacteria been incriminated as the causes of "sticky kits". However, mustelids are natural hosts of *S. delphini* group A and it has not been possible to link certain sero-groups of *E. coli* to pre-weaning diarrhea [4–6]. Mink astrovirus (MiAstV) and calicivirus were found to be associated with pre-weaning diarrhea [7] and rota- and coronavirus have been detected in mink kit feces in both healthy and "sticky" kits [5, 8]. Thus, the syndrome is still regarded as multifactorial and different studies have been carried out to identify risk factors in management, feed, milk composition and animals [2]. Henriksen [8] was of the opinion that some feed kitchens were associated with a higher frequency of the syndrome than other feed kitchens, and the morbidity increased with high humidity, temperatures, population density and poor hygiene. In other studies no significant effect of poor hygiene was present, but problems with "sticky kits" were significantly associated with diarrhea later in the growing season, and the problems had a tendency to recur at the farm the following year [9]. Studies on litter level revealed an almost four times increased risk of getting "sticky kits" in young wild type mink females compared to older females [10]. Also large, late born litters and litters from primiparous females were at a greater risk of having "sticky kits" [3, 10]. A higher frequency with pre-weaning diarrhea was seen on large farms compared to small farms and farms with occurrence of pre-weaning diarrhea had a lower feed consumption in late April and recurrent problems in the next season [11, 12]. In addition, females, which had been restricted fed for a prolonged period before birth, had a significant greater risk of having sticky kits/pre-weaning diarrhea in the kits [10]. Individual management practices for the farms include practices of litter equalization, introduction of new breeding dams, hygiene measures as well as biosecurity initiatives, which have not been fully studied. The aim of this study was to identify possible management risk factors on farm level concerning aspects of housing, hygiene, biosecurity and energy supply per female in late gestation for being a farm with outbreak of pre-weaning diarrhea. Secondarily, we also wanted to clarify the prescription patterns of antibacterials and some production efficiency parameters on farms with and without outbreaks of pre-weaning diarrhea.

Methods

Study design and participating farms

A case–control study was carried out from the 11th of May to weaning at the end of June 2015 on Danish commercial mink farms (n = 30). The first cases of pre-weaning diarrhea usually occur when mink kits are around two weeks of age, i.e. within the first 2 weeks of May. Since there was no surveillance system for this disease, and because farmers detected cases of diarrhea during their daily work, it was necessary for the investigation team to have pre-arranged agreements with a number of farmers (n = 53). Thus, from this group 15 farms, with a previous history of outbreak of pre-weaning diarrhea, called our investigation team for a visit when onset of pre-weaning diarrhea started, and these farms were designated "expected case farms". Concurrently, 15 farms, without a previous history of outbreaks of pre-weaning diarrhea, were randomly selected from the group of pre-arranged farms (n = 53) among farms, which received feed from the same feed kitchen in order to eliminate an effect of the feed composition and quality. These farms were designated "expected control farms". After June 2nd, no more farms contacted us concerning outbreaks. At weaning at the end of June, the percentage of affected litters recorded by the mink farmers was used to determine the final case–control status of the farms. Case farms (n = 14) were defined as farms having 13–77% affected litters during the period, whereas control farms (n = 16) were defined as farms with <8% affected litters. Thus, one expected control farm changed status and became a case farm, whereas two expected case farms appeared to have such limited problems (<8% affected litters), that they were re-categorized as control farms. The rest of the included farms (n = 27) kept their expected status. Since the incidence rate of pre-weaning diarrhea varies from year to year on farms, and the prediction of which farms will be affected is uncertain, sample size calculations were not possible.

Farm data

Farm data were obtained at visits on the farms and from face-to-face interviews with the mink farmers. The interviews were performed by using standardized questionnaires. Follow-up telephone interviews were made with the mink farmers after weaning. Farm data included: size of farm, production efficiency (fraction of barren females, total number of kits observed after birth, total number of weaned kits), composition of animals (color, age, newly introduced), housing (type of shed, types of litter material, use of wind shield, type of roof on the nest boxes, water source), management (man-hours used on nursing per 1000 females, litter equalization practice, replacement of litter material, use of feed additives, etc.), and hygiene and biosecurity initiatives (cleaning practice between and during seasons, change of clothes and boots for employers and visitors before entrance to the farm, hygiene practice when handling litters, access of dogs and cats to the farm, redistribution of feed left-overs, and flea prophylaxis). The variables farm size, percentage of 1-year old females, and percentage of females with mastitis recorded by the mink farmer were dichotomized. Likewise the color type composition was grouped into light (light and gray) or dark (black and brown). Cleaning of nest boxes and cages was recorded as performed if high pressure washer, water and soap or flaming were used.

Drinking water analysis

On each farm, a water sample from the drinking water system was collected from the end of two randomly selected mink sheds. The samples were stored, transported and analyzed according to the recommendations by Analyselaboratoriet, Dansk Pelsdyr Foder a.m.b.a., Denmark. The drinking water samples were categorized as above human limit value if one of the samples showed a total germ counts above 200/mL, fluorescence germ counts above 5/mL, coliform bacteria count above 0/100 mL, or thermo stabile coli count above 0/100 mL.

Feeding

The average feed energy supply per female was based on data from the feed kitchens. It was daily recorded how many kilograms of feed there had been delivered to the farm. The daily delivery in kilograms from week 14 to week 19 (corresponding to the late gestation period) was summed up per week and divided by the total number of animals (females and males if any) on the farm in that particular week. To compensate for differences in energy content in the feed from the supplying feed kitchens, results from regular quality test samples from each kitchen and feed plan were used to calculate the average energy content in a particular week. The results from the test samples were obtained from the Danish Fur Feed [13].

Antibiotic prescription

In Denmark, each farm has a six digit identity code in the Central Husbandry Register (CHR) [14]. This farm ID was used to merge data from different sources. Data on all prescriptions of antibacterial medicines from March 1 to July 1 2015 were extracted from the national veterinary prescription database, VetStat [15]. Vetstat is considered to cover more than 99% of the total amounts of antibacterials for veterinary use in Denmark (DANMAP 2001) [16]. In VetStat, each prescription is represented by a record, including information on date of purchase, product identity and quantity, farm ID, target animal species, target age group, target disease category, and the identity of the prescribing veterinarian.

All prescribed antibacterials exclusive those for topical use were included. In order to compare amounts of different kinds of antibacterials, the amounts of each antibacterial was converted into number of Defined Animal Daily Doses for treatment of 1 kg of mink ($DADD_{kg}$), as previously described [17].

Statistical analyses

The data were entered into MS Excel and transferred to SAS Enterprise Guide 7.1 (SAS Institute Inc.2014). Initially the coding and distribution was checked for each variable. Then bivariate analyses of all explanatory variables in relation to the case control status was performed and judged statistically by Student's t-test (for continuous variables) or Chi square/Fisher's exact test (for categorical variables) and judged epidemiologically by odds ratio (OR) estimation. Finally, multivariable analyses using the Mantel–Haenszel procedure and logistic analysis for all variables with a $P < 0.05$ in the bivariate analyses was performed. The reason for only including explanatory variables with a $P < 0.05$ was due to the small sample size of only 30 farms. The logistic analyses was conducted with proc logistic in SAS with the binary distributed case control status linked to the explanatory variables using the logit function ($\text{logit}(P) = \ln[p/(1-P)]$). Model fit was evaluated using the likelihood ratio test. We used manual model-building guided by a causal diagram with evaluation of confounding and interaction. We used the Type 3 Chi square test to evaluate significance of the contribution of each explanatory variable in the model.

Results

Descriptive analyses

Farm size varied between 890 and 16,327 females. There were no differences in the percentage of barren females in the two groups, no significant difference in number of kits/female (mated or breeding) and the average number of weaned kits/breeding female in the case group was 5.6 compared to 6.1 in the control group, which was not significant ($P = 0.2$).

The time used on care and treatment of the mink litters varied significantly. On case farms, 6.1 h/1000 females and on control farms 3.8 h/1000 females were spent ($P < 0.01$). Figure 2 illustrates the prescription pattern for antibacterials in case farms compared to control farms. Case farms were also prescribed more antibacterials per female (gestational unit) than control farms. The prescription was under 6 $DADD_{kg}$/breeding female for both case and control farms until 11th of May after which an increase was seen for both case and control farms. From 8th of June until weaning the prescription still increases but the rate was somewhat the same between the groups. For the whole period, case farms were prescribed 54 $DADD_{kg}$/breeding female compared to control farms which were prescribed 34 $DADD_{kg}$/breeding female.

Housing

The risk of being a case farm increased by farm size, i.e. if it was above the median ($OR = 5.5$, $P < 0.05$). No differences was found in type of shed, bedding material, type of roof on the nest boxes, use of wind shields on the nest boxes or in the drinking water source (private or public).

Composition of animals

Figure 3 illustrates the distribution of 1-year old females in relation to the frequency of affected litters. The odds of being a case farm increased with increasing proportion of 1-year old females ($OR = 5.9$, $P < 0.05$). There were no differences in the proportion of newly introduced animals or in the color compositions of the animals.

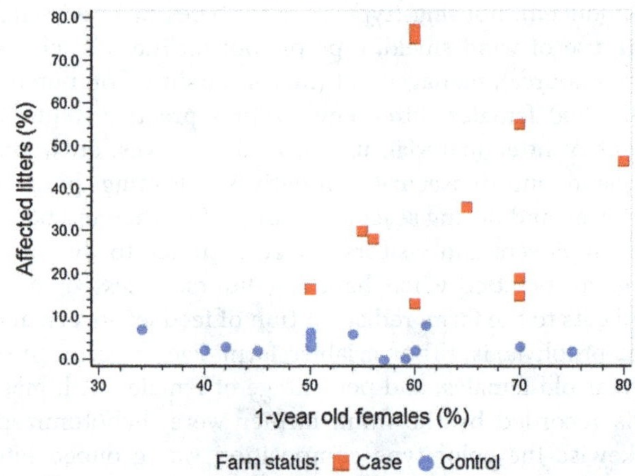

Fig. 3 Association between pct. 1-year old females and pct. affected litters with case control status

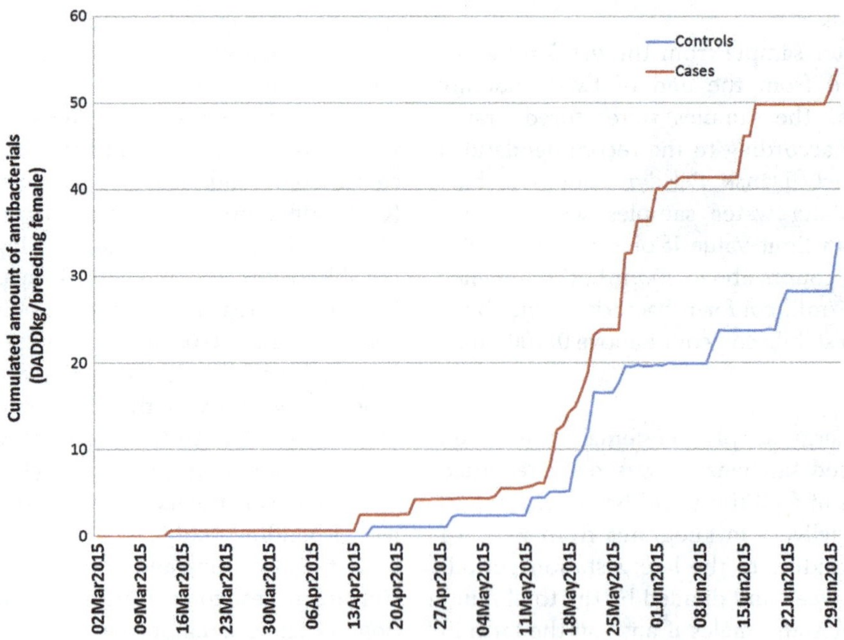

Fig. 2 Cumulated amount of prescribed antibacterials for case and control farms

Feeding

The average weekly energy delivered per female was lower in week number 17 in the case farms (839 kJ) compared to the control farms (957 kJ) ($P < 0.01$). In week number 18, the females on case farms received 758 kJ compared to females on control farms which received 842 kJ and the difference was significant ($P = 0.05$). In all the other weeks, females on case farms received less energy than females on control farms, but the difference was not significant. There was a tendency of general declining energy supply in the late gestation from week 14 to week 18 and then it increased again in week 19. Figure 4 shows the energy supply per female on a weekly basis and mean values are listed in Table 1.

The accumulated energy supply per female from week 14 to week 19 was 42,074 ± 5970 and 45,025 ± 3156 kJ for case and control farms, respectively ($P = 0.11$). The accumulated energy supply per female in week 17–18 was significantly lower ($P < 0.01$) in case farms compared to control farms with an accumulated energy per female of 11,183 ± 1580 and 12,597 ± 1185 kJ, respectively, for case and control farms.

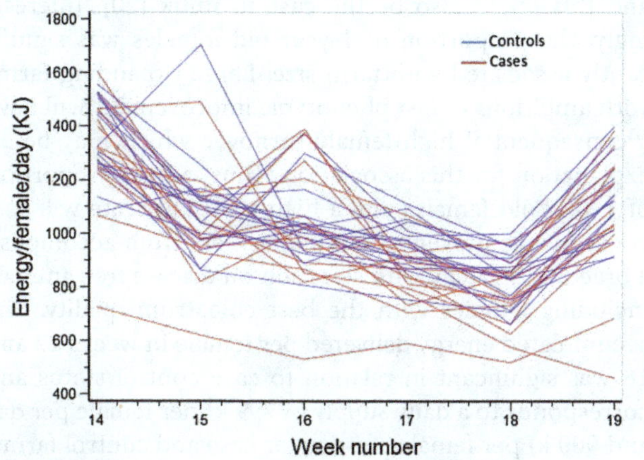

Fig. 4 Energy supply per female in April and May 2015 for case and control farms

Table 1 Feed energy supply per mink female per day (kJ)

Period	Case farms (n = 14)	Control farms (n = 16)
Week 14	1307 ± 219	1360 ± 150
Week 15	1023 ± 198	1099 ± 194
Week 16	1019 ± 235	1034 ± 143
Week 17**	839 ± 119	957 ± 95
Week 18*	758 ± 128	842 ± 99
Week 19	1063 ± 248	1139 ± 145

Mean values ± standard deviation

** $P < 0.01$; * $P = 0.05$

Management

No difference in how litter-equalization was used between case and control farms was found. Moreover, no difference was seen in how the mink farmers changed the nest bedding in healthy and diseased litters. None of the farms used water supplementation on the nest boxes during the early pre-weaning period or at the time of pre-weaning diarrhea.

Hygiene

Dogs' access to the farm area increased the risk ($OR = 9.3$, $P < 0.05$) of being a case farm. No associations were revealed in hygiene precautions such as use of boot cover, changing clothes before entering the farm or use of gloves or hand disinfectant between handling of mink litters in case farms compared to control farms. Neither could an association between farm status and the practice of redistribution of feed left-overs be seen. Drinking water quality was not a risk factor for farm status, and no association between flea prophylaxis and farm status was found.

The bivariate analyses are shown in detail in Additional file 1.

Multivariable analyses

Farm size was associated with the proportion of 1-year old females ($OR = 5.6$, $P < 0.05$) and large farms had an increased proportion of 1-year old females compared to small farms (Fig. 5). Hence, farm size was a confounder for the proportion of 1-year old females. Adjusted for farm size by Mantel–Haenszel analysis still gave a positive OR (=3.7), but it was no longer significant ($P = 0.32$).

The following four risk factors (1) access of dogs to the farm area (yes/no), (2) farm size (>/< median of 3461 females), (3) proportion of 1-year old females (>/<57%)

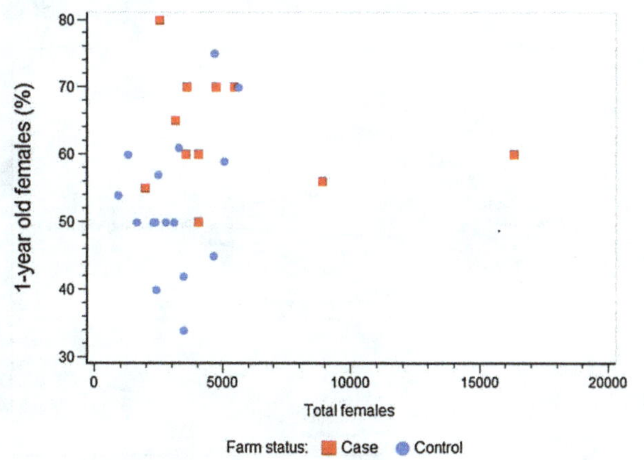

Fig. 5 Association between farm size and pct. 1-year old females with case control status

and (4) the accumulated energy supply per female in weeks 17–18 (>/<12,196 kJ) were chosen to multivariable analysis by logistic regression. Two models showed to be significant ($P < 0.05$) and one nearly significant ($P = 0.06$) (Fig. 6). In Model A comprising farm size and dogs' access to the farm area, the odds of being a case farm were higher for large farms compared to small farms, given dogs' access to the farms were held constant ($OR = 6.4$, $P < 0.05$). The odds of being a case farm were also higher for farms with dogs' access to farm area compared to farms, where dogs were not allowed to enter, ($OR = 10.7$, $P < 0.05$) if farm size were held constant. In model B comprising proportion of 1-year old females and dogs' access to the farm area, the odds of being a case farm increased if the farm had more than 57% 1-year old females compared to farms having less than 57% 1 year old females ($OR = 10$, $P < 0.05$), given dogs' access were held constant. The odds of being a case farm increased also if dogs were allowed access compared to farms where dogs didn't have access to the farm area ($OR = 19.6$, $P < 0.05$), given the proportion of 1-year old females were held constant. Model C comprised farm size and accumulated energy supply per female in weeks 17–18. There was an almost significant effect of farm size ($OR = 5.1$, $P = 0.06$) given the accumulated energy supply in weeks 17–18 were held constant. Farms supplying less than 12,196 kJ per female in weeks 17–18 also had a nearly significant increase in odds of being a case farm compared to farms giving more than 12,196 kJ per female ($OR = 5.1$, $P = 0.06$), when farm size were held constant.

Discussion

The case–control status could be explained by three multivariable models. A single model with more than two variables was not possible to fit due to too few observations.

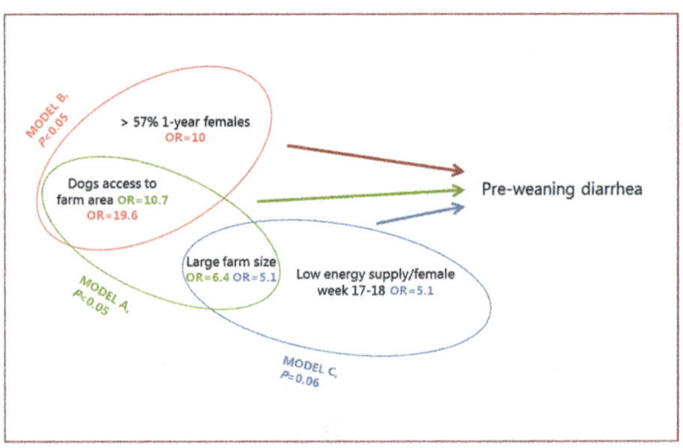

Fig. 6 Multivariable models for risk factors associated with case control status of pre-weaning diarrhea

Dogs' access to the farm area contributed to two of the models, which may reflect that dogs are carriers of microorganisms involved in the pre-weaning diarrhea syndrome. Another explanation is that dogs' access to the farm area was a proxy for other management of biosecurity and hygiene, meaning that farmers allowing dogs on the farm had a more relaxed approach to biosecurity and hygiene in general. Farm size was a risk factor in two of the multivariable models, which was also found in a study of pre-weaning diarrhea in pigs [18]. However herd size and herd density can be measured in different ways and the primary factor that produces the herd size effect may be found in management and environmental factors and can be protective as well [19]. The proportion of 1-year old females on the farm was a significant risk factor in bivariate analysis as well as in the multivariable analysis. This finding is in line with previous studies conducted on litter level [3, 10]. This might be explained by poorer nursing skills in the primiparous females or a poorer passive immunity transfer from young females to the kits compared to older females. A Norwegian study in dairy cows showed that cows in their fourth parity or more had significantly higher levels of IgG in the colostrum compared to cows in their first or second parity, and this might also be the case in mink [20]. Interestingly, the proportion of 1-year old females was significantly associated with farm size. Large expanding farms with ambitions of fast phenotypic improvement will have a consequential high female turnover which may be an explanation for this association. Thus, a high proportion of 1-year old females and a high morbidity rate will as a consequence prevent the mink farmers from accomplish a breeding strategy with selection on disease free animals including females with the best colostrum quality. The accumulated energy delivered per female in weeks 17 and 18 was significant in relation to case control status and corresponds to a daily supply of 799 kJ per female per day and 900 kJ per female per day for case and control farms, respectively. Hyperleptinemia in the pregnant mink may exert anorexigenic effects in the second but especially the last trimester resulting in a declining energy uptake and negative energy balance [21]. Some of the general declining energy consumption in the last gestation period is therefore due to a natural decline in appetite among the females. However there is no obvious reason why females on case farms should consume less than females on the control farms. Therefore, the mink farmers had restricted the minks' energy intake, perhaps in an attempt to get more active females prior to birth. The results is supported by other studies in which restricted feeding during the gestation period was found to be a risk factor for pre-weaning diarrhea in mink kits [10, 22]. Based on these studies, a critical limit of 879 kJ per female per day was suggested [23]. With considerable variation in weather, quality of insulation in nest boxes and management on the farms added to a tendency of increasing animal size, energy consumption and safety limits should continuously be evaluated. Mastitis as a triggering factor for "sticky kits" has been suggested [8].

Mastitis was indeed a concurrent problems in many of the farms, however mastitis was not found to be a necessary cause for the development of "greasy kits" [24]. Incidences of mastitis above 10% was a risk factor of being a case farm, but diagnosing "mastitis" was mainly done by the staff on the farm when appetite in the female ceased and imply difficulties owing to the fact that mastitis in mink often is subclinical [24]. Mastitis in the female may, however, still be a risk factor in a multifactorial disease complex, but further studies are needed to clarify this. Besides dogs' access to the farm area, no association to hygiene or biosecurity precautions was found. However, an explanation for the lack of proof for good practice of hygiene and biosecurity could be that the etiologic agents involved in pre-weaning diarrhea is very common in the animals during this period, and the cause should be searched for in a more generalized debility of the females and kits.

The pattern in antibacterial prescription showed that case and control farms were prescribed antibacterials before the onset on pre-weaning diarrhea, and the rapid increase from 11 to 18th of May until 8th of June corresponds very well with the period of outbreaks of pre-weaning diarrhea. The largest difference in prescription rate between the two groups was seen from 25th of May to 8th of June after which time outbreaks of pre-weaning diarrhea usually cease in Denmark [11, 25]. The fact that case farms were prescribed more antibacterials prior to the onset of pre-weaning diarrhea must reflect farm history based expectations of more problems on case farms compared to control farms. Prescription of antibacterials has increased during recent years in Danish mink farms and associated with herd size, season and the laboratory diagnosis of MiAstV [17]. The results from this study suggest that further investigation should focus on young females, and consultants of farms with recurrent problems of pre-weaning diarrhea should pay attention to parity profile and feeding strategies especially on large farms.

Conclusions

Associations between farm size, parity profile, energy supply in late gestation and farm status was revealed. Also dogs accessing the farm area was a risk factor. The study did not find any other associations in hygiene practices, housing or in management between case and control farms. Antibacterial prescription was higher and staff spent more time nursing and treating the animals on case farms compared to control farms.

Authors' contributions

JMB designed and planned the study, designed and conducted the interviews, collected data, performed all data analyses and drafted the manuscript. JFA participated in planning the study and the statistical and epidemiological analyses. CD participated in designing and conducting the face-to face interviews. VFJ collected and analyzed the data regarding antibacterial consumption. ASH, TS and HEJ participated in conceiving and planning the study. All authors read and approved the final manuscript.

Author details

[1] Department of Veterinary and Animal Sciences, Faculty of Health and Medical Sciences, University of Copenhagen, Ridebanevej 3, 1870 Frederiksberg C, Denmark. [2] National Veterinary Institute, Technical University of Denmark, Kemitorvet, 2800 Kongens Lyngby, Denmark. [3] Kopenhagen Diagnostics, Kopenhagen Fur, Langagervej 60, 2600 Glostrup, Denmark.

Acknowledgements

The authors would like to thank all the farmers participating in the study for the time and effort they put into the interviews and to the Danish feed kitchens providing data about feed consumption. Grateful acknowledgements should be given to the Danish veterinarians with relations to the participating farms for sharing their experiences about pre-weaning diarrhea and especially thanks to Anabelle Jakobsen participating and helping with the farm visits.

Competing interests

The authors declare that they have no competing interests.

Funding

The authors disclosed receipt of the following financial support for the research, authorship and/or publication of this article: this work was cofunded by Pelsdyrafgiftsfonden, Pelsdyrenes Forskningsfond and the Innovation Fund Denmark.

References

1. Svennekjær NC. Minksygdomme og aktuelle problemer i minkavlen (mink diseases and current problems in mink farming). Dansk Pelsdyravl. 1954;17:384–404.
2. Clausen TN, Dietz HH. Wet kits in mink: a review. Scientifur. 2004;28:87–90.
3. Olesen CR, Hansen M, Clausen TN. Fedtede hvalpe—risikofaktorer og årsagssammenhænge ("Sticky kits" risk factors and causality). Dansk Pelsdyravl. 1992;55:170–2.
4. Sledge DG, Danieu PK, Bolin CA, Bolin SR, Lim A, Anderson BC, et al. Outbreak of neonatal diarrhea in farmed Mink Kits (*Mustella vison*) associated with enterotoxigenic *Staphylococcus delphini*. Vet Pathol. 2010;47:751–7.
5. Jørgensen M, Scheutz F, Strandbygaard B. *Escherichia coli* and virus isolated from "sticky kits". Acta Vet Scand. 1996;37:163–9.
6. Guardabassi L, Schmidt KR, Petersen TS, Espinosa-Gongora C, Moodley A, Agersø Y, et al. Mustelidae are natural hosts of *Staphylococcus delphini* group A. Vet Microbiol. 2012;159:351–3.
7. Englund L, Chriél M, Dietz HH, Hedlund K-O. Astrovirus epidemiologically linked to pre-weaning diarrhoea in mink. Vet Microbiol. 2002;85:1–11.
8. Henriksen P. En oversigt over syndromet "Fedtede hvalpe" hos mink (A review of the syndrome "sticky kits" in mink). Dansk VetTidsskr. 1987;70:580–3.
9. Rattenborg E, Dietz HH, Chriél M. Variationen i forekomsten af mave-tarmlidelser hos mink på forskellige niveauer samt enkeltfaktorers betydning på farmniveau (Variation in prevalence of gastro-intestinal diseases

in mink on different levels and single factors influence on farm level). Annual Report, Kopenhagen Research, Kopenhagen Fur. 1997; 185–9.
10. Chriél M. Lad minktæverne selv bestemme! (Let the mink females decide themselves). Dansk Pelsdyravl. 1997;60:196–8.
11. Olesen CR, Clausen TN. Fedtede hvalpe Resultater fra Forsøgsfarmen Vest 1989 ("Sticky kits" results from the investigation farm West 1989). Annual Report, Kopenhagen Research, Kopenhagen Fur. 1989; 154–64.
12. Børsting E. Sole Minkfoders feltundersøgelser over fedtede hvalpe (Sole mink feed field study of sticky kits). Annual Report, Kopenhagen Research, Kopenhagen Fur. 1997; 169–78.
13. Den Frivillige Foderkontrol Database (Voluntary feed control data base). Dansk Pelsdyr Foder a.m.b.a., Århus N. 2016. http://www.danskpelsdyr-foder.dk/Default.aspx?ID=7. Accessed 1 Aug 2016.
14. Det Centrale Husdyrbrugsregister. Danish Veterinary and Food Administration, Copenhagen. 2015. https://chr.fvst.dk/chri/faces/frontpage?_adf.ctrl-state=sz650pga1_31. Accessed 1 May 2015.
15. VetStat. Danish Veterinary and Food Administration, Copenhagen. 2015. https://www.foedevarestyrelsen.dk/Leksikon/Sider/VetStat.aspx. Accessed 1 Aug 2016.
16. Stege H, Bager F, Jacobsen E, Thougaard A. VetStat—The Danish system for surveillance of the veterinary use of drugs for production animals. Prev Vet Med. 2003;57:105–15.
17. Jensen VF, Sommer HM, Struve T, Clausen J, Chriél M. Factors associated with usage of antimicrobials in commercial mink (*Neovison vison*) production in Denmark. Prev Vet Med. 2016;126:170–82.
18. Dewey CE, Wittum TE, Hurd HS, Dargatz D, Hill GW. Diarrhea morbidity and mortality in piglets 4–14 days of age. Swine Health Prod. 1995;3:105–12.
19. Gardner IA, Willeberg P, Mousing J. Empirical and theoretical evidence for herd size as a risk factor for swine diseases. Anim Health Res Rev. 2002;3:43–55.
20. Gulliksen SM, Lie KI, Sølverød L, Østerås O. Risk factors associated with colostrum quality in Norwegian dairy cows. J Dairy Sci. 2008;91:704–12.
21. Tauson A-H, Forsberg M, Chwalibog A. High leptin in pregnant mink (*Mustela vison*) may exert anorexigenic effects: a permissive factor for rapid Increase in food intake during lactation. Br J Nutr. 2004;91:411–21.
22. Møller SH, Chriél M. Health Effects of the feeding stategies in the pre-mating and gestation periods of mink. Scientifur. 2000;24:37–41.
23. Møller SH. Management of health in mink. A HACCP plan for energy allowance during winter and gestation in order to control sticky kits. Scientifur. 2004;28:50–7.
24. Clausen TN, Dietz HH. Mastitis in the lactating mink female (*Mustela vison* S.) and the development of "Greasy Kits". Acta Vet Scand. 2000;41:243–7.
25. Hammer AS, Ullman K, Czifra G. Diarre i dieperioden IV: Astrovirus hos minkhvalpe—virologiske og patologiske fund i fedtede hvalpe indsendt til diagnostisk undersøgelse (Diarrhea in the pre-weaning period IV—Astrovirus infection in mink kits—viral and pathological findings in sticky kits submitted for diagnostic examination). Annual Report, Kopenhagen Research, Kopenhagen Fur. 2006; 165–70.

13

Do cats with a cranial cruciate ligament injury and osteoarthritis demonstrate a different gait pattern and behaviour compared to sound cats?

Sarah Stadig[1*], B. Duncan X. Lascelles[2,3] and Anna Bergh[4]

Abstract

Background: Osteoarthritis (OA) is a common cause of chronic pain and dysfunction in older cats. The majority of cats with OA do not show signs of overt lameness, yet cats with orthopaedic disease are known to redistribute their body weight from the affected limb. OA can cause changes in the cat's behaviour, which is often misinterpreted as signs of aging. The aim of the present study was to investigate if cats with a previous cranial cruciate ligament (CCL) injury perform differently on the pressure mat and exhibit different behaviour compared to sound cats according to the owner´s subjective assessment. Ten cats with a previous CCL injury were assessed with a pressure mat system and their owners were asked to complete an assessment questionnaire. The results were compared to those of 15 sound cats, matched to have the same weight and body condition score.

Results: The front/hind limb index for peak vertical force (PVF) was significantly higher for CCL cats, and there was a decreased PVF and vertical impulse (VI) on the affected hindlimb compared to the unaffected one. The results indicate that cats with a previous CCL injury put less weight, on the affected hindlimb but for a longer time. There was a significantly higher owner assessment questionnaire score for the group of cats with CCL injury compared to sound cats.

Conclusions: Cats with a previous CCL injury have a different gait pattern compared to sound cats and a different behaviour according to owner subjective assessment. It is of great importance that further studies are performed to investigate the long term effects of CCL injury as a cause of pain and physical dysfunction, and its role in the development of OA in cats. Improved assessment tools for chronic pain caused by OA in cats are needed, both to facilitate diagnosis and to evaluate pain-relieving treatment.

Keywords: Feline, Cranial cruciate ligament, Pain questionnaire, Owner assessment, Pressure mat technique

*Correspondence: sarah.stadig@slu.se
[1] Department of Clinical Sciences, Faculty of Veterinary Medicine and Animal Husbandry, Swedish University of Agricultural Sciences, PO Box 234, S532 23 Skara, Sweden
Full list of author information is available at the end of the article

Background

Appendicular joint osteoarthritis (OA) is a frequently occurring disease in older cats [1–5]. As in other mammals, it causes chronic pain and physical disability. It is a challenge to diagnose OA in cats since they appear to have an innate ability to disguise injury and disease, particularly in unfamiliar surroundings, such as the clinical examination room [6, 7]. Furthermore, the cat demonstrates non-specific clinical signs, such as being less active [1, 3, 8–10]. These findings are often misinterpreted as signs of normal aging.

Currently, the diagnosis of OA in the cat is based on a combination of information from the cat owner, the cat´s medical history, clinical examination and radiography. The results from radiography are not always consistent with the clinical findings from the orthopaedic examination [2, 11, 12]. Despite this inconsistency, radiographic imaging is still considered the primary diagnostic instrument for suspected OA in cats [3, 13, 14].

The majority of cats with OA do not show signs of overt lameness [2, 3, 5, 11], yet orthopaedic disease is known to cause a redistribution of body weight from the affected limb [15–17]. The lack of overt signs of lameness in the majority of cats may be due to the fact that there is multiple limb involvement in the majority of cases. Despite this fact, studies have shown that kinetic data generated using a pressure mat system can detect cats with an asymmetric gait pattern that may be associated with appendicular OA [18, 19]. In addition, the information that the cat owner provides regarding behavioural changes has been shown to make an important contribution to the diagnosis of OA [8, 9, 20–22].

Most cases of feline OA appear to be primary or idiopathic and the actual cause or aetiology can only be established in a small number of cases [1, 2]. Hardie et al. suggested that observed cases of OA were likely secondary to undetermined previous factors such as dysplasia, chronic low grade trauma or malarticulation [3]. However, these conclusions appear to be based on the aetiology of OA in dogs and may not be applicable in the cat. For example, recent information in cats has indicated that they do not appear to suffer from fragmented coronoid process, the most common cause of elbow OA in dogs [23]. In human patients, obesity is regarded as a predisposing factor for OA [24, 25]. This has not been established in the cat, although there is one study showing that heavier cats were more likely to be taken to the veterinarian because of lameness [26].

In the feline stifle joint, injury to the cranial cruciate ligament (CCL) has been shown to lead to OA. Transection of the CCL in cats has been used as a model to study the mechanisms behind traumatic joint injury and the degenerative response, eventually leading to OA. The altered joint mechanics have been shown to cause adaptive changes in the articular cartilage [27, 28], the periarticular bone [29], the muscle mass [27] and the vertical ground reaction forces of the affected hindlimb [27, 30].

However, little is known concerning the aetiology, clinical features and the outcome of treatment in feline CCL injury. Most published information on feline CCL disease is in the form of case reports describing various surgical stabilization techniques [31–39]. Some authors suggest two aetiologically different groups of CCL injuries, traumatic and degenerative [40, 41] and discuss whether obesity is a cause or a result of an injury. Furthermore, there is an ongoing discussion regarding the relative roles of obesity and CCL injury in the development of stifle OA. Consequently, there is a need for additional studies on cats with CCL injury and eventually secondary OA.

The aim of the present study was to investigate if cats with previous CCL injury perform differently on the pressure mat compared to sound cats, and whether they show behavioural changes according to an owner assessment questionnaire. The hypotheses were:

1. Cats with a previous CCL injury have more asymmetrical front/hind symmetry indices for peak vertical force (PVF) and vertical impulse (VI), compared to sound cats.
2. Cats with a previous CCL injury have a decreased PVF and VI on the affected hindlimb compared to the unaffected hindlimb.
3. Cats with a previous CCL injury have a different way of distributing the pressure under the paws, compared to sound cats.
4. Cats with a previous CCL injury have a different behaviour, compared to sound cats.

Methods

The participating CCL cats were privately owned pet cats recruited from the patient data base at the local animal hospital. The sound cats were selected from a previous dataset [42]. The study was approved by the local Ethical Review Board on Animal Experiments (no. C23/15). Prior to inclusion each cat owner signed an informed client consent form.

Animals

Cats with previous CCL injury

The inclusion criteria for the study were as follows:

- Age between 1 and 12 years old, of either sex, and any breed other than Scottish fold, with a previous diagnosis of unilateral CCL injury.
- Have results from haematology and serum biochemistry analyses (haemoglobin, albumin, total protein,

alanine transaminase (ALT), alkaline phosphatase (ALP), urea and creatinine) that are within the reference intervals of a healthy reference population of cats.

Exclusion criteria were as follows:

- Cats with gait disturbances caused by diseases other than a previous CCL injury in the affected stifle joint.
- Palpatory findings on clinical and orthopaedic examination of the musculoskeletal system of a larger magnitude then that from the affected stifle joint.
- Cats that were on any treatment for OA or other disease, with either a registered pharmaceutical or a supplement or a diet containing substances with alleged effect on OA.

Normal controls

Fifteen sound cats were selected from a previous dataset [42] to match the weight and body condition score of the cats with previous CCL injury. They were determined as sound based on their medical history, that is, without any disease or injury that could interfere with the study, on the clinical and orthopaedic examination, and from the results of the owner assessment questionnaire and a symmetrical gait based on pressure mat registrations [42].

Outcome measures

One owner-administered clinical metrology instrument (referred to as owner assessment questionnaire) and gait analysis from a pressure mat was used as outcome measures.

Owner assessment questionnaire

The owner filled out Bennet and Morton's owner assessment questionnaire [8, 22]. It is designed to identify changes within four behavioural domains (mobility, activity, grooming and temperament). The cat-owner marks whether the behaviour is normal or abnormal. If it is abnormal the owner is asked to rate the severity of the problem from 1 to 10. The owner is also asked to rate the overall severity of the problem from 1 (mild) to 10 (severe). The maximum score is 50, indicating an abnormal behaviour.

Pressure mat technique

The kinetic data were collected using a pressure sensitive walkway (Walkway High Resolution HRV4; Tekscan, South Boston, Massachusetts, USA). The portable mat measures 1.95 × 0.45 m and consists of a low profile floor mat (0.57 cm thick). The walkway was connected to a laptop computer (Siemens Fujitsu Lifebook, Hewlett Packard EliteBook) and data were analyzed using specific software provided by the manufacturer (Walkway 7.02). The mat was placed against a wall and transparent plexiglas screens, each 1.0 m long, were placed along the other side of the mat. The walkway was covered with a 1.0 mm thick plastic mat to avoid the slick surface, extending 0.3 m on either side of the end-/starting points for the sensors. The actual end-points of the walkway were demarcated with white tape. Prior to commencing data acquisition the walkway sensors were equilibrated and calibrated as recommended by the manufacturer. The data acquisition parameter was set to a frequency of 60 Hz, and each data movie was accompanied by a simultaneous video capture of the pass.

Study protocol

The study was performed in a quiet examination room used for feline gait analyses. The owners completed the assessment questionnaire in the same room. The cat was weighed on an electronic scale and allowed to acclimatize to the surroundings for 5–10 min before walking on the mat. The cat was encouraged to walk on the mat by being called, using toys or treats, or by placing the transport carrier at the end of the mat. Data collection continued until five valid trials were attained. A trial was considered valid when the cat walked in a straight line, at a visually even pace and with the head facing straight forward.

A complete clinical and orthopaedic examination of the axial and appendicular skeleton, including evaluation of muscle symmetry, was carried out on each cat, after pressure mat data collection. It was performed by the same veterinarian (SS) each time, who also evaluated the cat´s body condition score (BSC) according to a 5-point system [43] and a 9-point system [44]. The evaluation was made by palpating the ribs, lumbar vertebra and abdominal fat pad according to the written instructions for each scoring system. The cat was also visually inspected from above and from the side to evaluate its contour and absence or presence of a waist. This was then compared to the illustrations on each scoring system. The evaluator calibrated herself against both scoring systems every day they were used. The cats were screened for neurological conditions that could cause pain, gait abnormalities or other symptoms. Every joint was palpated for periarticular thickening, joint effusion and pain response to palpation. The joints were also examined for range of motion and joint stability. The results from the examination of the joints is presented (Table 1) as the cumulative assessment of each joint, graded as mild, moderate or severe.

After this procedure was concluded, a blood sample was taken from the cats. If the haematology and serum biochemistry analyses were normal, the cats were sedated with a combination of medetomidine and butorphanol. The joints that were found to be affected on the

Table 1 Clinical characteristics of cats with previous cranial cruciate ligament injury

Cat no	Age	Weight at exam	Time since injury (months)	Treatment	Visual gait assessment	Cumulative assessment joint examination	Summary of radiographic findings
1	12	5	30	L: S	Mildly stiff gait hind	R elbow mild changes, L stifle severe, hip bilateral and R stifle moderate changes	R stifle* mild to moderate OA, R tarsometatarsal joint suspected OA, both coxofemoral joints mild to moderate OA, R shoulder joint moderate to severe OA, L shoulder joint mild OA
2	11	4.6	88	R: S	Mildly increased hyperextension stifle joints bilateral	R stifle moderate changes, L stifle mild changes	R stifle moderate OA, L stifle minute changes, possible OA, but uncertain finding
3	9	4.5	22	R: S	Moves with increased width between hindlimbs	L stifle moderate changes, R stifle mild changes	L stifle moderate to severe OA, R stifle mild OA
4	12	3.5	2	L: S	Mild hyperextension L stifle joint, 1° lameness LH	L stifle moderate changes	Only presurgical radiographs
5	8	5.9	48	L: C	Mildly stiff gait hind, 1° lameness LH	L stifle moderate changes	L stifle moderate OA
6	10	5.4	3	R: C	Mildly stiff gait hind	L stifle moderate changes, R stifle mild changes	L and R stifle mild to moderate OA
7	8	5.6	4	L: C	Mildly stiff gait hind	R stifle mild changes	R stifle soft tissue findings, no radiographic OA
8	10	5.3	18	L: S	LH: shorter stride and mild hyperflexion stifle joint	L stifle moderate changes	R stifle moderate to severe OA, L stifle small uncertain finding, not OA, R coxofemoral joint moderate OA
9	8	4.2	24	L: S	LH mild hyperflexion stifle joint, 1° lameness LH	L stifle moderate changes	L stifle severe OA
10	7	6.8	7	L: C	Mildly stiff gait hind	L stifle moderate changes	L stifle moderate OA

Grading of findings: mild, moderate, severe. Lameness graded 0–5 according to American Association of Equine Practitioners (AAEP)

C conservative treatment, *L* left, *LH* left hind, *OA* osteoarthritis, *R* right, *S* surgical treatment

*Left stifle was not radiographed

orthopaedic examination were radiographed. Sedation was reversed with atipamezole. The sound cats went through the same procedure as the cats with previous CCL injury, apart from the blood sampling and radiographic examination.

Data analyses

The symmetry indices for front/hind PVF were calculated by dividing the average PVF of the two front feet by the PVF of the two hind feet. The left/right symmetry indices were calculate (with PVF left hind/right hind as an example) by taking the average of the PVF of all left hind foot stances, divided by the PVF of all right hind foot stances. This was done according to the manufacturer´s instructions by the software program (Walkway 7.02). The data was evaluated for normal distribution using normal probability plots for the residuals. Data was log-transformed in some cases where skewness was detected from residual plots. The kinetic variables calculated were peak vertical force (PVF) and vertical impulse (VI). These were expressed as a percentage of total bodyweight (%BW) with approximate 95 % confidence intervals. Difference in gait parameters was investigated using the freely-available statistical software, R [45] mixed linear models, with health status as fixed factor and cat as random factor. Since there was no statistical difference depending on whether the cats had their CCL injury on the left or right hind, these data were analysed together. When analysing the distribution of the vertical forces within a paw, measurements of PVF (%BW) and VI (%BW*sec) were obtained by dividing the paw print into four equally sized areas: craniolateral, craniomedial, caudolateral and caudomedial (Fig. 1, for further details see [42]). Data regarding age, weight and BCS are presented as mean (±standard deviation). ANOVA was used to compare inter-cat variability. The correlation between the parameters age, weight and BCS was analysed using intraclass correlation-coefficient [46]. Difference in Bennett's questionnaire was tested using Mann–Whitney's test. The level of significance was set at $P < 0.05$.

Results

Clinical characteristics

The clinical characteristics of the cats with previous CCL injury are presented in Table 1. Of the 10 cats, 70 % were domestic shorthair and 30 % were purebred (one British shorthair, one European shorthair and one Siberian cat). Six cats were male and four female; all were neutered or spayed. The average age was 9.5 (±1.8) years and the mean weight 5.1 (±0.9) kg. They had a BCS with a mean of 3.8 (±0.4) on a 5-point system [43] and a BCS of 6.6 (± 0.8) on a 9-point system [44]. All cats with previous CCL injury had palpable periarticular thickening of the affected stifle joint. A decreased range of motion (8/10), and muscle atrophy proximally of the affected stifle joint (8/10), were common findings on clinical examination. Few cats had joint crepitus (1/10) or palpable joint effusion (2/10). Most of the cats showed signs of pain on manipulation of the affected stifle joint, either on palpation of the actual joint (3/10) or at the extremes of the range of motion (8/10).

Of the 15 sound cats, 60 % were domestic shorthair and 40 % were purebred, the latter consisting of one Somali, two Ragdolls, two Burmese and one Norwegian forest cat. Nine were neutered males, four were spayed females and two were intact females. The average age was 5.9 (±3.3) years and the mean weight was 4.8 (±0.9) kg. They had a body condition score (BCS) of 3.7 ± 0.5 on a 5-point system [43] and a BCS of 6.5 (±0.9) on a 9-point system [44]. The cats were matched regarding BCS in order to avoid the possibility that the findings from the pressure mat were induced by overweight or obesity.

The cats with a previous CCL injury were significantly older than the sound cats (9.5 ± 1.8 years, and 5.9 ± 3.3 years respectively; $P = 0.006$). There was no significant difference in weight or BCS between the two groups of cats. There was no correlation between body weight, BCS and any of the gait parameters. Out of the ten cats with CCL injury, six were surgically (S) treated and four were conservatively (C) treated. The surgical method used was the same for five of the cats, the stifle joint being stabilized by lateral retinacular suture technique. In the remaining cat the stifle joint was stabilized with both medial and lateral retinacular sutures. Independently of the chosen treatment, the owners of all cats were advised to keep them in a restricted area, to enforce rest and, for most cats, to try to avoid jumping. Nine out of the ten cats were treated with meloxicam, one cat was

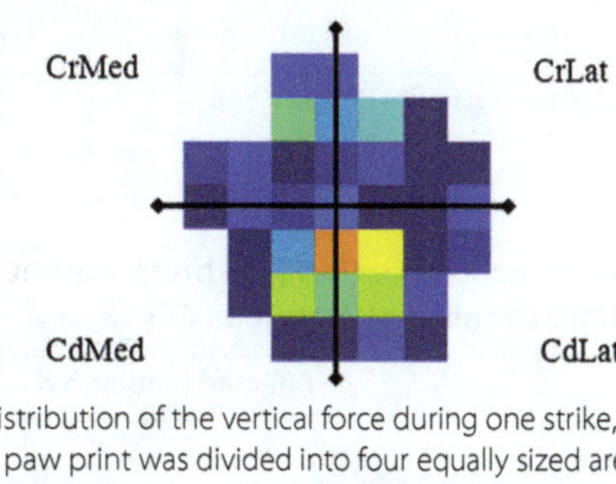

Fig. 1 Distribution of the vertical force during one strike, right front paw. The paw print was divided into four equally sized areas for analysis. Craniolateral (CrLat), Caudomedial (CdMed), Craniolateral (CrLat), Craniomedial (CrMed)

treated with tolfenamic acid in connection with the acute injury.

Pressure mat technique

Distribution of the vertical forces in the limbs

Variables from the pressure mat were analysed from two valid trails for each cat. These two trials were selected by looking at video captures and the pressure mat images on the software. The sound cats had a mean velocity of 0.68 (±0.16) m/s and the CCL cats had a mean velocity of 0.66 (±0.16) m/s. On average 10.9 (±2.0) strikes were analysed from the sound cats, and on average 11.4 (±2.8) strikes from the CCL cats. The results of the pressure distribution are presented in Tables 2 and 3. The affected limb is defined as the hindlimb with the predominant findings in the stifle joint at the orthopaedic exam, which is also the limb with the previous CCL injury. The unaffected limb is the hindlimb where the stifle joint has no or minor findings at the orthopaedic examination. The front/hind symmetry index for the variable PVF (%BW) was 1.4 (±0.1) for the cats with a previous CCL injury and 1.2 (±0.1) for the sound cats ($P = 0.001$). The symmetry index for the same variable on the contralateral front/hind limb pair, that is the limb pair on the opposite the side of the affected hind limb, was 1.68 (±0.29).

Distribution of the vertical forces in the paws

The results of pressure distribution within the paws are based on data from nine cats with previous CCL injury. The data from one cat were excluded due to polydactyly. The pressure distribution under the paws of the hindlimbs differed compared to sound cats (Fig. 2). There was no significant difference in VI (%BW). However, cats with a previous CCL injury had a significantly lower PVF (%BW) and a longer duration of stance phase, compared to sound cats. As previously reported, the cats with previous CCL injury increased the force in the vertical plane towards their forelimbs; however, the distribution within the front paws did not change significantly.

Owner assessment questionnaires

The maximum total score on the owner assessment questionnaire was 50. There was a significant difference in the total score between the cats with a previous CCL injury (9.9 ± 8.7) and the sound cats (1.1 ± 2.5) ($P < 0.031$).

Discussion

The hypotheses of the present study were essentially verified. Thus, cats with a previous CCL injury in the stifle joint showed:

- a higher front/hind symmetry index for PVF but not for VI,
- a decreased PVF and VI on the affected compared to the unaffected hindlimb,
- a different way of distributing the pressure under the paws, and
- a difference in behaviour according to the owner´s subjective assessment, compared to sound cats.

The redistribution of weight, from the affected to the unaffected limbs, registered in the present study may have several explanations. The asymmetry may be due to a mechanical factor, with a reduced ability to stabilise the stifle joint and thus a reduced willingness to put load on the affected hindlimb. This has been shown in both cats [27, 30] and dogs [47, 48] with CCL injuries. However, several factors probably contribute to the pressure asymmetry of the cats with previous CCL injury. Instability

Table 2 Peak vertical force (PVF) [% body weight (BW)] and vertical impulse (VI) (%BW*sec) for hindlimbs in cats with previous cranial cruciate ligament (CCL) injury and sound cats

Variable	Cats with CCL n = 10 (mean ± SD)	Sound cats n = 15 (mean ± SD)	P value
Peak vertical force (%BW)	22.4 ± 2.4	27.1 ± 3.6	0.0006
Vertical impulse (%BW*sec)	8.1 ± 1.7	8.2 ± 1.5	0.81

Data expressed as mean ± standard deviation (SD)

Table 3 Peak vertical force (PVF) [% body weight (BW)] and vertical impulse VI (%BW*sec) for the affected and the unaffected hindlimb of cats with previous CCL injury

Variable	Affected hindlimb n = 10 (mean ± SD)	Unaffected hindlimb n = 10 (mean ± SD)	P value
Peak vertical force (%BW)	21.9 ± 2.4	23.1 ± 2.3	0.0024
Vertical impulse (%BW*sec)	7.6 ± 1.5	8.8 ± 1.7	0.0009

Data expressed as mean ± standard deviation (SD)

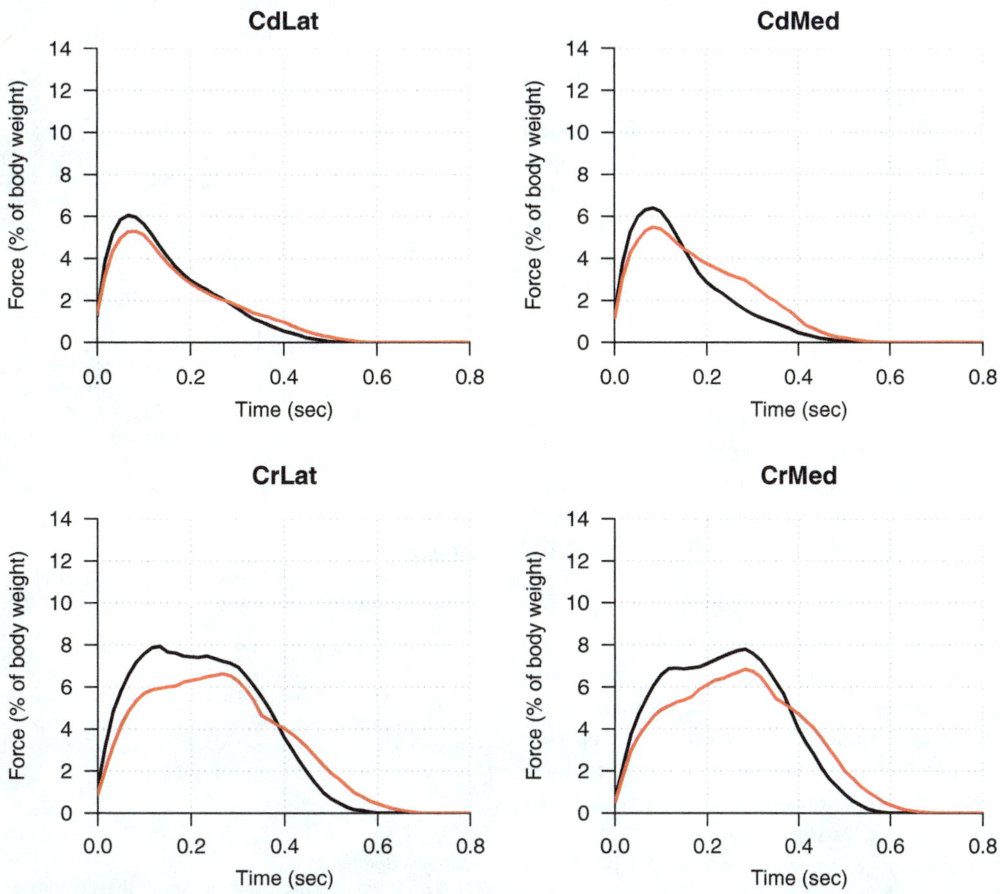

Fig. 2 Pressure distribution under the hind paws of 9 cats with a previous CCL injury (*red*) and 15 sound cats (*blue*). Vertical force [% body weight (BW)] vs time (sec) in each of the four quadrants of the hind paws. Craniolateral (CrLat), Caudomedial (CdMed), Craniolateral (CrLat), Craniomedial (CrMed)

of the stifle joint, muscle atrophy, altered proprioceptive ability and a modified gait pattern to avoid or minimise pain, are all likely to contribute. This is supported by the results from the clinical- and orthopaedic examination showing pain on manipulation, muscle mass atrophy and decreased joint range of motion. All the cats diagnosed with CCL were diagnosed by a positive drawer test in the stifle joint concerned. Since some cats had findings on the orthopaedic examination and/or radiographic findings in the contralateral stifle joint, it cannot be completely excluded that they had bilateral orthopaedic disease. Although the predominant findings from the orthopaedic exam were consistent with previous CCL injury, they were not always consistent with the radiographic findings. This discrepancy between clinical and radiographic findings is well known regarding OA. A limitation in studying feline osteoarthritis as a naturally occurring disease in privately owned cats, rather than experimentally induced OA, is that the cats are likely to have several joints affected by OA. The pressure mat has a limitation in detecting bilateral changes, but it is likely to detect alterations when looking at the distribution of the load on all four limbs.

Biomechanical disability and physical discomfort are both explanations for the differences in kinetic values, and the significant difference in PVF, however not in VI between the two groups. Our data suggest that cats with a previous CCL injury use the affected limb in such a way as to decrease the peak force, compensating with longer contact times compared to sound. The overall pressure will therefore be similar to that of sound cats, but it will be distributed differently over time. It is a natural reaction in order to reduce pain during the stance phase. This is also a likely explanation to the altered distribution of pressure within the paw. Our study showed a difference in the distribution of the vertical force between the affected and unaffected hindlimbs. Herzog et al. (1993) showed the same result in cats with transected CCL, registering the decrease in the ground reaction force of the affected hindlimb on a force plate [27]. However, in their study, the significant difference in weight distribution disappeared at 16 weeks after surgery. One possible explanation of the somewhat divergent results can be that their results were based on two cats of young age.

The owner assessment questionnaires showed a change in behaviour, with less physical activity compared to sound cats. The result from the questionnaire verifies that the cat owner can contribute with important information in the evaluation of normal and abnormal behaviour. However, further studies are needed to investigate the possibility of distinguishing between different levels of abnormality using the information obtained from the questionnaire.

The recruited cats with previous CCL injury were overweight, assessed by body condition scores. The present study cannot determine if the overweight was caused by, or was a consequence of, the OA. In order to reduce the measurement errors, the weights of the sound cats were matched to the one of the cats with previous CCL injury, since it is unknown if overweight in itself influences the gait pattern.

Currently, radiographic imaging is considered the primary diagnostic instrument for OA in cats, although the results might not be consistent with the findings from orthopaedic examination [3, 13, 14]. As in other species, cats can have radiological features of osteoarthritis and still have a pain-free joint, and it is possible to have osteoarthritis with severe damage to the synovial cartilage with no, or very few, radiographic signs [1, 9]. Our cats were recruited based on their medical history of CCL injury, and with a clinical suspicion of a secondary OA. Since risk factors for OA are old age and previous trauma, there is a possibility that the cats with a previous CCL injury had concurrent orthopaedic conditions that could have interfered with the results of the study. However, this is not likely, since the combined assessment during the study, with clinical and orthopaedic examination, owner assessment questionnaire, pressure mat registrations and radiographs, showed a unanimous result. Consequently, it is likely that the differences in the results of weight distribution and owner assessments are due to the cats' adaptation to biomechanical disability and/or joint pain caused by previous CCL injury and concomitant OA.

Conclusions

The present study show that cats with a previous CCL injury have different gait pattern and a difference in owner subjective assessment of behavior compared to sound cats. The cats redistributed their weight from the affected to the unaffected limbs. It is of great importance that further studies are performed to investigate the long term effects of CCL injury on pain and physical dysfunction and its role in the development of OA in cats. Improved assessment tools for chronic pain caused by OA in cats are needed, both to facilitate diagnostics and to evaluate pain relieving treatment.

Abbreviations

BCS: body condition score; BW: body weight; C: conservative treatment; CCL: cranial cruciate ligament; CdLat: caudolateral; CdMed: caudomedial; CrLat: craniolateral; CrMed: craniomedial; L: left; OA: osteoarthritis; PVF: peak vertical force; R: right; S: surgical treatment; SD: standard deviation; Sec: second; VI: vertical impulse.

Authors' contributions

SS and AB performed the design of the study, planned and performed the animal experiments. They also participated in analysis and interpretation of the results, drafted and submitted the manuscript. BDXL helped with planning of the experiment, interpreting the results and participated in drafting the manuscript. All authors read and approved the final manuscript.

Author details

[1] Department of Clinical Sciences, Faculty of Veterinary Medicine and Animal Husbandry, Swedish University of Agricultural Sciences, PO Box 234, S532 23 Skara, Sweden. [2] Comparative Pain Research, Department of Clinical Sciences, College of Veterinary Medicine, North Carolina State University, Raleigh, NC 27606, USA. [3] Center for Pain Research and Innovation, School of Dentistry, University of North Carolina, Chapel Hill, NC, USA. [4] Department of Anatomy, Physiology and Biochemistry, Faculty of Veterinary Medicine and Animal Husbandry, Swedish University of Agricultural Sciences, PO Box 7011, S750 07 Uppsala, Sweden.

Acknowledgements

The authors would like to thank all the cats that contributed to this study and their owners for allowing them. Thanks also to Dr. Mikael Andersson Franko for the statistical processing of the collected data, Professor Görel Nyman for continuous support, Dr. Charles Ley for radiographic expertise and Dr. Cecilia Ley for laboratory work and fruitful discussion. Thanks to Agria Insurance company for funding part of the study, through their competitive grants program.

Competing interests

The authors declare that they have no competing interests.

Declaration

Publication charges for this article were funded by the research platform Future Animal Health and Welfare at the Swedish University of Agricultural Sciences.

About this supplement

This article has been published as part of *Acta Veterinaria Scandinavica* Volume 58 Supplement 1, 2016: Animal obesity—causes, consequences and comparative aspects: current research. The full contents of the supplement are available online at http://actavetscand.biomedcentral.com/articles/supplements/volume-58-supplement-1.

References

1. Clarke SP, Bennett D. Feline osteoarthritis: a prospective study of 28 cases. J Small Anim Pract. 2006;47:439–45. doi:10.1111/j.1748-5827.2006.00143.x.

2. Godfrey DR. Osteoarthritis in cats: a retrospective radiological study. J Small Anim Pract. 2005;46:425–9.
3. Hardie EM, Roe SC, Martin FR. Radiographic evidence of degenerative joint disease in geriatric cats: 100 cases (1994–1997). J Am Vet Med Assoc. 2002;220:628–32.
4. Lascelles BD, Henry JB 3rd, Brown J, Robertson I, Sumrell AT, Simpson W, et al. Cross-sectional study of the prevalence of radiographic degenerative joint disease in domesticated cats. Vet Surg. 2010;39:535–44. doi:10.1111/j.1532-950X.2010.00708.x.
5. Slingerland LI, Hazewinkel HAW, Meij BP, Picavet P, Voorhout G. Cross-sectional study of the prevalence and clinical features of osteoarthritis in 100 cats. Vet J. 2011;187:304–9. doi:10.1016/j.tvjl.2009.12.014.
6. Bennett D, Zainal Ariffin SM, Johnston P. Osteoarthritis in the cat: 1. How common is it and how easy to recognise? J Feline Med Surg. 2012;14:65–75. doi:10.1177/1098612X11432828.
7. Kerwin S. Orthopedic examination in the cat: clinical tips for ruling in/out common musculoskeletal disease. J Feline Med Surg. 2012;14:6–12. doi:10.1177/1098612X11432822.
8. Bennett D, Morton C. A study of owner observed behavioural and lifestyle changes in cats with musculoskeletal disease before and after analgesic therapy. J Feline Med Surg. 2009;11:997–1004. doi:10.1016/j.jfms.2009.09.016.
9. Lascelles BD, Hansen BD, Roe S, DePuy V, Thomson A, Pierce CC, et al. Evaluation of client-specific outcome measures and activity monitoring to measure pain relief in cats with osteoarthritis. J Vet Intern Med. 2007;21:410–6.
10. Klinck MP, Frank D, Guillot M, Troncy E. Owner-perceived signs and veterinary diagnosis in 50 cases of feline osteoarthritis. Can Vet J. 2012;53:1181–6.
11. Clarke SP, Mellor D, Clements DN, Gemmill T, Farrell M, Carmichael S, et al. Prevalence of radiographic signs of degenerative joint disease in a hospital population of cats. Vet Rec. 2005;157:793–9.
12. Budsberg SC. Outcome assessment in clinical trials involving medical management of osteoarthritis in small animals. Vet Clin North Am Small Anim Pract. 1997;27:815–23.
13. Ettinger SJ, Feldman EC. Textbook of veterinary internal medicine: diseases of the dog and cat. St Louis, Mo: Elsevier; 2010.
14. Lascelles BDX. Feline degenerative joint disease. Vet Surg. 2010;39:2–13. doi:10.1111/j.1532-950X.2009.00597.x.
15. Carroll GL, Narbe R, Peterson K, Kerwin SC, Taylor L, DeBoer M. A pilot study: sodium urate synovitis as an acute model of inflammatory response using objective and subjective criteria to evaluate arthritic pain in cats. J Vet Pharmacol Ther. 2008;31:456–65. doi:10.1111/j.1365-2885.2008.00973.x.
16. Romans CW, Conzemius MG, Horstman CL, Gordon WJ, Evans B. Use of pressure platform gait analysis in cats with and without bilateral onychectomy. Am J Vet Res. 2004;65:1276–8. doi:10.2460/ajvr.2004.65.1276.
17. Romans CW, Gordon WJ, Robinson DA, Evans R, Conzemius MG. Effect of postoperative analgesic protocol on limb function following onychectomy in cats. J Am Vet Med Assoc. 2005;227:89–93.
18. Guillot M, Moreau M, Heit M, Martel-Pelletier J, Pelletier JP, Troncy E. Characterization of osteoarthritis in cats and meloxicam efficacy using objective chronic pain evaluation tools. Vet J. 2013;196:360–7. doi:10.1016/j.tvjl.2013.01.009.
19. Guillot M, Moreau M, d'Anjou MA, Martel-Pelletier J, Pelletier JP, Troncy E. Evaluation of osteoarthritis in cats: novel information from a pilot study. Vet Surg. 2012;41:328–35. doi:10.1111/j.1532-950X.2012.00976.x.
20. Benito J, Gruen ME, Thomson A, Simpson W, Lascelles BD. Owner-assessed indices of quality of life in cats and the relationship to the presence of degenerative joint disease. J Feline Med Surg. 2012. doi:10.1177/1098612X12453904.
21. Zamprogno H, Hansen BD, Bondell HD, Sumrell AT, Simpson W, Robertson ID, et al. Item generation and design testing of a questionnaire to assess degenerative joint disease-associated pain in cats. Am J Vet Res. 2010;71:1417–24. doi:10.2460/ajvr.71.12.1417.
22. Sul RM, Chase D, Parkin T, Bennett D. Comparison of meloxicam and a glucosamine-chondroitin supplement in management of feline osteoarthritis. A double-blind randomised, placebo-controlled, prospective trial. Vet Comp Orthop Traumatol. 2014;27:20–6. doi:10.3415/VCOT-12-11-0139.
23. Freire M, Meuten D, Lascelles D. Pathology of articular cartilage and synovial membrane from elbow joints with and without degenerative joint disease in domestic cats. Vet Pathol. 2014;51:968–78. doi:10.1177/0300985813516648.
24. Felson DT, Chaisson CE. Understanding the relationship between body weight and osteoarthritis. Baillieres Clin Rheumatol. 1997;11(4):671–81. doi:10.1016/S0950-357980003-9.
25. Schouten JSAG, Vandenouweland FA, Valkenburg HA. A 12 year follow-up-study in the general-population on prognostic factors of cartilage loss in osteoarthritis of the knee. Ann Rheum Dis. 1992;51:932–7. doi:10.1136/Ard.51.8.932.
26. Scarlett JM, Donoghue S. Associations between body condition and disease in cats. J Am Vet Med Assoc. 1998;212:1725–31.
27. Herzog W, Adams ME, Matyas JR, Brooks JG. Hindlimb loading, morphology and biochemistry of articular cartilage in the ACL-deficient cat knee. Osteoarthritis Cartilage. 1993;1:243–51.
28. Wu JZ, Herzog W, Epstein M. Joint contact mechanics in the early stages of osteoarthritis. Med Eng Phys. 2000;22:1–12.
29. Boyd SK, Muller R, Leonard T, Herzog W. Long-term periarticular bone adaptation in a feline knee injury model for post-traumatic experimental osteoarthritis. Osteoarthritis Cartilage. 2005;13:235–42. doi:10.1016/j.joca.2004.11.004.
30. Suter E, Herzog W, Leonard TR, Nguyen H. One-year changes in hind limb kinematics, ground reaction forces and knee stability in an experimental model of osteoarthritis. J Biomech. 1998;31(6):511–7.
31. Alexander JW, Shumway JD, Lau RE, Westfall GJ. Anterior cruciate ligament rupture. Feline Pract. 1977;7:38–9.
32. Allan RM. A modified Maquet technique for management of cranial cruciate avulsion in a cat. J Small Anim Pract. 2014;55:52–6. doi:10.1111/jsap.12125.
33. Cucuel JPE, Frye FL. Anterior cruciate ligament repair in a cat (a case report). Vet Med Sm Anim Clin. 1970;65:38.
34. Harasen G. Bilateral rupture of the cranial cruciate ligaments in a cat. Can Vet J. 1988;29:172.
35. Hoots EA, Petersen SW. Tibial plateau leveling osteotomy and cranial closing wedge ostectomy in a cat with cranial cruciate ligament rupture. J Am Anim Hosp Assoc. 2005;41:395–9. doi:10.5326/0410395.
36. Kilic N, Derincegoz OO. Surgical treatment of rupture of the anterior cruciate ligament in a cat caused by dog bite. Acta Sci Vet. 2012;40:1059.
37. Perry K, Fitzpatrick N. Tibial tuberosity advancement in two cats with cranial cruciate ligament deficiency. Vet Comp Orthop Traumatol. 2010;23:196–202. doi:10.3415/VCOT-09-02-0014.
38. Ryer KA. Rupture of the anterior cruciate ligament in a cat. Feline Pract. 1981;11:15–6.
39. Whiting PG, Pool RR. Intrameniscal calcification and ossification in the stifle joints of 3 domestic cats. J Am Anim Hosp Assoc. 1985;21:579–84.
40. Harasen GLG. Feline cranial cruciate rupture—17 cases and a review of the literature. Vet Comp Orthopaed. 2005;18:254–7.
41. Scavelli TD, Schrader SC. Nonsurgical management of rupture of the cranial cruciate ligament in 18 cats. J Am Anim Hosp Assoc. 1987;23:337–40.
42. Stadig SM, Bergh AK. Gait and jump analysis in healthy cats using a pressure mat system. J Feline Med Surg. 2014;. doi:10.1177/1098612X14551588.
43. German A, Martin L. Feline obesity. In: Encyclopedia of feline clinical nutrition. Aimargues, France: Royal Canin; 2008.
44. Laflamme D. Development and validation of a body condition score system for cats: a clinical tool. Feline Pract. 1997;25:13–8.
45. R Core Team. R: A language and environment for statistical computing. In: R Foundation for Statistical Computing. Vienna, Austria. 2013. http://www.r-project.org/. Accessed 21 Jan 2013.
46. Stanish WM, Taylor N. Estimation of the intraclass correlation-coefficient for the analysis of covariance model. Am Stat. 1983;37:221–4. doi:10.2307/2683375.
47. Ballagas AJ, Montgomery RD, Henderson RA, Gillette R. Pre- and postoperative force plate analysis of dogs with experimentally transected cranial cruciate ligaments treated using tibial plateau leveling osteotomy. Vet Surg. 2004;33:187–90. doi:10.1111/j.1532-950x.2004.04027.x.
48. Souza AN, Tatarunas AC, Matera JM. Evaluation of vertical forces in the pads of Pitbulls with cranial cruciate ligament rupture. BMC Vet Res. 2014;10:51. doi:10.1186/1746-6148-10-51.

14

Electrodiagnostic studies in presumptive primary hypothyroidism and polyneuropathy in dogs with reevaluation during hormone replacement therapy

Elżbieta Gabriela Giza*, Marta Płonek, Józef Marian Nicpoń and Marcin Adam Wrzosek

Abstract

Background: Peripheral neuropathy is the most common neurological manifestation of canine hypothyroidism. Data concerning electrodiagnostic studies in hypothyroid associated polyneuropathy in dogs are very limited and usually lack a reevaluation after hormone replacement therapy. The objective of this study was to perform a detailed, retrospective analysis of electromyographic (EMG), motor nerve conduction velocity (MNCV), F-wave and brainstem auditory evoked response (BAER) findings in 24 dogs with presumptive primary hypothyroidism and polyneuropathy with a comparison of the results before and after initiation of levothyroxine treatment with the assessment of the clinical outcome.

Results: The results obtained from hypothyroid dogs showed a significant reduction in MNCV at a proximal–distal and middle–distal stimulation, decreased amplitudes of compound muscle action potentials (CMAP), an increased CMAP duration and a prolonged distal latency prior to treatment. Fifty percent of the dogs had an increased F-wave latency. A normal BAER recording was found in 78 % of the hypothyroid patients without vestibular impairment. Bilaterally increased peak V latencies and increased interpeak I–V latencies were found in the remaining individuals. Dogs with concurrent vestibular impairment had ipsilaterally increased peak latencies with normal interpeak latencies and decreased amplitudes of wave I and II. A comparison of the findings before and after 2 months of treatment revealed a decrease in the pathological activity on EMG, an improvement of proximal, middle and distal CMAP amplitudes and an increase in the proximal–distal conduction velocity in all dogs. F-wave latency improved in 38 % of dogs. The BAER reexamination revealed a persistent prolongation of peak I, II, III and V latencies and decreased wave I amplitude on the affected side in all dogs manifesting vestibular signs. Conversely, in dogs without vestibular signs, the peak V and interpeak I–V latencies decreased to normal values after a given time of the treatment.

Conclusions: The results indicate a demyelinating and axonal pattern of polyneuropathy in dogs with suspected hypothyroidism. Most of the patients without vestibular signs showed neither peripheral nor central auditory pathway impairment, concurrent to the generalized neuropathy. The follow-up examination showed a very good clinical outcome and only partial improvement in electrophysiological assessment.

Keywords: Electrodiagnostic, BAER, Levothyroxine, Hypothyroidism, Polyneuropathy, Dog

*Correspondence: elzbieta.giza@up.wroc.pl
Department of Internal Medicine and Clinic of Horses, Dogs and Cats, Faculty of Veterinary Medicine, Wroclaw University of Environmental and Life Sciences, pl. Grunwaldzki 47, 50-366 Wroclaw, Poland

Background

Canine hypothyroidism is the most common endocrinopathy in mature, middle- to large-sized dogs and is characterized by a range of clinical manifestations [1, 2]. While the classical signs of this disease are well recognized, the correlation between hypothyroidism and neurologic dysfunction is less known [3]. Both central and peripheral neurological signs have been described in veterinary medicine [4]. Although the brain is considered relatively resistant to hypothyroidism in animals [5], seizures, disorientation, circling, coma and brainstem abnormalities, including central vestibular signs have been reported in hypothyroid dogs [3, 6, 7]. Peripheral nervous system syndromes, including cranial neuropathies (trigeminal, facial and vestibulocochlear nerve dysfunction), laryngeal paralysis, megaesophagus and, most frequently, generalized neuromuscular signs, have been reported in canine hypothyroidism [4, 7, 8].

The pathophysiology of polyneuropathy in hypothyroidism is not well understood [9]. Based on human studies, it is hypothesized that decreased metabolism in neurons may lead to impaired axonal transport and, in consequence, axonal atrophy [10, 11]. Another explanation for polyneuropathy is demyelination that is caused by the deposition of mucopolysaccharides in the cytoplasm of Schwann cells and connective tissue of the nerve [9, 12]. It may also be a result of vascular damage due to disturbances in the blood-nerve barrier [13, 14].

Polyneuropathy and myopathy associated with thyroid hormone deficiency in dogs may present as exercise intolerance, fatigue, a stiff gait, muscle atrophy, intermittent lameness, para- and tetraparesis [15–17]. Hypothyroid animals may have decreased proprioception, hypotonia and decreased to absent spinal reflexes [15]. According to previous reports, the clinical signs of peripheral nerve dysfunction and central vestibular disease in hypothyroid dogs typically resolve after 2 months of levothyroxine supplementation [6, 18, 19].

The electrodiagnostic findings in canine hypothyroidism with neurological manifestations include increased insertional activity and abnormal spontaneous activity during electromyography (EMG), reduction in the amplitudes of compound muscle action potentials (CMAP), a decreased motor nerve conduction velocity (MNCV) and brainstem auditory evoked response (BAER) abnormalities [6, 8, 9]. Most of these studies were carried out on a very small number of dogs (case reports and case series). A single electrodiagnostic test without reevaluation after levothyroxine supplementation was performed in the majority of cases, particularly if complete resolution of the clinical signs was achieved.

The purpose of this study was a retrospective evaluation of EMG, MNCV, F-wave and BAER findings in 24 dogs with presumptive naturally occurring hypothyroidism and peripheral neuropathy, and a comparison of the results before and after initiation of levothyroxine supplementation with the assessment of the clinical outcome.

Methods

Case selection

Electrodiagnostic recordings from 34 dogs referred for a neurological consultation to the Department of Internal Medicine with the Clinic of Horses, Dogs and Cats, Wroclaw University of Environmental and Life Sciences between February 2010 and February 2014, were analyzed retrospectively.

Group A consisted of 24 dogs with a presumptive diagnosis of hypothyroidism and polyneuropathy based on the following criteria: (1) a hypothyroid state with a high probability of primary hypothyroidism based on clinical findings, the hemato-biochemical blood profile and thyroid function test (decreased T4, fT4 and increased cTSH; if cTSH normal—the presence of other laboratory abnormalities and at least two extraneural clinical signs indicative of hypothyroidism), (2) neurological signs of progressive, generalized lower motor neuron impairment, (3) an electrodiagnostic evaluation, confirming peripheral neuropathy, (4) a positive clinical response to thyroid hormone replacement therapy (THRT), (5) an unremarkable abdominal ultrasound, chest x-rays, cerebrospinal fluid examination, (6) a normal head MRI in cases with cranial nerves deficits. In order to be included in the study, patients could not have a history of recent trauma or surgery, exposure to toxins or treatment with phenobarbital.

The age of the examined animals at presentation ranged between 5 and 12 years (average: 9 years, median 8.5 years) and included 9 males (1/9 neutered) and 15 females (11/15 spayed). Subgroup A1 consisted of 11 dogs that underwent an electrodiagnostic reexamination 2 months after starting THRT. The detailed data regarding the breeds of dogs, history and electrodiagnostic tests is given in Table 1.

Group B (control group) consisted of ten dogs that were initially admitted for a neurological examination, but were diagnosed with an orthopedic problem and were otherwise healthy. The age of the dogs was similar to those from group A, and ranged between 5 and 10 years (average 8 years, mean 7 years). This group consisted of 4 males and 6 females (4/6 spayed). The body weight ranged from 11 to 46 kg (mean 23 kg, median 26 kg). Hypothyroidism was excluded in this group based on normal blood test results. MNCV recordings, CMAP latencies, amplitudes and durations as well as BAER test recordings were documented. All the results were considered normal for the given age, size and limb length of the dogs based on a comparison with a previous report [20].

Table 1 Results of the clinical and electrodiagnostic evaluations in individual hypothyroid dogs before and after treatment

Dog No.	Breed	Age [years] sex	Motor deficits BT, other signs	Motor deficits AT, other signs	EMG		MNCV[m/s]				Expected F-wave lat.[ms]	F-wave lat.[ms] BT	F-wave lat.[ms] AT
					BT	AT	Proximal–distal		Middle-distal				
							BT	AT	BT	AT			
1	Bernese M. Dog	8 ♀	3	1	4	3	26	28	20	24	21.6	24.1	24
2	Golden Retriever	7 ♂	2, Vestib.	1	3	2	31	42	30	31	20.6	26.8	22
3	Golden Retriever	11 ♀	2	1	3	2	32	34	28	28	18.6	21.3	21.1
4	Labrador Retriever	6 ♀	3, Vestib.	1	4	3	35	44	31	34	19.6	32.2	30.1
5	Labrador Retriever	11 ♀	2	1	4	2	35	38	33	35	20.3	29.3	29.4
6	Irish Setter	5 ♀	2	1	3	2	39	40	36	36	21.3	29.5	24.7
7	Flat-coat. Retriever	12 ♀	2	1	3	2	41	48	36	39	19.6	20.2	NP
8	Mongrel (35 kg)	11 ♂	3	1	4	2	44	46	39	41	19.0	20.1	NP
9	Mongrel (15 kg)	10 ♀	3	1	3	1	44	48	41	42	16	16.5	NP
10	Wire Fox Terrier	12 ♂	2	1	3	1	46	55	41	44	15.1	18.9	16.5
11	WHWT	11 ♀	3	1	3	1	47	58	45	46	12.7	16.2	15.9
12	Labrador Retriever	9 ♂	2	0	3	NP	45	NP	42	NP	NP	NP	NP
13	Irish Setter	11 ♂	2	0	3	NP	45	NP	39	NP	21.6	23	NP
14	German Shepherd	7 ♂	2, Vestib.	0	3	NP	46	NP	43	NP	NP	NP	NP
15	Golden Retriever	8 ♀	2	0	3	NP	48	NP	47	NP	18.6	20.4	NP
16	Eng. Cocker Spaniel	6 ♀	2, Vestib.	0	3	NP	48	NP	44	NP	14.7	15	NP
17	Golden Retriever	7 ♂	1	0	3	NP	48	NP	43	NP	NP	NP	NP
18	Mongrel (20 kg)	8 ♀	1, Vestib.	0	3	NP	49	NP	47	NP	NP	NP	NP
19	Min. Schnauzer	11 ♂	1	0	3	NP	50	NP	45	NP	NP	NP	NP
20	Min. Poodle	12 ♀	1	0	3	NP	50	NP	44	NP	NP	NP	NP
21	Dachshund	8 ♀	1	0	2	NP	52	NP	48	NP	11	11.9	NP
22	Golden Retriever	6 ♀	1	0	2	NP	53	NP	46	NP	18.6	18.5	NP
23	Golden Retriever	9 ♂	1	0	2	NP	53	NP	48	NP	NP	NP	NP
24	Maltese	10 ♀	1	0	2	NP	54	NP	47	NP	NP	NP	NP

Dogs are ranked in ascending order, according to proximal–distal MNCV before the treatment. The ranking is separate for cases No. 1–11 (group A1) and for the remaining 13 cases

NP not performed, *BT* before treatment, *AT* after treatment [2 months], *WHWT* west highland white terrier

Clinical examination

All dogs were examined clinically, orthopedically, and neurologically. Motor function was evaluated and motor deficits were classified according to the following scale: Grade 0—normal motor function and muscle strength, Grade 1—mild motor deficits, muscle weakness, ambulatory paresis; Grade 2–moderate deficits, non-ambulatory paresis and Grade 3—severe deficits, complete loss of strength, plegia. A basic laboratory workup for neuromuscular disease according to Cuddon [9], including a hemato-biochemical blood profile and urinalysis was performed in all dogs. The thyroid function tests included measurements of total thyroxine (T4) (normal range 1.4–4.5 μg/dl), free thyroxine (fT4) by equilibrium dialysis (normal range 8–40 pmol/L), and serum canine thyroid stimulating hormone (cTSH) concentrations (normal range 0.01–0.50 ng/mL).

The electrophysiological examination was carried out at an ambient temperature of 22 °C with the use of the Nicolet Viasys Healthcare portable electrodiagnostic equipment and the version 11.0 of the Viking Quest software. Prior to testing, dogs were premedicated with a combination of medetomidine at a dose of 20 μg/kg and butorfanol at a dose of 0.1 mg/kg administered in the triceps brachii muscle. The electrodiagnostic examination was performed under general anesthesia using propofol at an induction dose of 1–4 mg/kg and a maintenance dose of 0.1–0.4 mg/kg/min, respectively.

The EMG was performed in all dogs in both groups by intramuscular insertions of a standard concentric needle electrode into the appendicular and axial muscles, with the monopolar ground electrode placed subcutaneously on the animal's flank. A semi-quantitative numerical scale by Kimura [21] was modified and adopted for the purpose of this study to evaluate the severity of EMG changes (Table 2).

The MNCV study and F-wave assessment were performed with the use of: (1) two stimulating needle electrodes, (2) a concentric recording needle electrode, placed in the plantar interosseous muscle and (3) a ground electrode, placed between the stimulating and recording electrodes. The MNCV measurements were obtained in dogs in both groups in the sciatic/tibial nerves using a single supramaximal electrical stimulus with a 0.1 ms (ms) duration at three stimulation points according to Walker et al. [22]: proximal—caudal to the greater trochanter of the femur; middle—at the level of stifle and caudal to the distal end of the femur; and distal—above the hock, lateral to the gastrocnemius tendon of the tuber calcanei. The recordings of the MNCV and CMAP latency, duration and amplitude were analyzed and compared between groups A and B. The same variables were analyzed in group A1, before and 2 months after initiating THRT. The F-wave evaluation was based on the measurement of the latency of the recorded F-waves in comparison to the expected minimum F-wave latency calculated according to the following formula $3.45 + 0.33 \times \text{limb length (cm)}$ for the sciatic/tibial nerve [20]. The limb length was measured on an extended limb from the level of the greater trochanter of the femur to the distal tip of the 3rd digit. Responses were elicited by 16 stimuli and the smallest latency period before the F-wave complex was measured.

Table 2 Modified semi-quantitative numerical scale for the electromyographic evaluation of the degree of pathological potentials

Grade	Description
0	No pathological potentials
1	Very rare denervation potentials
2	Sporadic pathological activity recorded in two or more places
3	Frequent pathological activity recorded regardless of the position of the needle electrode
4	Abundant pathological activity recorded regardless of the position of the needle electrode

The BAER test was performed in both groups of dogs using a previously described technique [20]. Briefly, standard subcutaneous needle-electrodes were placed in the mastoid reference (M), where the recording electrode was positioned at the vertex, the reference electrode was placed at the base of the ear and the ground electrode was placed at the midline of the 1st cervical vertebra. The auditory stimulus (1000 sweeps) was emitted through tubal insert ear phones at a 90 dB nHL intensity to the tested ear. A masking noise of 60 dB was simultaneously applied to the contralateral ear. All recordings were performed in rarefaction polarity, with a frequency setting of 11 Hz. The analysis of the BAER recording, obtained from the both ears in each individual, included an identification of waves I–V, measurement of their amplitudes and latencies and the determination of the I–V interpeak latency (IPL). All those variables were compared between the dogs in group A and B. In case of abnormal BAER recordings at the first examination, the comparison of the results before and after the initiation of the therapy was additionally performed in each individual. The BAER examination was preceded by an otoscopic examination.

The follow-up examination, which included a reevaluation of the clinical and neurological status as well as carrying out thyroid function tests was performed approximately 1 month after starting THRT at a dose of 20 μg/kg twice daily (BID) in all dogs in group A. The dosage was further adjusted according to the clinical response, the results of laboratory tests and clinical findings. Electrodiagnostic reevaluation was performed 2 months after initiating the THRT and was always conducted by this same examiner for the respective cases. Detailed information on the individual cases is presented in Table 1.

The results of the electrodiagnostic measurements were subjected to statistical analysis, using Excel 6.0 software and StatSoft Inc Statistica 10 software. The non-parametric Mann–Whitney U test was used to compare non-parametric values in the hypothyroid and control group. Student's t test was used to compare parametric data before and after starting levothyroxine treatment. $P < 0.05$ was considered significant.

Results

Clinical and electrodiagnosting findings prior to levothyroxine supplementation

All of the 24 dogs in group A (hypothyroid) were presented with generalized weakness and hyporeflexia. Lethargy was noted in 16/24, excess weight in 14/24, bradycardia in 8/24 and typical dermatological signs in 5/24. Motor deficits were evaluated as Grade "1" in 8/24 dogs, Grade "2" in 11/24 individuals and Grade "3" in 5/24 canine patients (Table 1). Five hypothyroid patients additionally manifested signs of peripheral vestibular dysfunction (head tilt, horizontal nystagmus, vestibular strabismus). The duration of clinical signs varied from 1 to 12 weeks (median 6 weeks, mean 5 weeks) with a slow progression of generalized weakness in all dogs. According to the owners' reports, the motor deficits were acutely exacerbated in seven individuals prior to the consultation. The onset of vestibular signs was also acute in all cases.

The diagnosis of hypothyroidism in group A was based on laboratory findings including decreased tT4 (24/24), decreased fT4 (22/24) and increased cTSH in 15/24. All dogs with normal cTSH (9/24) had moderate to severe fasting hypercholesterolemia, 7/9 dogs had fasting hypertriglyceridemia, 4/9 were presented with normocytic anemia, 2/9 had mildly increased aspartate aminotransferase and creatinine kinase activity. In total, 22/24 dogs in group A had hypercholesterolemia, 18/24 had hypertriglyceridemia, 7/24 had anemia and 6/24 dogs had a mildly increased aspartate aminotransferase and creatinine kinase activity.

The EMG examination in group A revealed increased insertional activity in 14/24 dogs, multifocal patterns of fibrillation potentials (FPs) in all 24 patients and positive sharp waves in 18/24 dogs. The changes were noticeable in all four limbs in all dogs in group A. The abnormal activity was equally appreciated in the proximal and distal parts of the front and hind limbs. Additional FPs were present in the axial muscles of eight dogs. The severity of individual EMG changes for each individual is shown in Table 1. The MNCV study in the hypothyroid group revealed a statistically significant reduction in the conduction velocity at the proximal–distal (26–54 m/s) and middle-distal stimulation (20–48 m/s) when compared to the control group (Table 3). The detailed analysis of CMAP parameters revealed a prolonged distal latency, decreased CMAP amplitudes and an increase in the CMAP duration at all stimulation points in group A (Table 3). The F-wave was recorded in 16 dogs from group A (Cases No. 1–11, 13, 15, 16, 21, 22). The F-wave latency was increased by more than 2 ms in eight patients (50 %) when compared to the expected F wave latency calculated for each dog (cases 1–6, 10, 11) (Table 1).

The BAER examination was performed in 14 patients in group A, including five dogs with vestibular signs.

Table 3 Comparison of motor nerve conduction variables in hypothyroid dogs and healthy controls before and after treatment

Group parameter	Group A (hypothyroid) [n = 24]	Group B (control) [n = 10]	P value	Group A1 before THRT [n = 11]	Group A1 after THRT [n = 11]	P value
MNCV prox-dist [m/s]	44.2 ± 7.6	65.4 ± 2.5	*<0.05*	38.2 ± 6.9	45.7 ± 6.2	*<0.05*
MNCV mid-dist [m/s]	40.1 ± 7.3	60.8 ± 2.2	*<0.05*	34.5 ± 7.1	36.2 ± 6.3	0.57
Latency prox [ms]	9.2 ± 1.7	7.8 ± 0.4	0.31	–	–	–
Latency mid [ms]	7.1 ± 1.6	5.8 ± 0.3	0.25	–	–	–
Latency dist [ms]	6.1 ± 1.1	3.0 ± 0.4	*<0.05*	5.6 ± 1.1	5.5 ± 1.2	0.89
Amplitude prox [mV]	5.7 ± 2.3	10.2 ± 1.2	*<0.05*	4.5 ± 1.1	7.6 ± 1.3	*<0.05*
Amplitude mid [mV]	6.3 ± 2.3	12.4 ± 2.3	*<0.05*	5.6 ± 1.6	8.8 ± 1.6	*<0.05*
Amplitude dist [mV]	7.7 ± 1.5	14.1 ± 2.5	*<0.05*	7.4 ± 1.2	11.0 ± 1.4	*<0.05*
Duration prox [ms]	9.2 ± 2.7	4.7 ± 0.5	*<0.05*	11.2 ± 2.6	9.9 ± 2.1	0.2
Duration mid [ms]	9.1 ± 2.1	4.9 ± 0.6	*<0.05*	10.7 ± 2.0	9.7 ± 1.6	0.19
Duration dist [ms]	8.7 ± 2.5	4.2 ± 0.7	*<0.05*	9.9 ± 2.0	9.3 ± 1.9	0.45

Statistically significant differences are indicated in italics. THRT thyroid hormone replacement therapy

Dogs No. 2, 4, 14, 16 and 18, manifesting vestibular dysfunction, had increased peak I, II, III and V latencies with a normal I–V IPL and decreased amplitudes of wave I and II on the affected side when compared to group B (Table 4). The BAER recordings in 7/9 hypothyroid dogs without clinical vestibular dysfunction did not differ significantly from the control group regarding the analyzed parameters. The remaining two dogs (No. 7 and 13) had bilaterally increased peak V latencies and increased I–V IPL latencies. Dog No. 7 had unilaterally decreased amplitudes in the entire waveform (Table 4).

The results of the clinical, neurological and laboratory investigations in group B (control group) were within normal limits. The EMG examination of the control limbs showed electrically silent muscles with normal insertional activity. MNCV at the proximal–distal stimulation ranged from 62 to 71 m/s and from 57 to 64 m/s at the middle-distal stimulation site. The comparison of nerve conduction studies in dogs from group A and B is shown on Fig. 1. F wave latency values did not exceed expected latency values by more than 2 ms. The results of the BAER are presented in Table 4.

Table 4 Comparison of the BAER results between the control group and hypothyroid dogs with and without vestibular signs before and after initiating treatment with levothyroxine

	Latency [ms]				Interpeak latency	Amplitude [μV]			
	I	II	III	V	I–V	I	II	III	V
Group B (n = 10)									
Range	1.9–2.22	2.72–3.06	3.38–3.76	4.32–4.79	2.42–2.57	2.5–3.2	1.8–2.3	0.8–1.2	1.6–2.1
Mean	2.1	2.93	3.55	4.61	2.52	2.9	2.1	1.1	1.9
Group A not vestibular[a] (n = 7)									
Range	2.0–2.26	2.88–3.07	3.35–3.74	4.4–4.8	2.4–2.6	2.6–3.1	1.7–2.4	0.6–1.1	1.5–1.9
Mean	2.15	2.99	3.48	4.68	2.54	2.9	2.1	0.8	1.8
Group A vestibular (n = 5) BT									
Ipsilateral									
Range	*2.45–2.58*	*3.15–3.27*	*3.84–4.0*	*4.99–5.3*	2.54–2.68	*0.9–1.8*	*1.1–1.5*	0.6–0.9	1.4–1.8
Mean	*2.47*	*3.18*	*3.91*	*5.13*	2.59	*1.5*	*1.3*	0.7	1.7
Contralateral									
Range	2.2–2.3	2.85–3.05	3.44–3.8	4.48–4.82	2.3–2.62	2.3–2.9	1.7–2.2	0.6–1.0	1.5–2.0
Mean	2.24	2.94	3.63	4.72	2.53	2.7	2.0	0.8	1.8
Group A vestibular (n = 5) AT									
Ipsilateral									
Range	2.36–2.58	3.15–3.23	3.85–3.9	4.9–5.13	2.5–257	1.4–2.2	1.5–2.0	0.7–10	1.4–1.9
Mean	2.51	3.18	3.89	5.09	2.55	1.8	1.7	0.8	1.7
Contralateral									
Range	2.2–2.44	2.84–3.05	3.41–3.83	4.46–4.9	2.23–2.52	2.4–2.8	1.7–2.1	0.6–1.0	1.5–2.1
Mean	2.29	2.92	3.66	4.75	2.45	2.6	1.9	0.8	1.8
Dog No. 7 BT									
L	2.22	2.92	3.81	*5.14*	*2.92*	2.3	1.7	0.7	1.7
R	2.21	3.03	3.83	*5.25*	*3.04*	*1.5*	*1.1*	*0.3*	*1.1*
Dog No. 7 AT									
L	2.2	2.91	3.77	4.81	2.61	2.4	1.7	0.8	1.7
R	2.21	3.04	3.8	4.83	2.62	1.7	1.4	0.6	1.5
Dog No. 13 BT									
L	2.05	3.09	3,76	*5.28*	*3.23*	2.5	2.1	1.1	2.0
R	2.08	3.1	3.79	*5.35*	*3.27*	2.4	2.2	1.0	1.8
Dog No. 13 AT									
L	2.04	2.81	3.7	4.59	2.54	2.5	2.3	1.1	1.7
R	2.05	2.89	3.75	4.62	2.58	2.5	2.0	0.9	1.9

Significant differences are indicated in italics. [a] excluding cases No. 7 and 13. *BT* before treatment, *AT* after treatment [2 months], *L* left ear, *R* right ear

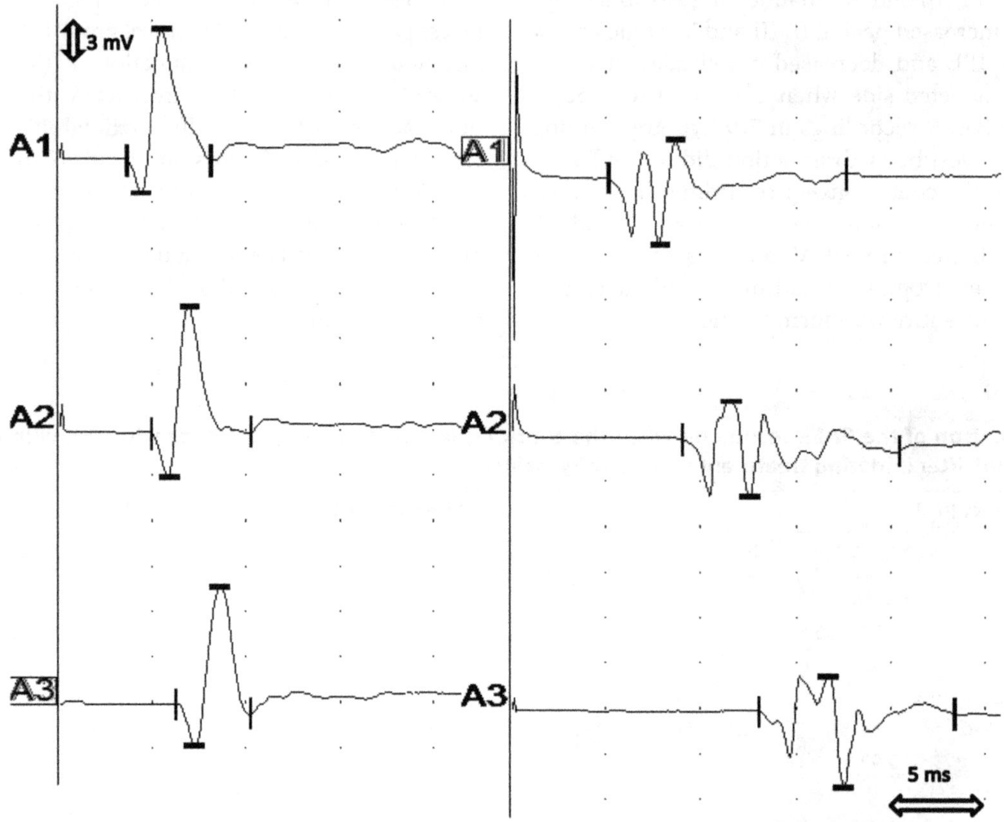

Fig. 1 The comparison of nerve conduction studies in dogs from group A and B. The recording on the left was obtained from an 8-year-old mixed-breed dog from group B. The MNCV was 61–64 m/s and it was considered normal. The recording on the right was obtained from a 7-year-old Golden Retriever with suspected primary hypothyroidism. The MNCV was decreased to 30–31 m/s. *Decreased* CMAP amplitudes and *increased* CMAP duration (temporal dispersion) at all stimulation points were observed (*distal* A1, *middle* A2, *proximal* A3)

Clinical and electrodiagnosting findings after initiation of levothyroxine supplementation

In group A, the first follow-up clinicopathological examination was performed 1 month after starting the levothyroxine treatment. At that time, all the studied dogs were more alert and active. The neurological evaluation revealed improvement in motor function by at least one Grade in 19/24 dogs. Dogs that showed no improvement after 1 month of the therapy and had a decreased tT4 level (No. 4 and No. 8) were administered a double levothyroxine dose (40 μg/kg BID). Dogs No 1, 5 and 9 had a tT4 level at a normal–low range. Because those dogs did not show a noticeable neurological improvement, levothyroxine supplementation was increased to 30 μg/kg BID. Dog No. 19 had a mildly increased serum tT4 concentration. Therefore, the levothyroxine dosage was decreased to 15 μg/kg BID.

Two months after initiating THRT, the results of the follow-up thyroid function tests and clinical examination were within normal limits in all 24 dogs. All overweight dogs lost weight. However, eight of them still exceeded recommended body mass. The majority of the vestibular signs resolved. Three dogs had a mild, persistent head tilt (No. 2, 16, 18). A full recovery of the motor function (Grade "0") was achieved in 13/24 dogs (No. 12–24). Eleven dogs that were initially scored as Grade "3" in 5 cases and Grade "2" in 6 cases (No. 1–11 in Table 1) showed an improvement to Grade "1" (ambulatory tetraparesis). This group was subjected to electrodiagnostic reexamination and named A1.

The EMG examination showed decreased pathological activity in all dogs. This improvement was from Grade "4" to "3" in 2/11 dogs, from Grade "4" to "2" in 2/11 dogs, from Grade "3" to "2" in 4/11 individuals and from Grade "3" to "1" in 3/11 dogs, as shown in Table 1. The analysis of the MNCV recordings showed statistically significant improvement of the proximal, middle and distal CMAP amplitudes and the proximal–distal conduction velocity when compared to the results before treatment (Table 3). The middle–distal conduction velocity, CMAP latencies and durations did not differ significantly before and after starting treatment in group A1 (Table 3). The F-wave was reexamined in the eight dogs that had a prolonged F-wave latency at the first examination (No. 1–6 and 10, 11). After a 2 month THRT therapy, there was no significant improvement in the F-wave latency in 5/8 dogs. The F-wave latency reached the normal value in 2/8 dogs. In one individual (dog No. 6), the latency shortened markedly, but the value still exceeded the expected F-wave latency by >2 ms (Table 1).

The BAER examination was repeated in five individuals with vestibular signs (dogs No. 2, 4, 14, 16 18) and two other dogs with an abnormal BAER recording during the first examination (No. 7 and 13) after 2 months of THRT. The second test revealed persistent prolongation of peak I, II, III and V latencies and a decreased wave I amplitude on the affected side in all dogs manifesting vestibular signs. The amplitude of wave II increased significantly in this group after replacement therapy (Table 4). In dogs without vestibular signs (No. 7 and 13), the peak V latencies and I–V IPL reached normal values after initiating therapy. Amplitudes in Dog No. 7 that were decreased prior to therapy increased markedly when measured at the second time point. However, they were lower than those obtained from the contralateral ear (Table 4).

Discussion

Diagnosis of polyneuropathy in hypothyroidism

Insufficient secretion of thyroid hormones is considered as a possible cause of polyneuropathy in 2–4 % of human patients [23]. Neurological abnormalities have been described in 6–29 % of dogs with naturally occurring hypothyroidism [1]. Peripheral neuropathy is the best documented neurologic manifestation of this disease in canine patients [8, 18]. However, a definitive diagnosis of canine primary hypothyroidism is complex [2]. The serum cTSH concentration has a high specificity for the diagnosis of hypothyroidism in dogs (more than 90 %) when the baseline serum T4 or fT4 concentration is concurrently low [24]. However, 20–40 % of dogs with primary hypothyroidism have normal cTSH levels, which gives the test low sensitivity [2]. A similar percentage of dogs with normal cTSH levels and decreased T4 and fT4 was present in our study (37.5 %). Caution should be taken in diagnosing hypothyroid neuropathy based only on a concurrent presence of low thyroid hormone levels [9]. Therefore, the presence of typical, extraneural clinical signs and accompanying hypercholesterolemia was required in this study to strengthen the suspicion of primary hypothyroidism in cases with normal cTSH. Despite the fact that a large number of additional tests was performed in order to rule out most systemic diseases, the nonthyroidal illness syndrome cannot be entirely excluded. Furthermore, we cannot exclude the possibility that symptoms in some dogs with acquired polyneuropathies of non-thyroidal etiology may resolve over a 2-month period. Hence, chronic inflammatory demyelinating polyneuropathy and distal denervating disease [9] may have been unintentionally included in the study.

The results indicate both a demyelinating and axonal pattern of polyneuropathy in dogs with a thyroid hormone deficiency. It is usually difficult to unequivocally distinguish between primary axonal and primary demyelinating polyneuropathy (i.e., neuropathy with extensive demyelination is often accompanied by slight axonal degeneration) [21]. Hypothyroid human patients have features of both axono and myelinopathy with a predominance (52–57 %) of demyelinating abnormalities in nerve conduction studies [11, 23, 25]. A prolonged CMAP and F-wave latency, a decrease in the nerve conduction velocity and temporal dispersion indicate demyelinating changes in our patients. Decreased CMAP amplitudes and EMG findings, which were also found in our study, stand for axonal involvement [26]. However, they may also indicate myopathy, especially in cases with elevated aspartate aminotransferase and creatine kinase activity [27]. In a study performed by Rossmeisl [27], a subclinical myopathy was the only electrodiagnostic finding in chronically hypothyroid dogs. No evidence of polyneuropathy, either clinical, or electrodiagnostic, was found in nine dogs with experimentally induced hypothyroidism. It has been suggested that immunological dysregulation contributes to peripheral nerve impairment in naturally-occurring hypothyroidism [27].

Electrodiagnostic exam during the course of levothyroxine treatment

After initiation of levothyroxine supplementation, a range of electrophysiological findings have been described in human patients. According to Kececi et al. [25], polyneuropathy in hypothyroid patients can be reversed within 3 months using THRT. Significant improvement in MNCV, motor distal latency and amplitude values were reported. Nemni et al. [28] described complete recovery in the clinical status and a significant improvement in motor and sensory NCV, distal latency and amplitude in two patients following a 3 months replacement therapy. A similar improvement was observed after 6 months of supplementation in the remaining two patients. On the other hand, other authors demonstrated that nerve conduction studies did not show significant improvement, even after long-term replacement therapy [11, 23]. The reports regarding electrodiagnostic studies after replacement therapy in veterinary medicine are very limited. Budsberg et al. [15] noted a complete resolution of pathological EMG activity in three out of four dogs and partial improvement in the remaining dog after 2 months of levothyroxine supplementation. Similarly, Jaggy et al. [8]

reported a complete improvement of EMG activity and MNCV variables in one hypothyroid dog with LMN signs 2 months after initiating replacement therapy. Our study showed that regardless of the clinical outcome, only some electrodiagnostic variables (CMAP amplitudes, proximal–distal MNCV and EMG) improved significantly after 2 months of replacement therapy in group A1.

Hypothyroidism and BAER

Thyroid hormone deficiency has also been associated with auditory and vestibular system dysfunction in human [29] and canine patients [6, 8]. Vestibular signs may be the only clinical manifestation of concurrent, underlying polyneuropathy [8]. Vestibulocochlear nerve impairment can be associated with or occur independently of peripheral neuropathy [9]. All dogs in our study were presented with generalized polyneuropathy and 21 % of them manifested peripheral vestibular signs before treatment. The BAER findings, including ipsilaterally delayed peak latencies with a normal interpeak latency and markedly decreased wave I amplitude, which did not improve after treatment, are suggestive of vestibulocochlear neuropathy. The unilateral, isolated cranial nerve deficit may possibly be associated with a myxedematous compression of the nerve (in this case vestibulocochlear) as it exits through the foramen of the cranium [9]. The BAER examination in hypothyroid dogs without vestibular manifestation was within normal limits in 78 % of cases. The remaining individuals had bilaterally prolonged peak V latency and the I–V interpeak latency, indicating central conduction dysfunction. Jaggy et al. [8] reported that two hypothyroid dogs presenting with generalized LMN dysfunction had concurrent BAER abnormalities (bilaterally prolonged latencies or lack of response) without presenting vestibular signs. Thornton and Jarvis [29] reported a significant reduction in the amplitudes of waves III and V and an increase in the I–V interpeak latency (iPL) in the BAER in hypothyroid human patients. They stated that those abnormalities may be explained by the low body temperature of those individuals rather than retrocochlear involvement. In our study, the body temperature of the patients was within normal limits. Hence, we cannot concur with this explanation. However, the thyroid hormone is known to control protein synthesis and myelin production in the central auditory pathway [30]. In addition, T4 also acts as a neurotransmitter in the central nervous system [30]. This may be an explanation for central conduction dysfunction that was detected using the BAER in our patients. It has been suggested that BAER abnormalities and coexistent polyneuropathy in the course of acquired hypothyroidism may also be explained by segmental demyelination [6].

A two-month levothyroxine treatment resulted in a significant clinical improvement of the peripheral vestibular signs in our patients. A very good clinical outcome in dogs with vestibular disease and hypothyroidism was also reported by others [6, 8]. However, a mild, persistent head tilt was observed within 2 months of THRT in 77 % of the canine patients reported by Jaggy et al. [8] and 60 % of the dogs in our study.

Based on the BAER reexamination, we found that only partial improvement was achieved 2 months after the treatment initiation. In other veterinary reports, the complete resolution of BAER abnormalities was achieved after 6 weeks of treatment in one dog [6], and 3–5 months in two dogs [8].

Conclusions

The results of the electrodiagnostic assessment in dogs with presumptive hypothyroidism and polyneuropathy showed features of both demyelination and axonal damage in the peripheral nerves. Most of the patients without vestibular signs showed neither peripheral nor central auditory pathway impairment, concurrent to the generalized neuropathy. The follow-up examination showed a very good clinical outcome and only partial improvement of the electrophysiological test results.

Abbreviations

BAER: brainstem auditory evoked response; BID: twice daily; CMAP: compound muscle action potential; cTSH: canine thyroid stimulating hormone; EMG: electromyography; FPs: fibrillation potentials; fT4: free thyroxine; IPL: interpeak latency; MNCV: motor nerve conduction velocity; MS: millisecond; T4: total thyroxine; THRT: thyroid hormone replacement therapy.

Authors' contributions

EG performed the clinicopathological and electrodiagnostic investigation, collected and analyzed the data and is the main author of the manuscript. MP helped to draft the manuscript and performed statistical analysis and English proofreading. JN revised the manuscript and helped with statistical analysis and data interpretation. MW coordinated the study, performed the clinicopathological and electrodiagnostic investigation and revised the manuscript. All authors have read and approved the final manuscript.

Competing interests

The authors declare that they have no competing interests.

References

1. Scott-Moncrieff JC. Clinical signs and concurrent diseases of hypothyroidism in dogs and cats. Vet Clin North Am Small Anim Pract. 2007;37:709–22.
2. Scott-Moncrieff JC. Hypothyroidism. In: Feldman EC, Nelson RW, Reusch C, Scott-Moncrieff JC, editors. Canine and Feline endocrinology. Makati City: Elsevier; 2015. p. 77–135.
3. Bertalan A, Glass EN, Kent M, de Lahunta A. Hypothyroid-associated neurologic signs in dogs. Vet Med. 2013;108:242–50.
4. Bischel P, Jacobs G, Oliver JE. Neurologic manifestations associated with hypothyroidism in four dogs. J Am Vet Med Assoc. 1988;192:1745–7.
5. Rudas P, Ronai ZS, Bartha T. Thyroid hormone metabolism in the brain of domestic animals. Dom Anim Endocrinol. 2005;29:88–96.

6. Higgins MA, Rossmeisl JH, Panciera DL. Hypothyroid associated central vestibular disease in ten dogs: 1999–2005. J Vet Intern Med. 2006;20:1363–9.
7. Coates JR. Neurologic manifestations of hypothyroidism. Canine Pract. 1997;22:27–8.
8. Jaggy A, Oliver JE, Ferguson DC. Neurological manifestations of hypothyroidism: a retrospective study of 29 dogs. J Vet Intern Med. 1994;8:328–36.
9. Cuddon PA. Aquired canine peripheral neuropathies. Vet Clin North Am Small Anim Pract. 2002;32:207–49.
10. Cruz MW, Tendrich M, Vaisman M, Novis SA. Electroneuromyography and neuromuscular findings in 16 primary hypothyroidism patients. Arq Neuropsiquiatr. 1996;54:12–8.
11. El-Salem K, Ammari F. Neurophysiological changes in neurologically asymptomatic hypothyroid patients: a prospective cohort study. J Clin Neurophysiol. 2006;23:568–72.
12. Murray IPC, Simpson JA. Acroparaesthesia in myxoedema. A clinical and electromyographic study. Lancet. 1958;28:1360–3.
13. Khedr EM, El Toony LF, Tarkhan MN, Abdella G. Peripheral and central nervous system alterations in hypothyroidism: electrophysiological findings. Neuropsychobiol. 2000;41:88–94.
14. Quattrini A, Nemni R, Marchettini P, Fazio R, Iannaccone S, Corbo M, Canal N. Effect of hypothyroidism on rat peripheral nervous system. NeuroReport. 1993;4:499–502.
15. Budsberg SC, Moore GE, Klappenhach K. Thyroxin-responsive unilateral forelimb lameness and generalized neuromuscular disease in four hypothyroid dogs. J Am Vet Med Assoc. 1993;11:1859–60.
16. Suraniti AP, Gilardoni LR, Lial MGR, Echevarria M, Marcondes M. Hypothyroid associated polyneuropathy in dogs: report of six cases. Braz J Vet Res Anim Sci. 2008;45:284–8.
17. Fors S. Neuromuscular manifestations of hypothyroidism in dogs. EJCAP. 2007;17:173–8.
18. Indrieri RJ, Whalen LR, Cardinet GH, Holliday TA. Neuromuscular abnormalities associated with hypothyroidism and lymphocytic thyroiditis in three dogs. J Am Vet Med Assoc. 1987;190:544–8.
19. Srikala D, Satish Kumar K, Tirumala Rao DS. Clinico-therapeutic management of thyroxine responsive polyneuropathies in dogs. Intas Polivet. 2011;12:96–9.
20. Cuddon PA. Electrodiagnosis in veterinary neurology: Electromyography, Nerve Conduction Studies and Evoked Responses. Colorado: Veterinary Specialists of Northhern Colorado; 2000.
21. Kimura J. Electrodiagnosis in diseases of nerve and muscle: principles and practice. 3rd ed. Oxford: Oxford University Press; 2001.
22. Walker TL, Redding RW, Braund KG. Motor nerve conduction velocity and latency in dog. Am J Vet Res. 1979;40:1433–9.
23. Nebuchennykh M, Løseth S, Mellgren SI. Aspects of peripheral nerve involvement in patients with treated hypothyroidism. Eur J Neurol. 2010;17:67–72.
24. Peterson ME, Melian C, Nichols R. Measurement of serum total thyroxine, triiodothyronine, free thyroxine, and thyrotropin concentrations for diagnosis of hypothyroidism in dogs. J Am Vet Med Assoc. 1997;211:1396–402.
25. Kececi H, Degirmenci Y. Hormone replacement therapy in hypothyroidism and nerve conduction study. Clin Neurophysiol. 2006;36:79–83.
26. Johnsen B, Fuglsang-Frederiksen A. Electrodiagnosis of polyneuropathy. Neurophysiol Clin. 2000;30:339–51.
27. Rossmeisl JH. Resistance of the peripheral nervous system to the effects of chronic canine hypothyroidism. JVIM. 2010;24:875–81.
28. Nemni R, Bottacchi E, Fazio R, Mamoli A, Corbo M, Camerlingo M, Galardi G, Erenbourg L, Canal N. Polyneuropathy in hypothyroidism: clinical, electrophysiological and morphological findings in four cases. J Neurol Neurosurg Psychiatry. 1987;50:1454–60.
29. Thornton ARD, Jarvis SJ. Auditory brainstem response findings in hypothyroid and hyperthyroid disease. Clin Neurophysiol. 2008;119:786–90.
30. Di Lorenzo L, Foggia L, Panza N, Calabrese MR, Motta G, Tranchino G, et al. Auditory brainstem response in thyroid diseases before and after therapy. Horm Res. 1995;43:200–5.

15

Bacteriological etiology and treatment of mastitis in Finnish dairy herds

Johanna Vakkamäki[1*], Suvi Taponen[1], Anna-Maija Heikkilä[2] and Satu Pyörälä[1]

Abstract

Background: The Finnish dairy herd recording system maintains production and health records of cows and herds. Veterinarians and farmers register veterinary treatments in the system. Milk samples for microbiological analysis are routinely taken from mastitic cows. The laboratory of the largest dairy company in Finland, Valio Ltd., analyzes most samples using real-time PCR. This study addressed pathogen-specific microbiological data and treatment and culling records, in combination with cow and herd characteristics, from the Finnish dairy herd recording system during 2010–2012.

Results: The data derived from 240,067 quarter milk samples from 93,529 dairy cows with mastitis; 238,235 cows from the same herds served as the control group. No target pathogen DNA was detected in 12% of the samples. In 49% of the positive samples, only one target species and in 19%, two species with one dominant species were present. The most common species in the samples with a single species only were coagulase-negative staphylococci (CNS) (43%), followed by *Staphylococcus aureus* (21%), *Streptococcus uberis* (9%), *Streptococcus dysgalactiae* (8%), *Corynebacterium bovis* (7%), and *Escherichia coli* (5%). On average, 36% of the study cows and 6% of the control cows had recorded mastitis treatments during lactation. The corresponding proportions were 16 and 6% at drying-off. For more than 75% of the treatments during lactation, diagnosis was acute clinical mastitis. In the milk samples from cows with a recorded mastitis treatment during lactation, CNS and *S. aureus* were most common, followed by streptococci. Altogether, 48% of the cows were culled during the study. Mastitis was reported as the most common reason to cull; 49% of study cows and 18% of control cows were culled because of mastitis. Culling was most likely if *S. aureus* was detected in the milk sample submitted during the culling year.

Conclusions: The PCR test has proven to be an applicable method also for large-scale use in bacterial diagnostics. In the present study, microbiological diagnosis was unequivocal in the great majority of samples where a single species or two species with one dominating were detected. Coagulase-negative staphylococci and *S. aureus* were the most common species. *S. aureus* was also the most common pathogen among the culled cows, which emphasizes the importance of preventive measures.

Keywords: Bovine mastitis, Bacteriology, PCR, Treatment, Culling

Background

During recent decades, considerable structural changes have occurred in the dairy industry in many countries. In Finland, the total number of dairy farms has decreased substantially but average herd size and numbers of farms with automatic milking systems (AMS) have increased [1–3]. With increasing herd size, good management practices and care of the cows become ever more important [4, 5]. Despite decades of mastitis control programs in countries with an intensive dairy industry, mastitis continues to be the most common and economically important disease of dairy cows. It considerably affects milk production, animal welfare, and food safety [6–8]. Today's consumers make increasing demands for adequate animal welfare as well as food quality and safety, which also must be taken into account on modern dairy farms [9].

*Correspondence: johanna.vakkamaki@helsinki.fi
[1] Department of Production Animal Medicine, Faculty of Veterinary Medicine, University of Helsinki, Paroninkuja 20, 04920 Saarentaus, Finland
Full list of author information is available at the end of the article

Mastitis results from intramammary infection (IMI), mostly caused by various bacterial species. Knowledge on the bacteriological etiology of IMI is important for efficient mastitis control and treatment [10, 11]. Distribution of the pathogens causing IMI varies among countries and herds. The most common causes of IMI are the major pathogens *Escherichia coli*, *Staphylococcus aureus*, and environmental streptococci, and the minor pathogens coagulase-negative staphylococci (CNS) [12–15]. Previous studies on the microbiological etiology of mastitis or IMI were mainly based on sampling selected herds in different countries. In Finland, national surveys with a random sample from all Finnish dairy herds were published [16]. In a previous Finnish study, Koivula et al. [17] used a smaller, culture-based bacteriological database of similar type as in this study. Some studies investigated the relationship between herd factors, such as general management, milking technique or production type, and distributions of mastitis-causing bacterial species in the herds [15, 18–20]. To our knowledge, studies combining pathogen-specific bacteriological mastitis data, treatment and culling records, and cow and herd characteristics from large national databases have not been carried out.

The Finnish dairy herd recording system has long traditions: it began in 1898 [21]. In 2015, the recording system covered 74% of dairy herds and 81% of dairy cows [22]. In herds belonging to this system, production records, including milk yield, milk protein content, milk fat content and milk somatic cell count (SCC), are recorded for every cow. The national health monitoring of dairy herds, constituted during the early 1980s, keeps health records for every Finnish cow. Veterinarians and farmers register all veterinary treatments per cow or herd in this system. The Nordic dairy herd health recording system is globally unique. In many countries, mastitis treatments are not recorded or are recorded at herd level only, or in connection with a specific health project. Unfortunately, the completeness of the records for clinical mastitis in Finland, according to a study carried out in 2008, was only 56%, which was lower than in the other Nordic countries [23].

In Finland, milk samples for bacteriology are routinely taken in most cases of mastitis [24]. The laboratory of the largest dairy company in Finland, Valio Ltd., analyzes the majority of these samples: 78% of Finnish dairy producers send milk samples to this laboratory (Personal communication Kristiina Sarjokari, Valio Ltd., 2016). Since 2010, a multiplex real-time polymerase chain reaction (PCR) assay has been used for the microbiological analyses.

Our first aim was to use a large microbiological database of quarter milk samples from mastitic dairy cows to study the bacteriological etiology of mastitis in Finland. Our second aim was to study treatment and culling records for the cows in the study herds collected from the databases of the Finnish dairy herd recording system. Detailed analysis of the relationships between pathogen-specific IMI and different cow- and herd-specific factors are presented in Taponen et al. [25]. The present study provides information about a PCR assay used for routine microbiological diagnostics of mastitic milk samples.

Methods

Microbiological data

Microbiological diagnoses of quarter milk samples from mastitic cows analyzed at the laboratory of Valio Ltd. during 2010, 2011 and 2012 were received from the database of Valio Ltd. For microbiological analyses, PathoProof™ Mastitis PCR Complete-12 assay (Thermo Fisher Scientific, Waltham, MA, USA) was used, which contained oligonucleotides for the staphylococcal β-lactamase gene (*blaZ*) and for the following microbial species or groups of species: *Corynebacterium bovis*, *Enterococcus* spp., including *Enterococcus faecalis* and *Enterococcus faecium*, *E. coli*, *Klebsiella oxytoca* and *Klebsiella pneumoniae*, *Serratia marcescens*, *Staphylococcus* spp., including all relevant CNS, *S. aureus*, *Streptococcus agalactiae*, *Streptococcus dysgalactiae*, *Streptococcus uberis*, and *Trueperella pyogenes* and *Peptoniphilus indolicus*. In March 2012, the test kit was changed to PathoProof™ Mastitis PCR Complete-16 assay, which also includes *Mycoplasma* (*M.*) spp., *Mycobacterium bovis*, *Prototheca* spp., and yeasts.

The reason for milk sampling was evidence of clinical or subclinical mastitis (elevated milk SCC) in the quarter. Milk sample was taken by herd staff or a visiting veterinarian using an aseptic technique [26]. In this study, a cow with a quarter milk sample with DNA of at least one target pathogen species in the PCR assay was considered to have IMI. These cows comprise the study group. Only samples with microbial DNA of one microbial species alone were included in calculation of the proportions of different pathogens. The control group comprised all other cows from the same herds: those for which no milk samples were sent for microbiological analysis to the laboratory of Valio Ltd.

Bacteriological data for 2010–2012 consisted of microbiological results from 240,067 quarter milk samples (Table 1). Samples were taken from 93,529 dairy cows in 4725 dairy herds. The control group consisted of 238,235 cows from the same dairy herds. In the analyses carried out on an annual basis, the same cow may appear several times.

Milk and health recording data

Milk and health recording data of the cows were received from the databases of the Finnish dairy herd recording system, and the Finnish cattle health monitoring system.

Table 1 Number of quarter milk samples, cows sampled (study group) and control cows (no milk samples submitted) in 2010, 2011 and 2012

		2010	2011	2012	Total number of samples
Samples		64,630	84,413	91,024	240,067
Samples with one target pathogen		31,731	44,037	41,743	117,511
				Total number of cows	Total number of individual cows
Cows in the study group	32,723	41,949	45,582	120,254	93,529
Cows in the control group	177,409	177,205	180,427	535,041	238,235
Total number of cows	210,132	219,154	226,009	655,295	331,764

The data include information on individual cows for breed, age, parity, annual milk, fat and protein yield, results of test milking six to twenty-four times a year, the number of feeding days, date of diagnosis and treatment for mastitis (clinical, subclinical) or dry cow therapy (DCT), and date and reason for culling. The data also provide herd-specific information, such as that for milking and housing system and production type (organic vs. conventional) for 93% of the cows in the dataset.

In Finland and other Nordic countries, only veterinarians are permitted to prescribe antimicrobials for use in animals. According to Finnish legislation, veterinarians record treatment of a cow after administering products with a withdrawal period, such as antimicrobials. Treatment records are regularly submitted to the central cattle health database. In subclinical or mild clinical mastitis, herd staff often take a milk sample and send it for microbiological analysis and contact their veterinarian after receiving the microbiological result. Mastitis treatment in such cases may be prescribed without the veterinarian visiting the farm, and the herd staff should record the treatment for that cow. Veterinary-supervised cases are recorded using four different codes for mastitis during lactation: acute clinical, subclinical, chronic, and unspecified mastitis, and one code for DCT [27]. Herd staff use three additional codes to record treatment of mastitis: mastitis during lactation, DCT for mastitis, and DCT for prevention. Finnish legislation concerning antimicrobial treatments of production animals changed after the onset of this study. Dairy farmers now have limited access to antimicrobials to treat some predefined diseases like subclinical mastitis, on certain conditions. These herds have to belong to herd health recording system and have regular visits of a supervising veterinarian. Microbiological results of milk samples shall be available before treatment of mastitis.

The data were organized and analyzed using SAS 9.4 (SAS Institute Inc., Cary, NC, USA) and SPSS 22 (IBM SPSS Statistics, Armonk, NY, USA) software. Differences in the treatment records for mastitis between the study group and the control group were tested using a Chi square test.

Results

Characteristics of cows and herds

In our data, 61.9% of cows were Nordic Red (NR), also known as Finnish Ayrshire, 36.6% Holstein (HOL), and 1.8% Finncattle, Jersey, or different crossbreds. The mean parity was 2.4 in NR and 2.2 in HOL cows (range 1–15). The proportions of parities 1, 2, 3 and ≥4 were 33.8, 26.5, 18.4, and 21.3%, respectively. The average annual milk production of the cows was 8598 kg per cow, 8323 kg for NR and 9154 kg for HOL cows.

Most herds were in conventional production systems and only 1.9% of the cows were on organic farms. 1.6% of both NR and HOL cows were in organic production, but for Finncattle the proportion was 7.7%. The average herd size was 44.7, 46.5, and 48.0 in 2010, 2011, and 2012, respectively. The minimum number of cows in a herd was three for all years, but the maximum number increased from 444 in 2010 to 498 in 2012. The proportions of free-stalls and AMS increased during the study period. In the entire period, 51.8% of the cows were housed in tie-stall barns, 46.6% in different types of free-stall barns, and 1.6% in barns with different mixed systems. In total, 52.0% of the cows were milked with a pipeline milking system in tie stalls, 30.4% in a milking parlor, 17.0% with AMS, and 0.6% with a bucket milking machine in tie stalls.

Microbiological results of the milk samples

DNA of some target pathogen species or group of species was detected in 87.6% of the quarter milk samples. 12.4% of the samples were negative, i.e. did not contain DNA of any target species. In 49% of the samples, DNA of only one target species or group of species, and in 25.2% two species or group of species, were detected. In samples with DNA of two bacterial species, a dominant species (>90% of the total target DNA in the sample) was present in 66.2% of the samples. In 13.4% of all samples, DNA of more than two bacterial species was found. In these samples, the number of target species or group of species detected in the sample was as follows: 3 in 9.2%, 4 in 2.9%, 5 in 0.9%, 6 in 0.3%, 7 in 0.07%, and 8 or 9 in less than 0.02%. One milk sample contained DNA from 10 target species or group of species.

The most common bacteria detected in milk samples were CNS and *S. aureus*. Results for milk samples with DNA of only one microbial species or group of species are shown in Table 2. Mean cycle threshold (Ct) values, reflecting the amount of pathogen DNA in the sample, ranged between 21.9 and 33.1 (Table 2). The staphylococcal *BlaZ* gene was found in 27.5% of samples with DNA of CNS and in 26.9% of samples with DNA of *S. aureus*.

In milk samples with two bacterial species or groups of species detected, with one dominant species, the most common dominant species were CNS (40.2%), *Str. dysgalactiae* (16.7%), *S. aureus* (14.4%), *Streptococcus uberis* (10.0%) and *T. pyogenes/P. indolicus* (5.3%). The most common species present in the sample together with the previously listed dominant species were *C. bovis* (29.6%), CNS (18.4%), yeasts (11.6%), *T. pyogenes/P. indolicus* (10.9%) and *S. aureus* (7.7%).

Table 2 Number and proportion of samples with DNA of a target bacterial species or group of species detected alone in 117,511 quarter milk samples analyzed in the laboratory of Valio Ltd. in Finland during 2010–2012 using PathoProofTM Mastitis PCR Assay, and the mean cycle threshold (Ct) values

Pathogen	N	%	Mean Ct value[a]
CNS	50,836	43.3	31.5
Staphylococcus aureus	24,754	21.1	28.0
Streptococcus uberis	10,572	9.0	26.6
Streptococcus dysgalactiae	9292	7.9	27.0
Corynebacterium bovis	8510	7.2	31.9
Escherichia coli	5562	4.7	29.3
Trueperella pyogenes/Peptoniphilus indolicus	2921	2.5	26.0
Yeasts	1812	1.5	31.3
Enterococcus spp.	1722	1.5	30.7
Klebsiella spp.	836	0.7	28.9
Streptococcus agalactiae	501	0.4	25.6
Serratia marcescens	149	0.1	33.1
Prototheca sp.	34	0	32.7
Mycoplasma spp.	7	0	21.9
Mycoplasma bovis	3	0	27.1
Total	117,511	100	

[a] Ct value reflects the amount of pathogen DNA in the sample: the lower Ct value, the more DNA

Mastitis treatments

In total, 53,993 cows in the study group and 63,843 cows in the control group received treatment for mastitis, received DCT, or received both. The proportion of cows in the study and control groups treated for clinical or subclinical mastitis, or with DCT, and the number of treatments per cow are presented in Table 3. The proportions of cows treated during lactation and with DCT were significantly higher in the study group than in the control group ($p < 0.001$). Quarter milk samples for bacteriology were submitted to the laboratory on average from 56.4% of the cows with a recorded treatment during lactation during the same year; this percentage increased during the study period from 47.4 to 64.4%.

Proportions of different mastitis diagnoses of the study group cows among the veterinary-supervised mastitis treatments reported in the health recording system in 2012 were as follows: acute clinical mastitis 75.2%, subclinical mastitis 9.6%, chronic mastitis 2.0%, unspecified mastitis 7.4%, and mastitis noted by herd staff 5.7% (mastitis during lactation). The respective figures in the control group were 77.7, 8.7, 2.1, 7.4 and 4.1%. Cows in the study group and treated after diagnosis of acute clinical mastitis, had most often the following species or group of species in their milk sample during the treatment year: CNS (22.6% of the cows), *S. aureus* (22.5%), *Str. uberis* (9.99%), *Str. dysgalactiae* (9.02%), *E. coli* (5.5%), and *C. bovis* (3.6%). For cows in the study group and treated for subclinical mastitis during the year, the order of the species was the same, with the exception of *E. coli* and *C. bovis:* The proportion of cows having *C. bovis* was higher than that of *E. coli*. The share of cows having CNS was 31.5%.

Culling of cows

Altogether 48.1% of the individual cows were culled during the 3-year study period. The reason for culling was reported for 88.5% of those cows. Among the reported reasons, the main causes were mastitis (23.6%) and poor fertility (19.0%). In the study group, mastitis was reported as the reason for culling for 49.1% of the culled cows for which the culling reason was reported. In the control group, the respective proportion was 18.2%. Table 4 shows the numbers and proportions of cows culled due to mastitis. The pathogens detected most often in the milk samples of the culled cows are also presented in the table.

Discussion

This study reports bacteriological results from bovine intramammary infections using information from more than 240,000 quarter milk samples analyzed with real-time PCR. Finland is to our knowledge the only country

Table 3 Proportion of cows in the study group and control group treated during lactation or at drying-off (dry cow therapy) or both. Number of treatments per cow during the study year is also shown

Year	Cows treated during lactation		Cows treated at drying-off	Cows treated both during lactation and at drying-off	
	Cows, %	Treatments per cow	Cows, %	Cows, %	Treatments per cow
Study group					
2010	31.0[a]	1.31	9.4[c]	6.8[e]	2.48
2011	29.4[a]	1.28	9.6[c]	6.6[e]	2.45
2012	27.7[a]	1.27	9.2[c]	5.8[e]	2.40
Average	29.3	1.29	9.4	6.4	2.44
Total number of treated cows	35,074		11,287	7632	
Control group					
2010	6.7[b]	1.23	5.2[d]	1.0[f]	2.35
2011	5.4[b]	1.21	5.1[d]	0.7[f]	2.32
2012	4.1[b]	1.19	4.6[d]	0.6[f]	2.31
Average	5.4	1.21	5.0	0.8	2.33
Total number of treated cows	28,976		30,762	4105	

Significance of difference: a, b, c, d, e, f, $p < 0.001$

Table 4 Number and proportion of the cows culled with mastitis as the reported culling reason in the study group and the control group, and the most common pathogens detected alone in the milk samples of the cows in the study group during the same year

	2010		2011		2012	
	Number of culled cows	%	Number of culled cows	%	Number of culled cows	%
Study group	3048	50.1[a]	4461	49.6[a]	4599	47.9[a]
CNS	581	19.1[b]	949	21.3[b]	866	18.8[b]
Staphylococcus aureus	888	29.1[b]	1383	31.0[b]	1239	26.9[b]
Streptococcus uberis	210	6.9[b]	336	7.5[b]	294	6.4[b]
Streptococcus dysgalactiae	168	5.5[b]	303	6.8[b]	221	4.8[b]
Corynebacterium bovis	143	4.7[b]	225	5.0[b]	197	4.3[b]
Escherichia coli	148	4.9[b]	238	5.3[b]	222	4.8[b]
Control group	7825	19.9[a]	6953	18.0[a]	6455	16.8[a]

[a] Proportion of cows from the total number of cows culled and culling reason reported in study group and in control group, respectively

[b] Proportion of cows having the respective pathogen in their milk sample from the total number of culled cows in study group

where PCR testing has largely replaced conventional culturing in routine microbiological diagnostics of quarter milk samples from mastitic cows [28, 29]. The PCR method used here identifies a wider range of target pathogens than commonly revealed by routine conventional culturing [24]. The uniform diagnostic method used and the large numbers of samples allowed us to make confident inferences on the microbiological etiology of mastitis in Finland.

The majority of the milk samples contained DNA of some target species or group of species. The proportion of negative target DNA samples, 12.4%, was lower than the proportion of "no growth" samples in studies using conventional bacteriology, which generally has ranged from 20 to 40% [13, 15, 17, 29]. This is at least partly explained by the capacity of the PCR method to detect also DNA of growth-inhibited or dead microbes [30]. The samples with DNA of some target species were largely easy to interpret because in 49.0% of the samples DNA of only one target species or group of species was detected. This agrees with previous reports where the same PCR test was used with smaller materials [24, 28]. In samples with DNA of two bacterial species (25.2%), a dominant species, being the likely causal agent of IMI, was found in 66.2% of the samples. Thus, in 75% of all samples, the causal pathogen could be identified and the result was unequivocal. These results can be considered diagnostically valid [24]. In 13.4% of the samples, DNA of more than two bacterial species was detected, up to ten species in one sample. Currently, reporting of PCR results differs from that for conventional culturing in that all target species detected in the sample in DNA quantities above the cycle threshold cut-off for the test are reported whereas in culturing, samples with three or more species growing on the plate are discarded, the plate being considered contaminated [26]. Sporadic colonies of minor pathogens or common contaminants on a plate with growth of a major mastitis pathogen are commonly ignored [24]. The same interpretation system could be applied also in PCR diagnostics [31]. In general, PCR testing has proven to be a fast, sensitive and reliable test suitable for routine mastitis bacteriology [24, 28, 32]. An advantage of the PCR test is the comprehensive panel of pathogens, and uniform procedure and interpretation, in contrast to bacteriological culturing, where performance and procedures of laboratories may differ [33]. High costs of molecular methods such as PCR may still limit their use for mastitis diagnostics in many countries.

Our pathogen distributions (Table 2) can be compared with those from previous studies even though others used conventional culture methods. In the present study, the most common bacterial species in the samples with DNA of only one target species or group of species were CNS (43.3%), followed by *S. aureus* (21.1%). The proportion of CNS agrees with previous findings in the Finnish national survey, where 49.6% of the isolates were CNS [16], but is much higher than in another Finnish study by Koivula et al. [17], who reported that CNS caused 18% of clinical and 24% of subclinical mastitis. In the study by Pitkälä et al. [16], the samples were taken from all quarters of all cows in the herds and thus the findings for bacterial infection were mainly associated with subclinical mastitis or teat end colonization. Our high proportion of CNS may partly be explained by the sensitivity of the PCR assay as compared with conventional culturing [24]. The high average Ct value for samples with CNS, generally indicating little DNA in the samples, also supports this view (Table 2).

The most common bacteria found in the milk samples of cows with recorded treatment of clinical mastitis were CNS and *S aureus,* with equal shares. The amount of CNS detections in milk samples (in total) was double compared to that of *S. aureus* detections (Table 2), showing that most *S. aureus* detections but only part of CNS detections lead to treatment of clinical mastitis. CNS are considered to be minor pathogens but are able to cause clinical mastitis, mostly mild [34]. It is possible that with changes in the dairy industry CNS currently cause more clinical mastitis than before, but another more likely explanation may be that herd staff are sensitive to react to mastitis with mild or transient clinical signs, aiming to keep bulk milk SCC low. Clinical mastitis is a broad term that includes all cases with any visible clinical sign, including mild changes in the milk appearance or consistency [35]. The high proportion of CNS in our study was not surprising because they have become very common IMI- and mastitis-causing agents in Finland and many other countries [15, 36, 37].

In our study, the proportion of *S. aureus* (21%) was higher than in the Finnish national survey (10%) [16]. It was similar to the proportion reported for clinical mastitis in Sweden [38], but high compared with studies from other countries [12, 15, 39, 40]. The high proportion of *S. aureus* recorded here means that this pathogen continues to be extensively responsible for mastitis problems in Finnish dairy herds. The proportions of *Str. uberis* (9.0%), *Str. dysgalactiae* (7.9%) and *E. coli* (4.7%) were similar to the results of Koivula et al. [17]. It is difficult to compare our proportion of *C. bovis* (7.2%) with that for other studies, in particular with those on clinical mastitis, because *C. bovis* is seldom reported. In the national survey, its proportion was over 34%, but then all cows and quarters in the study herds were sampled [16]. In samples with two bacterial species with one dominant species the most common concomitant species detected were *C. bovis,* CNS, yeasts, and *T. pyogenes/P. indolicus.* All these species are potential contaminants that originate from the teat end or barn environment, and their presence in milk samples is mostly of no clinical importance.

A clear difference between our results and those from other studies is the much higher proportion of environmental pathogens in many other countries. In studies from the UK, *Str. uberis* were the species most commonly isolated, followed by *Enterobacteriaceae* [12, 14]. In another countries, environmental streptococci were the most common finding in clinical mastitis [13, 39]. *Str. agalactiae* was rarely detected in this study (382 cows). These samples originated mainly from a few large herds: 57% of the samples were from herds with more than 99 cows and 27% from herds of 69–99 cows. Many samples came from the same cows: 22% of *Str. agalactiae*-positive cows had at least two positive samples (one to five positive samples) (data not shown). The herds with sampled cows were probably included in eradication programs. We conclude that proportions of mastitis-causing bacterial species always differ among countries and herds due to different environmental and management factors [13, 18, 41].

The Finnish cattle health monitoring system is mainly based on records of diagnoses and treatments made by veterinarians [42]. In contrast to the situation in many other countries, in Finland, as in all Nordic countries, antimicrobials are prescription-only medicines and strictly controlled by veterinarians. The current Finnish legislation on medical treatment of animals emphasizes the importance of microbiological diagnosis before any antimicrobial treatment of dairy cattle. In most cases when herd staff identifies a cow with clinical mastitis they contact their veterinarian who visits the farm. In cases of subclinical and mild clinical mastitis, herd staff first take a milk sample and then contact their veterinarian. Such cases do not necessarily receive antimicrobial treatment. In our study, on average 35.7% of the cows in the study group and 6.2% of the control cows had a recorded mastitis treatment during lactation. The significant difference between the sampled study cows and the control cows was expected.

In Finland, based on the numbers of milk samples, total number of dairy cows and antimicrobial consumption figures, it can be estimated that a milk sample for bacteriology is taken in a majority of mastitis cases [43]. We found that quarter milk samples were submitted to the laboratory on average for nearly 60% and, in the last study year, over 60% of the cows with a recorded treatment during lactation. It must be pointed out that the recording completeness for veterinary-supervised cases of mastitis in Finland has not been 100%, but according to a Nordic study only 56% (95% confidence interval 48–64%) [23]. Consequently, treatment records may be missing from our data, although disease reporting for dairy cows probably has become more complete since 2008 when the study of Wolff et al. [23] was carried out. Disease recordings are now done through the national herd health system Naseva [44] with which control of treatments has improved.

Control cows with a recorded treatment were either treated without taking a milk sample or the sample was taken but not analyzed in the laboratory of Valio Ltd. In Finland, veterinarians sometimes use triplate agars for rapid diagnosis of acute clinical mastitis and the results are generally not recorded [45]. It is still likely that mastitis cases diagnosed and sampled by farmers and treated via a veterinary prescription may remain unrecorded; this is supported by the low figure for treatments recorded with the specific code for notes of herd staff for treatment (data not shown). Many cows are repeatedly treated. The average number of treatments per cow was 1.3 and treatments may further accumulate for some of the cows.

The number of cows with recorded treatments for subclinical or chronic mastitis during lactation was low, which complies with the Finnish guidelines for mastitis treatment, where it is generally advised to postpone treatment of subclinical mastitis during lactation until drying-off, and treatment of chronic mastitis is not recommended [46]. Another possibility is that these treatments, often given by herd staff after veterinary prescription, are not reported. DCT was administered on average to 9.4% of the study cows and to 5.0% of control cows, and respectively 6.4 and 0.8% of the cows had been treated both during lactation and with DCT. Based on the consumption figures for intramammary products in Finland, approximately 22% of cows receive DCT [43]. Thus a considerable part of the treatment records for DCT are missing from our data. Figures for proportions of cows treated both during lactation and at drying-off were unexpectedly low. In general, DCT is recommended for cows that have had mastitis during lactation [46], but seemingly this advice is not followed on Finnish dairy farms.

Identification of the causal agent of IMI is important for mastitis management and treatment, but the routine is still rare in many countries and herds. For instance, in the Netherlands, only 34% of farmers submit milk samples for microbial analysis from cows with clinical mastitis and 22% from those with subclinical mastitis [10]. Prevention strategies in the herds should be pathogen-specific because problems caused by different bacteria need different approaches [11]. Treatment of mastitis should be based on microbiological diagnosis to avoid inefficient or unnecessary use of antimicrobials [14, 47, 48]. Even simple on-farm diagnostics, which only classifies mastitis-causing agents into Gram-negative and Gram-positive, has proven to be useful and reduced treatment costs [49, 50].

In the study group, mastitis was the reason for nearly half of the culled cows; in the control group the respective proportion was lower, as expected. Culling because of mastitis generally represents premature culling, which constitutes one-fifth of the costs of clinical mastitis in Finland [8]. The comparison of the shares of the pathogens in Tables 2 and 4 indicates that *S. aureus* was more common among culled cows than in the whole sample data. Thus, presence of *S. aureus* means increased risk of culling the cow. This may reflect the often poor outcome for treatment of mastitis caused by *S. aureus* [51]. The shares of the rest five pathogens presented in Table 4 were similar or lower among culled cows than in the whole dataset indicating that only *S. aureus* is a real risk factor for culling due to mastitis. However, more detailed studies on pathogen-specific diagnoses and treatment data using our large database will be carried out.

Conclusions

In Finland, quarter milk samples are routinely taken from cows with mastitis. Most are analyzed using a PCR-test which has proven to be an applicable method also for large-scale use in bacterial diagnostics. In the present study, microbiological diagnosis was unequivocal in the great majority of samples in which only one species or two species with one dominating were detected.

The reporting of results with more than two species detected should be improved to make the interpretation easier. CNS and *S. aureus* were the most common species detected in the milk samples whereas the proportion of environmental pathogens was lower than in many other countries. *S. aureus* was also the most common pathogen among the culled cows, which emphasizes the importance of preventive measures. Mastitis treatments are probably often based on bacterial diagnosis, but the activity of dairy farmers to submit milk samples for bacterial analysis could be further increased. With pathogen-specific treatments, inefficient and unnecessary use of antimicrobials can be decreased, which also improves food safety.

Authors' contributions

SP, AMH and ST planned the study. JV, AMH, and ST performed analysis of the data. All authors participated in drafting the manuscript and read and approved the final manuscript.

Author details

[1] Department of Production Animal Medicine, Faculty of Veterinary Medicine, University of Helsinki, Paroninkuja 20, 04920 Saarentaus, Finland. [2] Natural Resources Institute Finland (Luke), Koetilantie 5, 00790 Helsinki, Finland.

Acknowledgements

This study was funded by the Finnish Ministry of Agriculture and Forestry, the Walter Ehrström Foundation, and the Finnish Foundation of Veterinary Research. We also wish to thank Valio Ltd. for financing the study and for allowing us to use their bacteriological database, and ProAgria for providing us data from the Finnish dairy herd recording systems.

Competing interests

The authors declare that they have no competing interests.

References

1. Luke. Natural Resources Institute Finland. Economydoctor. Structural development of agriculture. Forecast of structural development; 2016a. http://www.luke.fi/en/services. Accessed May 2016.
2. Luke. Natural Resources Institute Finland. Statistics. Number of Livestock; 2016b. http://stat.luke.fi/en/number-of-livestock. Accessed May 2016.
3. Manninen E. 2014 a record year for milking robot sales (In Finnish). Maito ja Me. 2015;2:55. https://issuu.com/maitojame/docs/maito-ja-me-2-2015. Accessed Jan 2016.
4. Ouweltjes W, Beerda B, Windig JJ, Calus MPL, Veerkamp RF. Effects of management and genetics on udder health and milk composition in dairy cows. J Dairy Sci. 2007;90:229–38.
5. Cicconi-Hogan KM, Gamroth M, Richert R, Ruegg PL, Stiglbauer KE, Schukken YH. Associations of risk factors with somatic cell count in bulk tank milk on organic and conventional dairy farms in the United States. J Dairy Sci. 2013;96:3689–702.
6. Halasa T, Huijps K, Østerås O, Hogeveen H. Economic effects of bovine mastitis and mastitis management: a review. Vet Q. 2007;29:18–31.
7. Oltenacu PA, Broom DM. The impact of genetic selection for increased milk yield on the welfare of dairy cows. Anim Welf. 2010;19:39–49.
8. Heikkilä AM, Nousiainen JI, Pyörälä S. Costs of clinical mastitis with special reference to premature culling. J Dairy Sci. 2012;95:139–50.
9. Cardoso CS, Hötzel MJ, Weary DM, Robbins JA, von Keyserlingk MA. Imagining the ideal dairy farm. J Dairy Sci. 2016;99:1663–71.
10. Griffioen K, Hop GE, Holstege MM, Velthuis AG, Lam TJ, 1Health4Food-Dutch Mastitis Diagnostics Consortium. Dutch dairy farmers' need for microbiological mastitis diagnostics. J Dairy Sci. 2016;99:5551–61.
11. Ruegg P. New perspectives in udder health management. Vet Clin N Am-Food Anim Pract. 2012;28:149–63.
12. Badley AJ, Leach KA, Breen JE, Green LE, Green MJ. Survey of the incidence and aetiology of mastitis on dairy farms in England and Wales. Vet Rec. 2007;160:253–8.
13. Olde Riekerink RGM, Barkema HW, Kelton DF, Scholl DT. Incidence rate of clinical mastitis on Canadian dairy farms. J Dairy Sci. 2008;91:1366–77.
14. Milne MH, Barrett DC, Fitzpatrick JL, Biggs AM. Prevalence and aetiology of clinical mastitis on dairy farms in Devon. Vet Rec. 2002;151:241–2.
15. Levison LJ, Miller-Cushon EK, Tucker AL, Bergeron R, Leslie KE, Barkema HW, et al. Incidence rate of pathogen-specific clinical mastitis on conventional and organic Canadian dairy farms. J Dairy Sci. 2016;99:1341–50.
16. Pitkälä A, Haveri M, Pyörälä S, Myllys V, Honkanen-Buzalski T. Bovine mastitis in Finland 2001-Prevalence, distribution of bacteria, and antimicrobial resistance. J Dairy Sci. 2004;87:2433–41.
17. Koivula M, Pitkälä A, Pyörälä S, Mäntysaari EA. Distribution of bacteria and seasonal and regional effects in a new database for mastitis pathogens in Finland. Acta Agric Scand A. 2007;57:89–96.
18. Barkema HW, Schukken YH, Lam TJGM, Beiboer ML, Benedictus G, Brand A. Management practices associated with the incidence rate of clinical mastitis. J Dairy Sci. 1999;82:1643–54.
19. Dufour S, Fréchette A, Barkema HW, Mussell A, Scholl DT. Invited review: effect of udder health management practices on herd somatic cell count. J Dairy Sci. 2011;94:563–79.
20. Piepers S, Peeters K, Opsomer G, Barkema HW, Frankena K, De Vliegher S. Pathogen group specific risk factors at herd, heifer and quarter levels for intramammary infections in early lactating dairy heifers. Prev Vet Med. 2011;99:91–101.
21. Koivisto T, Seppälä J. Sata vuotta karjantarkkailua 1898-1998. (In Finnish). Helsinki: Maaseutukeskusten liiton julkaisuja 929. ProAgria Keskusten Liitto; 1998.
22. ProAgria. Results of the Finnish dairy herd recording system 2015. (In Finnish); 2016. https://www.proagria.fi/sites/default/files/attachment/lypsykarjan_tuotosseurannan_tulokset_2015.pdf. Accessed May 2016.
23. Wolff C, Espetvedt M, Lind AK, Rintakoski S, Egenvall A, Lindberg A, et al. Completeness of the disease recording systems for dairy cows in Denmark, Finland, Norway and Sweden with special reference to clinical mastitis. BMC Vet Res. 2012;8:1.
24. Hiitiö H, Riva R, Autio T, Pohjanvirta T, Holopainen J, Pyörälä S, et al. Performance of a real-time PCR assay in routine bovine mastitis diagnostics compared with in-depth conventional culture. J Dairy Res. 2015;82:200–8.
25. Taponen S, Liski E, Heikkilä A-M, Pyörälä S. Factors associated with intramammary infection in dairy cows caused by coagulase-negative staphylococci, *Staphylococcus aureus*, *Streptococcus uberis*, *Streptococcus dysgalactiae*, *Corynebacterium bovis* and *Escherichia coli*. J Dairy Sci. 2017;100:493–503.
26. Hogan J, González R, Harmon R, Nickerson S, Oliver S, Pankey J, et al. Laboratory handbook on bovine mastitis. Madison: National Mastitis Council; 1999.
27. Faba. Veterinary treatment codes for cows (In Finnish and Swedish). http://www.faba.fi/fi/tietopankki/terveystarkkailu. Accessed May 2016.
28. Koskinen MT, Wellenberg GJ, Sampimon OC, Holopainen J, Rothkamp A, Salmikivi L, et al. Field comparison of real-time polymerase chain reaction and bacterial culture for identification of bovine mastitis bacteria. J Dairy Sci. 2010;93:5707–15.
29. Verbeke J, Piepers S, Supré K, De Vliegher S. Pathogen-specific incidence rate of clinical mastitis in Flemish dairy herds, severity, and association with herd hygiene. J Dairy Sci. 2014;97:6926–34.
30. Taponen S, Salmikivi L, Simojoki H, Koskinen MT, Pyörälä S. Real-time polymerase chain reaction-based identification of bacteria in milk samples from bovine clinical mastitis with no growth in conventional culturing. J Dairy Sci. 2009;92:2610–7.
31. Hiitiö H, Simojoki H, Kalmus P, Holopainen J, Pyörälä S, Taponen S. The effect of sampling technique on the PCR-based bacteriological results of bovine milk samples. J Dairy Sci. 2016;99:6532–41.

32. Keane OM, Budd KE, Flynn J, McCoy F. Increased detection of mastitis pathogens by real-time PCR compared to bacterial culture. Vet Rec. 2013;173:268.
33. Pitkälä A, Gindonis V, Wallin H, Honkanen-Buzalski T. Interlaboratory proficiency testing as a tool for improving performance in laboratories diagnosing bovine mastitis. J Dairy Sci. 2005;88:553–9.
34. Simojoki H, Salomäki T, Taponen S, Iivanainen A, Pyörälä S. Innate immune response in experimentally induced bovine intramammary infection with *Staphylococcus simulans* and *S. epidermidis*. Vet Res. 2011;42:1.
35. International Dairy Federation. Suggested interpretation of mastitis terminology. Bull Int Dairy Fed. 2011:448.
36. Pyörälä S, Taponen S. Coagulase-negative staphylococci-emerging mastitis pathogens. Vet Microbiol. 2009;134:3–8.
37. Tenhagen BA, Hansen I, Reinecke A, Heuwieser W. Prevalence of pathogens in milk samples of dairy cows with clinical mastitis and in heifers at first parturition. J Dairy Res. 2009;76:179–87.
38. Unnerstad HE, Lindberg A, Waller KP, Ekman T, Artursson K, Nilsson-Öst M, et al. Microbial aetiology of acute clinical mastitis and agent-specific risk factors. Vet Microbiol. 2009;137:90–7.
39. Sampimon O, Barkema HW, Berends I, Sol J, Lam TJGM. Prevalence of intramammary infection in Dutch dairy herds. J Dairy Res. 2009;76:129–36.
40. Oliveira L, Hulland C, Ruegg PL. Characterization of clinical mastitis occurring in cows on 50 large dairy herds in Wisconsin. J Dairy Sci. 2013;96:7538–49.
41. Breen JE, Green MJ, Bradley AJ. Quarter and cow risk factors associated with the occurrence of clinical mastitis in dairy cows in the United Kingdom. J Dairy Sci. 2009;92:2551–61.
42. Rintakoski S. Epidemiological evaluation of the Nordic health registers for dairy cows-data transfer, validation and human influence on disease recordings. Helsinki: University of Helsinki; 2013. http://urn.fi/URN:ISBN:978-952-10-9488-0. Accessed May 2016.
43. Pyörälä S, Kaartinen L, Simojoki H, Kivilahti-Mäntylä K. Use of intramammary antimicrobials in Finland-towards lower consumption and targeted treatment of mastitis. Proceedings XXVII World Buiatrics Congress, June 3–8 2012, Lisbon. OC 14, p. 85.
44. ETT. Animal health ETT; 2017. http://www.ett.fi/sisalto/ett-english. Accessed Feb 2017.
45. Erkkilä S, Simojoki H, Pitkälä A. Praktisoivat eläinlääkärit hallitsevat päivystysviljelyn (In Finnish). Suom Eläinlääkäril (Finnish Vet J). 2007;113:608–12.
46. Evira. Recommendations for the use of antimicrobial agents in the treatment of the most significant infectious diseases in animals. Helsinki: Finnish Food Safety Authority Evira; 2016. https://www.evira.fi/globalassets/tietoa-evirasta/julkaisut/julkaisusarjat/elaimet/mikrobilaakkeiden_kayttosuositukset_fi-004.pdf. Accessed Oct 2016.
47. Ruegg P. Risks, realities and responsibilities associated with mastitis treatments. In NMC Regional Meeting, Ghent, Proceedings; 2014. p. 29–35.
48. Britten AM. The role of diagnostic microbiology in mastitis control programs. Vet Clin N Am-Food Anim Pract. 2012;28:187–202.
49. Lago A, Godden SM, Bey R, Ruegg PL, Leslie K. The selective treatment of clinical mastitis based on on-farm culture results: I. Effects on antibiotic use, milk withholding time, and short-term clinical and bacteriological outcomes. J Dairy Sci. 2011;94:4441–56.
50. Cameron M, McKenna SL, MacDonald KA, Dohoo IR, Roy JP, Keefe GP. Evaluation of selective dry cow treatment following on-farm culture: risk of postcalving intramammary infection and clinical mastitis in the subsequent lactation. J Dairy Sci. 2014;97:270–84.
51. Barkema HW, Schukken YH, Zadoks RN. Invited review: the role of cow, pathogen, and treatment regimen in the therapeutic success of bovine *Staphylococcus aureus* mastitis. J Dairy Sci. 2006;89:1877–95.

16

Risk assessment of sheep welfare at small-scale slaughter in Nordic countries, comparing with large-scale slaughter

Jan Hultgren[1*], Bo Algers[2], Sophie Atkinson[3], Kristian Ellingsen[4], Sofia Eriksson[5], Kjartan Hreinsson[6], Lotta Nordensten[7], Heidi Valtari[8] and Cecilie Marie Mejdell[4]

Abstract

Background: During the pre-slaughter period, animals experience novel environment and procedures which may cause reduced welfare and suffering. Over the last decades, the slaughter industry has restructured into fewer and larger abattoirs, implying potential risks of transport stress, injuries, and impaired animal welfare. Since recently, however, there is growing interest in small-scale slaughter to supply locally or regionally produced meat. Risk managers at all levels thus need to assess animal welfare risks also at small-scale operations. This study aimed to assess risks of poor animal welfare at small-scale lamb slaughter (≤5000 sheep/year and ≤70 sheep/day) in Norway, Iceland, Sweden and Finland, and to compare these risks to large-scale industrial slaughter. Assessment was done applying an individual expert opinion approach during a 2-day workshop. Nine experts in lamb slaughter procedures, behaviour, physiology, health, scoring schemes and/or risk assessment provided estimates of exposure, likelihood of negative consequences following exposure, and intensity and duration of negative consequences for 71 hazards. The methods applied mainly adhered to the risk assessment guidelines of the European Food Safety Authority. The list of hazards was modified from an earlier study and distributed to the experts before the assessment. No other literature was reviewed specifically for the purpose of the assessment.

Results: The highest risks to animal welfare identified in both small- and large-scale slaughter were related to inadequate conditions during overnight lairage at the slaughter plant. For most hazards, risk estimates were lower in small-scale slaughter. The reverse was true for splitting of groups and separation of one sheep from the group.

Conclusions: Small-scale slaughter has a potential for improved sheep welfare in comparison with large-scale industrial slaughter. Keeping the animals overnight at the slaughterhouse and prolonged fasting before slaughter should be avoided. Solutions include continuing education and training of stockpersons and, especially in large-scale slaughter, application of existing techniques for efficient transport logistics that minimise stress.

Keywords: Abattoir, Animal welfare, Expert opinion, Hazard, Stress

Background

During the pre-slaughter period, animals experience novel environment and procedures which may cause reduced welfare and suffering. Since several decades the slaughter industry in many countries has restructured into fewer and larger plants, resulting in longer transports of live animals. This implies an increased risk of impaired animal welfare, as well as meat quality, in sheep and other farm animals, due to stress and injuries [1]. Small-scale slaughter (SS) and mobile on-farm slaughter have attracted interest as means of supplying locally produced meat to consumers [2]. In Sweden small-scale slaughter has increased during the last decade, and 28 new SS plants were approved between 2006 and 2010 [3], which can partly be explained by subsidies to reduce fees for veterinary inspections.

*Correspondence: jan.hultgren@slu.se
[1] Department of Animal Environment and Health, Swedish University of Agricultural Sciences, P. O. Box 234, 53223 Skara, Sweden
Full list of author information is available at the end of the article

In 2013, 2.1 million sheep were slaughtered in the studied countries, of which 57 % in Norway, 29 % in Iceland, 12 % in Sweden, and 2.4 % in Finland [4]. There were five SS plants (here defined as ≤5000 sheep/year and ≤70 sheep/day), including one mobile unit, and 21 large-scale slaughter (LS, larger than SS) plants for sheep in Norway in 2014 [5]. In Iceland, the first SS plant for sheep was established in 2014. In Sweden, 75 out of totally 82 sheep slaughter plants processed less than 5000 animals in 2014 [6].

Despite positive public expectations, SS may present challenges to both animal welfare and meat quality due to high per-animal costs for investments in appropriate handling facilities, equipment and labour, dependence on the skills of a few stockpersons, lack of established work routines, and limited capacity for e.g. fresh water and cooling in mobile slaughter. There is a need for decision-makers at all levels, from abattoir managers to the European Commission, to assess whether such risks in SS and mobile slaughter differ from those identified in industrial LS. Research is needed to allow producer organisations and the food industry to develop quality assurance programmes and for competent authorities to develop and approve official animal welfare control schemes.

Risk assessment is a set of rational and probability-based methods, applicable to a variety of situations. Guidelines for risk assessment applied to food safety and the control of contagious disease have been presented by the Codex Alimentarius and the World Organisation for Animal Health (OIE). The term "hazard" usually denotes an infectious agent or risk factor potentially causing aversive effects, while "risk" is a function of the probability of occurrence of a hazard and its consequences in case of occurrence. The Animal Health and Animal Welfare Panel of the European Food Safety Authority (EFSA) has issued guidelines for risk assessment of animal welfare [7].

In a graduation project in Veterinary Medicine, Eriksson [8] made a pilot risk assessment of sheep welfare in SS, identifying and characterising important hazards, and collecting preliminary exposure data from seven Swedish SS abattoirs and one Norwegian mobile slaughter plant. Skog Eriksen et al. [9] compared a mobile slaughterhouse with a conventional stationary plant and found animals in the mobile facility to display fewer physiological and behavioural signs of stress. The present work aimed to assess risks of poor animal welfare at SS of lambs in Norway, Iceland, Sweden and Finland, and to compare these risks to industrial LS, using risk assessment and expert opinion.

Methods

Data collection

Twenty-two experts (including scientific researchers with varying experience in industry consultancy [n = 15], administrative officials of animal welfare, food control or academic institutions [n = 3], industry consultants [n = 1], quality assurance auditors [n = 1], clinical veterinary practitioners [n = 1], and slaughter plant managers [n = 1]) were invited to a 2-day workshop in Sweden 2012 to estimate risks of poor animal welfare at sheep slaughter. They were identified as knowledgeable and experienced in four areas of expertise; sheep slaughter procedures in general; behavioural, physiological and health-related responses in sheep; scoring schemes in general; or risk assessment in general. In connection with the invitation the experts were asked to fill out and send in a self-evaluation sheet, scoring their own level of knowledge or experience in each of the four areas of expertise as 4 = "very high", 3 = "relatively high", 2 = "relatively low" or 1 = "very low". Seventeen experts completed the self-evaluation and nine of them (all authors of this paper) agreed to participate in the workshop, including scientific researchers (n = 5), administrative officials of animal welfare, food control or academic institutions (n = 3), and clinical veterinary practitioners (n = 1). All participating experts were known to have practical experience in lamb slaughter, and at least three of them had extensive experience in small-scale slaughter.

The risk assessment was based on individual elicitation of expert opinion in a theoretical exercise. The methods mainly adhered to the guidelines presented by EFSA [7]. The list of hazards was modified from the report by Eriksson [8] and distributed to the workshop participants before the assessment. Detailed instructions were given at the beginning of the workshop. The experts were asked to make all initial assessments individually, i.e. without consulting the other workshop participants, based on their personal experiences and views. Totally 71 hazards were assigned to seven different steps of the slaughter process: unloading and driving to lairage; lairage; driving from lairage to stunning; waiting in stunning box; stunning with captive bolt; stunning with electricity; and bleeding (Additional file 1). Examples of hazards were, (1) during unloading and driving to lairage: stressful handling, long distance, and inappropriate flooring, (2) during lairage: mixing of groups, insufficient bedding, and overnight lairage, (3) during driving from lairage to stunning: stressful handling, inappropriate light, and separation from group, (4) during waiting in stunning box: single sheep, restraint, and spare weapon being kept unloaded in other room, (5) during stunning with captive bolt: poor gun maintenance, incorrectly placed shot, and no restraint, (6) during stunning with electricity: insufficient tong contact, prolonged tong application, and no restraint, and (7) during bleeding: long stun-to-stick interval and insufficient sticking. Animals were assumed to be stunned by either a penetrating captive bolt or electricity. The same hazard list was used in SS and LS. SS was defined as farm-based or handicraft-type slaughter of 5000 or less sheep per plant each year, with a maximum line speed of 70 animals per day. In contrast, LS denoted industrial-type slaughter with a larger number of sheep per year or higher maximum line speed than SS.

Apart from the report by Eriksson [8], no literature was reviewed specifically for the purpose of risk characterisation; it was assumed that the experts had sufficient knowledge of the exposure to different hazards and their effects on animals being slaughtered, and all data were thus provided by the experts during the workshop. No data were collected from slaughter plants. For each hazard and for SS and LS separately, each expert estimated hazard exposure, as well as intensity, duration and likelihood of negative effects given exposure to the hazard, and uncertainty of negative effects based on scientific literature. Hazard exposure expressed the probability of a sheep being exposed to the hazard during slaughter. Likelihood was the probability that a sheep, when exposed to the hazard, would experience the negative effects associated with it. Exposure and likelihood were expressed by three percentages each: the lowest possible (best-case), the most-likely and the highest possible (worst-case) probability. The intensity of the negative effects associated with the hazard was scored as 1 = "negligible": no or almost no pain, malaise, frustration, fear or anxiety, i.e. the animal behaving normally and quietly, 2 = "mild": minor pain, etc., some physiological changes, and moderate behavioural changes, e.g. commotion, increased movement or attentive postures, 3 = "moderate": some pain, etc., some change in motor behaviour, e.g. occasional attempts to escape, and occasional vocalisation, 4 = "severe": explicit pain, etc., dramatic change in motor behaviour, e.g. violent jumping, attempts to escape or resistance to being restrained, and vocalisation, or 5 = "critical": fatal effect, with death occurring either immediately or after some time. Duration of the negative effects was scored as 1 (<1 min), 2 (1–5 min), 3 (5–30 min), 4 (30–120 min), or 5 (≥120 min). It was assumed that this period could extend into one or several of the following steps of the slaughter process, up to the point of death.

Expert uncertainty was represented by the range between highest and lowest exposure and likelihood values. Bibliographic uncertainty was scored by the experts (based on their knowledge about available literature) as 1 = "negligible": solid and complete data available, with strong evidence in multiple references with most authors coming to same conclusions, or considerable and consistent field experience, 2 = "limited": some or only incomplete data available, with evidence provided in small number of references, authors' or experts' conclusions vary, or limited evidence from field observations, or solid and complete applicable data from other species, or 3 = "moderate": scarce or no data available, with evidence provided in unpublished reports, or few observations and personal communications, and/or authors' or experts' conclusions vary considerably.

All in all, the experts were thus asked to complete 1278 spreadsheet entries (two slaughter systems, each with 71 hazards and nine quantities for each hazard). The experts made the scoring on their own laptops using an Excel (Microsoft Corp., Redmond, WA, USA) spreadsheet which was distributed during the workshop. When needed, the procedure was clarified by the principal investigator (first author).

At the end of the first workshop day, all initial estimates were collected and combined by the principal investigator. Medians among the experts were calculated for all quantities. Medians with a standard deviation among expert scores above 0.3 (for exposure and likelihood) or 1.3 (for intensity and duration) were identified as uncertain due to disagreement between experts. On the second workshop day, all values and medians were presented anonymously to the expert group, i.e. without revealing the data source. The exact meaning and implications of hazards and estimates were discussed once more, with emphasis on hazards where there were particularly large differences in interpretation among experts, thus reducing misinterpretation. After the workshop, the experts were allowed to revise and adjust their personal scores for estimates where disagreement or errors had been found. The adjusted scoring sheets were collected by e-mail up to 48 days after the workshop. Logical errors, resulting from adjusting either the lowest, most-likely or highest value of exposure or likelihood without being able to make the necessary adjustments to other values, were corrected by adjusting the original value(s) to maintain the logical order from the lowest to the highest value. For example, if adjustment resulted in a lowest, most-likely and highest exposure of 25, 65 and 50 % after adjusting the most-likely value, the highest exposure was changed to 65 %. Based on the adjusted estimates, new medians were calculated for the final data analysis.

Finally, the experts were asked to describe the slaughter practices in their home countries to the best of their knowledge.

Statistical analysis

Based on the medians of all nine experts, aggregated magnitude (unitless) was calculated for each hazard as: (intensity × duration − 1)/24. Similarly, aggregated risk (unitless) was calculated as: magnitude × exposure × likelihood/10,000. In this way, both magnitude and risk ranged, theoretically, from 0 to 1. The lowest possible, most-likely and highest possible risks were calculated separately, assuming exposure and likelihood to be independent. A PERT probability distribution was fitted to describe the aggregated risk associated with each hazard. From these distributions, the ranges (difference between highest and lowest) were calculated and the interquartile ranges (IQR; Q3–Q1) were estimated by Latin hypercube simulation in the @Risk 5.5 add-into Excel (Palisade Corp., Ithaca, NY, USA) with 100,000 iterations. The ranges were interpreted as aggregate measures of personal uncertainty regarding the risk. Aggregated magnitude, most-likely risk, risk IQR and risk range were used to make comparisons between hazards, different steps in the slaughter process and slaughter systems; estimates were summarised as minimum, median and maximum values among the hazards included in each step.

The relationship between aggregated magnitude and most-likely risk was investigated by Spearman rank correlation in JMP 9 (SAS Institute Inc., Cary, NC, USA) in SS and LS. Likewise, the relationship between SS and LS was investigated by Spearman rank correlation for aggregated magnitude and most-likely risk. The significance level was set to 0.05.

To investigate how much of the variation in different quantities resided at expert level in different slaughter systems, i.e. how much was due to differences between experts rather than between hazards within expert, eighteen two-level linear mixed models were constructed in JMP, one for each quantity and slaughter system. In all models, hazard was included as the only fixed effect and expert identity as a random effect.

Results

Self-evaluation and risk assessment

The score sum of the self-evaluation concerning the four expertise areas ranged among the participants from 6 to 15 (median 12.5). The expert with the highest sum reported a very high level of knowledge or experience in three of the expertise areas (slaughter procedures, scoring schemes, and risk assessment), while the expert with the lowest sum reported a very low score in two areas (behaviour-physiology-health, and scoring schemes). None of the participants reported a very low score for expertise in lamb slaughter procedures in general. For remaining expertise areas, scores ranged from very low to very high.

At the end of the first workshop day, the experts had completed 633 entries (99 %) for SS, and 588 entries (92 %) for LS, as well as at least 87 and 62 %, respectively, of the 71 hazard entries for any quantity. All experts had completed all entries of 60 hazards (84 %) in SS and 23 hazards (32 %) in LS. Hence there were enough data to calculate medians for all hazards and quantities in both slaughter systems. In no case the number of experts that contributed to a median was less than seven. However, a bibliographic uncertainty score of 3 invalidated the aggregated risk estimate for *large group driving* from lairage to stunning (Additional file 1) in LS. When the expert estimates were aggregated, 24 % (SS) and 23 % (LS) of all 568 medians (excluding bibliographic uncertainty) were considered to be uncertain due to disagreement between experts.

After the workshop, 51 entries (9.0 %) in SS and 44 entries (7.8 %) in LS were adjusted by the participants. The overall percentage of entries adjusted varied among the experts between 0.6 and 13 %. The hazards for which entries were most commonly adjusted in SS were *restraint by shoulders and head* during stunning with captive bolt (30 %) and *spare weapon kept unloaded in same room* during waiting in stunning box (28 %) (Additional file 1). In LS, the hazards with most adjustments were *prolonged tong application* during stunning using electricity (36 %), *no restraint at electrical stunning* (34 %) and *manipulation before sticking*, i.e. animal chained and hung, or moved and placed horizontally before sticking (33 %). Adjustments were made both upwards and downwards; the mean change was 0.001 score points in SS and 0.009 score points in LS for intensity and duration, and 0.8 and 1.1 percentage units for other estimates, respectively. Between 0 and 30 (mean 5.2) illogical probability values per expert were corrected. After all adjustments, the percentage of uncertainty due to disagreement between experts was reduced to 9.7 % of median values in SS and 11 % in LS. Particularly large disagreement was found for three groups of values. First, most-likely likelihood estimates varied between 0–5 and 90–100 % for *large group driving* to stunning, *repeated re-shot* and *insufficient sticking* in SS. Second, most-likely exposure values varied between 10 and 100 % for *manipulation before sticking* in LS. Third, most-likely likelihood values varied between 0–10 and 95–100 % for *large group unloading, large group driving* to stunning, *single sheep* while waiting for stunning, *restraint by wool* while waiting, *spare weapon kept unloaded in other room, spare weapon kept unloaded in same room, single re-shot, repeated re-shot, restraint by neck only* during stunning with captive bolt, *restraint by shoulders only* during electrical stunning, and *insufficient sticking* in LS. Aggregated estimates of magnitudes and most-likely risks after adjustments are shown in Additional file 1.

Table 1 gives descriptive statistics of aggregated magnitude and risk in different slaughter process steps. There were considerable differences between the steps. Magnitude was highest during lairage and lowest during stunning with electricity. Most-likely risk was highest during lairage and lowest during bleeding in SS or during stunning with captive bolt in LS.

Table 1 Summary of welfare magnitudes and risks in different steps of slaughter

Process step	Measure	Small-scale			Large-scale		
		Min.	Median	Max.	Min.	Median	Max.
Unloading and driving to lairage (13 hazards)	Magnitude	0.042	0.13	0.33	0.042	0.13	0.27
	ML[a] risk	0.0042	0.0075	0.03	0.0056	0.023	0.078
	Risk, IQR[b]	0.0025	0.0058	0.018	0.0036	0.013	0.041
	Risk range[c]	0.009	0.021	0.07	0.013	0.047	0.15
Lairage (14 hazards)	Magnitude	0.083	0.33	0.58	0.083	0.33	0.69
	Risk, ML	0.013	0.027	0.13	0.010	0.048	0.18
	Risk, IQR	0.0087	0.018	0.057	0.0097	0.030	0.078
	Risk, range	0.033	0.064	0.20	0.037	0.11	0.32
Driving from lairage to stunning (14 hazards)	Magnitude	0	0.13	0.21	0.042	0.13	0.21
	Risk, ML	0	0.016	0.065	0.0075	0.021	0.06
	Risk, IQR	0	0.011	0.021	0.0057	0.012	0.025
	Risk, range	0	0.038	0.078	0.021	0.045	0.089
Waiting in stun box (10 hazards)	Magnitude	0.083	0.13	0.29	0.083	0.21	0.29
	Risk, ML	0.0044	0.010	0.053	0.0026	0.014	0.083
	Risk, IQR	0.0022	0.0070	0.023	0.0023	0.011	0.036
	Risk, range	0.0079	0.026	0.083	0.0088	0.039	0.13
Stunning with captive bolt (9 hazards)	Magnitude	0.042	0.13	0.29	0.083	0.13	0.29
	Risk, ML	0	0.005	0.038	0	0.0005	0.0095
	Risk, IQR	0.0001	0.0033	0.020	0.0002	0.0008	0.0072
	Risk, range	0.0007	0.012	0.071	0.0013	0.0031	0.026
Stunning with electricity (8 hazards)	Magnitude	0.042	0.10	0.13	0.083	0.094	0.13
	Risk, ML	0.0006	0.0032	0.007	0.005	0.012	0.028
	Risk, IQR	0.0002	0.0019	0.0049	0.0024	0.0063	0.015
	Risk, range	0.0008	0.0078	0.018	0.0088	0.023	0.054
Bleeding (3 hazards)	Magnitude	0	0.13	0.125	0	0.13	0.13
	Risk, ML	0	0.0025	0.005	0	0.0048	0.015
	Risk, IQR	0	0.0024	0.0045	0	0.0033	0.0092
	Risk, range	0	0.0093	0.017	0	0.012	0.033
Totally (71 hazards)	Magnitude	0	0.13	0.58	0	0.13	0.69
	Risk, ML	0	0.010	0.13	0	0.018	0.18
	Risk, IQR	0	0.0072	0.057	0	0.012	0.078
	Risk, range	0	0.027	0.20	0	0.044	0.32

Statistics of estimated magnitudes and risks of poor sheep welfare at small-scale and large-scale slaughter in Norway, Iceland, Sweden and Finland. Hazards arranged in seven process steps, specifying minimum, median and maximum values by process step. Aggregated data from nine experts 2012

[a] Most-likely

[b] Inter-quartile range

[c] Maximum–minimum

Figures 1 and 2 show hazards with particularly high aggregated magnitudes and most-likely risks in SS. *Prolonged insufficient feed* and *prolonged insufficient water* (Additional file 1) had the highest magnitudes (both 0.58). *Overnight lairage* and *splitting of group* during lairage and *separation from group* during driving to stunning had the highest risks (0.13, 0.070 and 0.065, respectively). In LS, *prolonged insufficient feed* and *prolonged insufficient water* had the highest magnitudes (0.58 and 0.69, respectively) and *overnight lairage* had the highest risk (0.18) (Fig. 3). There was a strong to moderate correlation between aggregated magnitude and most-likely risk in both SS (Spearman *rho* $= 0.65$; $P < 0.0001$) and LS (*rho* $= 0.43$; $P = 0.0002$).

The magnitudes of *overnight lairage* in SS or LS and *insufficient feed* in LS were only moderate but due to high exposure the corresponding estimated risks were high (Fig. 3). The opposite was true for prolonged insufficient feed and water in LS, with high magnitudes but moderate risks. Overall differences in most-likely risk estimates

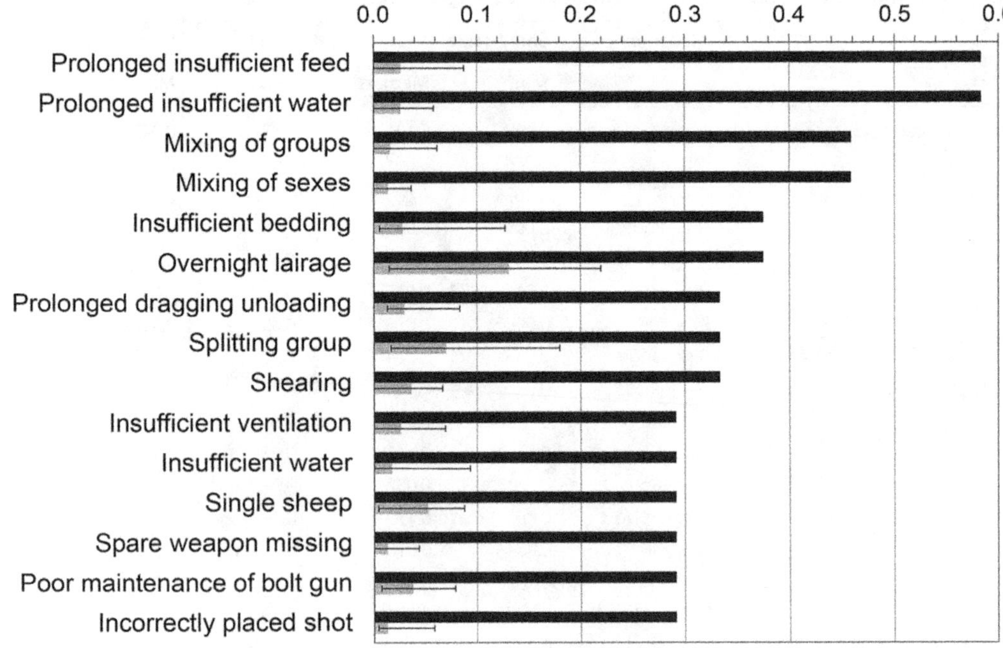

Fig. 1 Hazards ranked by welfare magnitude at small-scale slaughter. Sheep welfare hazards at small-scale slaughter in Norway, Iceland, Sweden and Finland; the 15 highest magnitude estimates (sorted by magnitude; *black bars*) and most-likely risk estimates (*grey bars*; *error bars* indicating risk range); aggregated data from nine experts 2012

between SS and LS and between slaughter process steps were generally accompanied by corresponding differences in personal uncertainty, as expressed by risk IQR and risk range. Risk IQR (Fig. 4) and range (not shown in figure) were larger when the estimated risk was high. However, there was no obvious association between scores for bibliographic uncertainty and personal uncertainty regarding risks as expressed by IQR of risk distributions.

There were strong to moderate correlations between SS and LS for magnitude (Spearman *rho* = 0.90; $P < 0.0001$) and most-likely risk (*rho* = 0.55; $P < 0.0001$). On average, magnitudes were 8 % lower and risks were 40 % lower in SS than in LS. When comparing SS to LS, *splitting of group* during lairage was associated with a higher magnitude in SS, while *overnight lairage* and *prolonged insufficient water* had lower magnitudes (Fig. 5). Most-likely risks were higher in SS for *splitting group*, *separation from group* during driving to stunning and *single sheep* while waiting in stunning box, but lower for *insufficient bedding* and *insufficient feed* during lairage and *noise waiting* in stunning box (Fig. 6).

Estimates from the linear mixed models of expert values are presented in Table 2. Coefficients of variation were similar for SS and LS, and the highest values were found for intensity and duration. For all parameters, variance components for experts were larger in SS than in LS (1.04–7.86 times larger). The highest percentage was found for uncertainty in SS and the lowest for most-likely exposure in LS.

Slaughter practices in different countries

The participating experts estimated that less than 10 % of the sheep slaughtered in the studied countries were processed at SS, with the highest percentages in Sweden and Finland. For Norway, there were three SS plants in service, including one mobile unit, that electrical head-only stunning was most commonly used (captive bolt in the mobile plant; electricity head-to-back in a few plants), and that overnight lairage was practised frequently. In Iceland, there were no SS or mobile plants and electrical head-only stunning was used primarily. In Sweden, it was estimated that there were around 55 SS plants but no mobile plant. Captive bolt stunning was used in approximately 80 % of the SS plants and head-only electrical stunning in the remaining 20 %. Electrical head-only stunning was used in all LS plants. In Finland, there were around 59 SS plants but no mobile unit, and both captive bolt and electrical stunning were used. In summary, around 6 % of the sheep slaughtered in Norway, Sweden and Finland were processed at SS plants, and approximately two-thirds of these animals were stunned by captive bolt and the remaining third by electricity, most commonly applied across the head of the animals. At

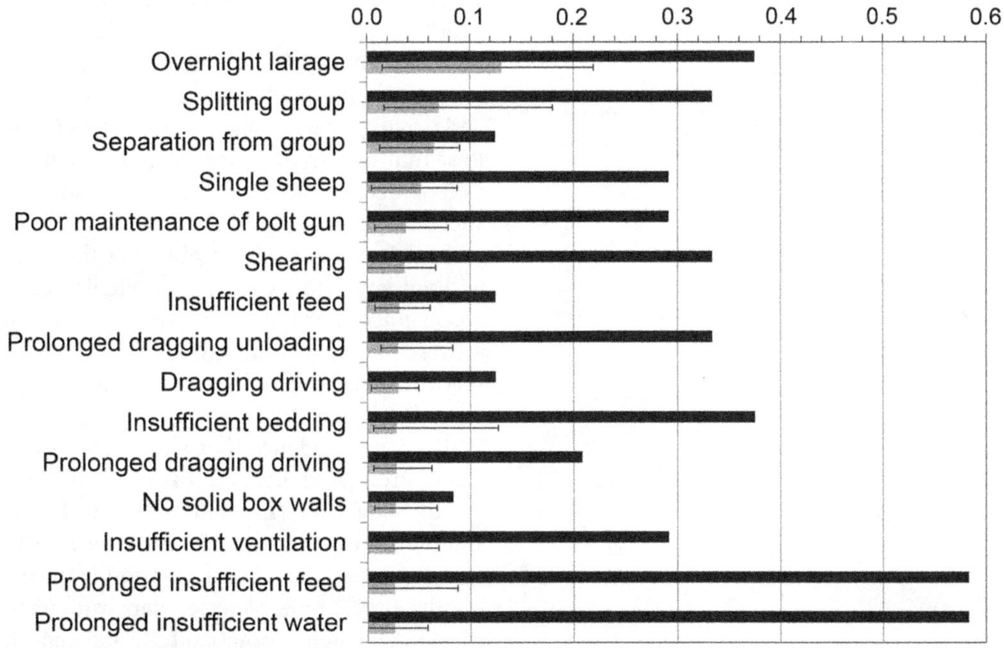

Fig. 2 Hazards ranked by welfare risk at small-scale slaughter. Sheep welfare hazards at small-scale slaughter in Norway, Iceland, Sweden and Finland; the 15 highest most-likely risk estimates (sorted by risk; *grey bars*; *error bars* indicating risk range), and magnitude estimates (*black bars*); aggregated data from nine experts 2012

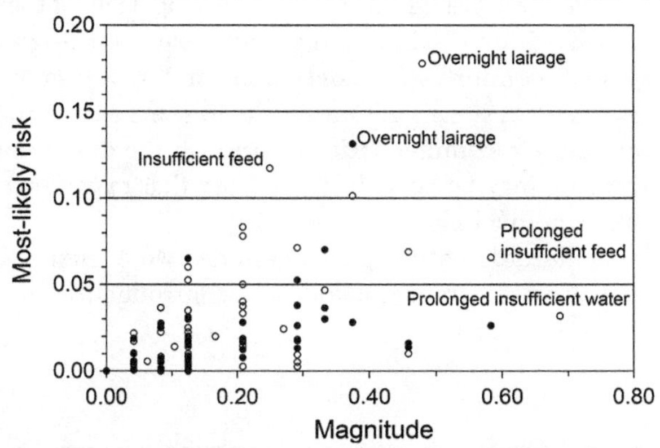

Fig. 3 Welfare magnitudes and risks. Relationship between estimates of magnitude and most-likely risk of poor sheep welfare for different sheep welfare hazards at small-scale (*black dots*) and large-scale slaughter (*white dots*) in Norway, Iceland, Sweden and Finland; aggregated data from nine experts 2012

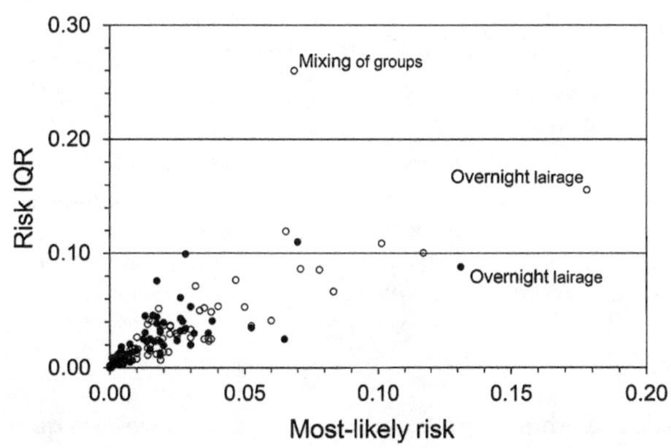

Fig. 4 Welfare risks and their interquartile ranges. Relationship between estimates of most-likely risk and interquartile range (IQR) of risk probability distributions of poor sheep welfare (IQR indicating aggregated personal uncertainty regarding the risk) for different sheep welfare hazards at small-scale (*black dots*) and large-scale slaughter (*white dots*) in Norway, Iceland, Sweden and Finland; aggregated data from nine experts 2012

least in Norway, shearing is traditionally done at the abattoir, but increasingly commonly it is done after killing.

Discussion

There was a strong association between SS and LS for aggregated magnitudes, indicating that the hazards were ranked very similarly in the two slaughter systems, while risk estimates were less strongly associated. The magnitudes were comparable in SS and LS, while the risks were considerably lower in SS, mainly due to lower exposure to the hazards. In both SS and LS, hazards to which the animals are exposed during lairage were associated with the highest magnitude and

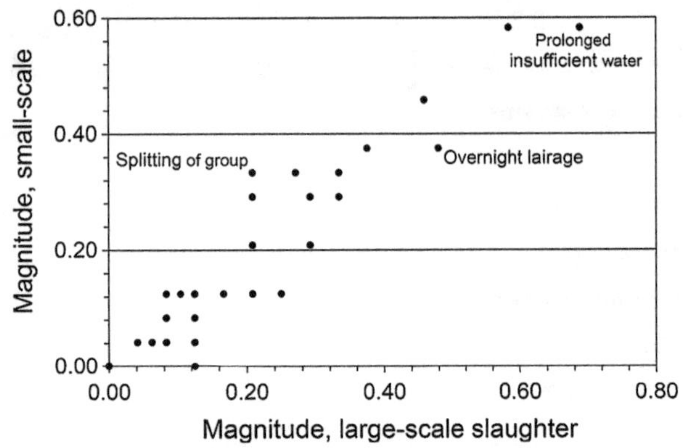

Fig. 5 Welfare magnitudes at large-scale and small-scale slaughter. Relationship between magnitude estimates for different sheep welfare hazards at small-scale and large-scale slaughter in Norway, Iceland, Sweden and Finland; aggregated data from nine experts 2012

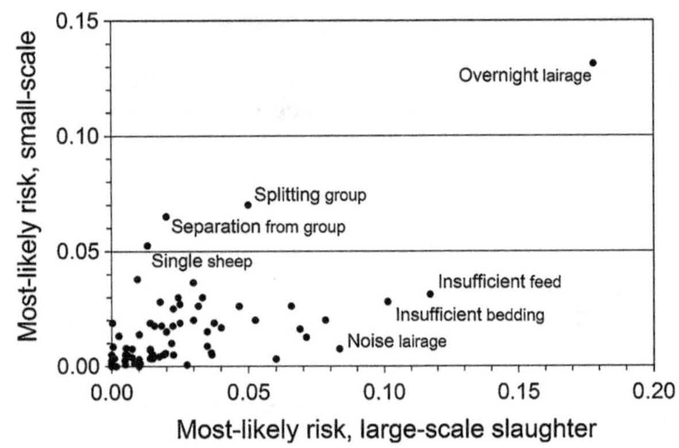

Fig. 6 Welfare risks at large-scale and small-scale slaughter. Relationship between most-likely risk estimates for different hazards to sheep welfare at small-scale and large-scale slaughter in Norway, Iceland, Sweden and Finland; aggregated data from nine experts 2012

risk estimates, compared to other steps of the slaughter process.

In both SS and LS, the highest magnitudes were found for prolonged insufficient feeding (>16 h) during lairage, and prolonged insufficient watering (>8 h) during lairage. Research on physiological effects of temporary deprivation of feed and water is diverging. Fisher et al. [10] found sheep in different body conditions to adapt to up to 30 h of feed deprivation by mobilising their energy reserves without any evidence of metabolic depletion such as low blood glucose or high meat pH. Inaccessibility of feed for a short period of time (possibly 12–16 h) thus does not seem to have large physiological implications, although the animals may experience some degree of hunger. There is also some evidence that sheep have an ability to withstand prolonged periods of water restriction. According to Silanikove [11] and Jacob et al. [12], the plasma volume and body water balance can be maintained by drawing water into the circulation from the rumen during the first 2 days of water deprivation. In some countries, it is standard practice to fast sheep for a prolonged period before and after transport to slaughter. The main reason for this seems to be a reduced risk of faecal contamination of the fleece and carcass during transport and dressing. Furthermore, New Zealand's Occupational Safety and Health Service [13] recommends that weaned lambs and ewes are fasted prior to shearing, leaving them without feed for 12–32 h and without water for 8–24 h, to avoid discomfort, stress, defecation and urination during handling at shearing. Our results to some extent contradict these recommendations, although the discomfort at shearing may be very different from that experienced during handling before slaughter [14].

Other hazards with high magnitudes were mixing of animals from different transports and introduction of an

Table 2 Summary of linear mixed models of welfare quantities

Quantity	Small-scale		Large-scale	
	R^2	Expert variance (% of total)	R^2	Expert variance (% of total)
Lowest possible exposure	0.39	0.0031 (15)	0.43	0.0042 (11)
Most-likely exposure	0.47	0.0039 (11)	0.48	0.00063 (1.4)
Highest possible exposure	0.54	0.012 (21)	0.53	0.0040 (6.3)
Intensity	0.64	0.21 (29)	0.59	0.16 (22)
Duration	0.59	0.12 (15)	0.62	0.034 (5.0)
Lowest possible likelihood	0.48	0.037 (38)	0.45	0.030 (35)
Most-likely likelihood	0.40	0.024 (28)	0.37	0.022 (27)
Highest possible likelihood	0.37	0.017 (25)	0.32	0.016 (22)
Bibliographic uncertainty	0.53	0.22 (46)	0.37	0.14 (30)

Coefficients of determination (R^2) and expert variance components from linear mixed models of quantities related to sheep welfare risks at small-scale and large-scale slaughter in Norway, Iceland, Sweden and Finland; aggregated data from nine experts 2012 adult ram into the group during lairage. When groups of sheep unfamiliar to each other are mixed, they keep to their own groups for several weeks before full integration occurs [15].

In terms of risk, overnight lairage was associated with the highest estimate in SS, almost twice as high as the second highest estimate, although the magnitude was moderate. Existing research on effects of abattoir lairage time on animal welfare is limited and results are inconsistent. Some studies show that lairage after transport potentially allows animals to decrease the concentrations of stress hormones, restore muscle glycogen concentrations and reduce dehydration [1, 16]. Other studies suggest that lairage conditions themselves may prevent animals from resting and recovering from feed and water restriction [17]. Overnight lairage received a considerably lower risk estimate in SS than in LS, but also a somewhat lower magnitude, possibly indicating that the lairage conditions were considered to be superior in SS.

In Europe and North America, sheep are usually slaughtered on the day of arrival to the abattoir, whereas in e.g. Australia, New Zealand and China sheep are more typically slaughtered the day after arrival [18]. In the Nordic countries, sheep farms are often small and located at some distance from the abattoir. Hence, it may be difficult to collect enough sheep to start LS in the early morning without overnight lairage. However, research has shown that this is usually a result of poor logistics [19]. The application of modern logistics technology, such as specialised software and central coordination of contracted vehicles, has been shown to allow for higher efficiency, better animal welfare and lower emissions in Swedish farm animal transport [20].

Beside overnight lairage, main risks identified in SS included splitting of groups during lairage, separation of one sheep from the group during driving to stunning, and isolating single sheep while waiting for stunning. These hazards were associated with only low to moderate risk estimates in LS. In SS, the groups are smaller than in LS, implying that a larger proportion of sheep will experience being the first animal taken out or the last one left in a group. Sheep react on being isolated from their flock mates by agitation, escape (or immobilisation), vocalisation and a physiological stress response [21, 22]. Baldock and Sibly [23] found that isolation from the flock resulted in a stronger stress response than transportation did. In contrast, Hargreaves and Hutson [14] did not detect changes in heart rate, plasma cortisol or haematocrit as a stress response to 4 min of isolation, and suggested that individual handling and familiarity with the procedure may have attenuated this response. Isolation is less stressful if the sheep are able to see other sheep nearby [24].

In LS, particularly high risk estimates were obtained for insufficient feeding (no feed available for >2 h), insufficient bedding (hard, wet or dirty flooring), and mechanical noise (sound levels of >75 dB from metal fittings or ventilation) during lairage. The importance of bedding quality to maintain welfare depends on whether lairaged sheep are newly sheared; not fully fleeced ewes show a preference for a soft lying surface with low thermal conductivity [25]. Hall et al. [26] found that excess noise during transportation had effects on salivary cortisol, heart rate and behaviour.

Eriksson [8] classified hazards as of "high", "lower" or "negligible" risks and found overnight lairage to be associated with relatively high risks in comparison with other hazards, which is in agreement with our risk assessment. The author found dragging or pulling of animals by wool, horns, ears or tail for >10 % of the time when driving from lairage to stunning to be the main risk. Algers et al. [27] presented no risk estimates for hazards in sheep slaughter, and did not mention overnight lairage as a hazard. EFSA [28] concluded that research is needed to develop methods for restraining single sheep with minimal stress to the animal prior to stunning and methods to maintain good electrical contact with the stunning equipment, but did not make a complete hazard identification. Neither Algers et al. [27], nor EFSA [28] addressed SS or mobile slaughter specifically.

Clearly, many of the hazards included in this study are related to the competence and skills of the abattoir stockpersons and the slaughter line speed. For example, insufficient feeding and incorrect grouping of animals may be caused by human shortcomings. Likewise, a lower line speed allows stockpersons to care for individual animals and take extraordinary time-consuming measures when required. The amount of distress that sheep suffer during handling is likely to be affected by the quality of the stockperson [29–31], and the time available for appropriate handling of animals [32]. EFSA [33] concluded that an inability to understand animal needs, infrequent inspection to assess whether animal needs are being met, inspections where animals cannot be properly observed or too many animals per stockperson can all lead to poor management decisions that may impact on sheep welfare. In addition, behavioural reactivity to human handling may be affected by previous handling [34] and breed.

Typically, risk assessment produces separate estimates of magnitude and risk for each hazard, with limited possibilities to account for interaction between hazards, as discussed by EFSA [7]. In reality, multiple interactions are usually present. For example, simultaneous exposure to separation from flock mates, stressful handling and high noise levels may produce a larger decrease in welfare than is indicated by the three separate magnitude and risk estimates. According to Hutson and Grandin [31], it is likely that sheep flock more tightly together if they are fearful. Stress may also accumulate during the slaughter process, and stress caused by hazards in early steps may increase susceptibility to hazards appearing later on. For example, animals exposed to overnight lairage, prolonged fasting or rough handling when arriving at the abattoir are probably more vulnerable to welfare hazards in connection with stunning. The present study did not consider interactions between hazards or cumulative effects.

For some hazards, the scientific evidence of exposure and adverse effects on sheep at slaughter is scarce, making risk assessment difficult. Furthermore, the current study relied completely on the expertise and experience of nine experts who contributed with individual estimates of exposure to hazards, and intensity, duration and likelihood of negative effects. Another group of experts may have generated different estimates, due to different levels of knowledge, experience and personal values. It is obvious that pre-conceived personal preferences for SS may have biased the comparison with LS. However, the 22 experts invited to the workshop were among the most knowledgeable persons in the studied countries, and nine of them provided the data.

The results also depend on the way hazards were specified and explained at the workshop, and how they were interpreted and conceived by the participants. It is not unlikely that some of the large disagreements between experts were due to misunderstanding or misconception although, during the workshop, care was taken to discuss different hazards and types of estimates in order to reach a common understanding. The experts were allowed to adjust their estimates for quantities with a high degree of disagreement, which was shown to increase agreement and can be expected to have improved the quality of final estimates. Still, even after these adjustments, major disagreements were found for a number of hazards regarding likelihood values in SS and both exposure and likelihood estimates in LS. Although none of these differences concerned hazards with particularly high magnitude or risk estimates, they show that experts may disagree strongly if they are allowed to express personal opinions. This underlines that selection and elicitation of experts is a delicate task which requires great care to enable reliable results. Furthermore, in consensus assessment, disagreements may probably be hidden by opinions that are expressed forcefully by the most dominant individuals in a group of experts.

The current risk assessment applies to all sheep processed by SS or LS in Norway, Iceland, Sweden and Finland. Estimates of exposure, intensity, duration and likelihood were averaged over all conceivable slaughter plants in the four countries. In practice, the circumstances, and thus the animal welfare risks, may vary heavily between different plants and regions, due to differences in sheep breeds, farming structure, slaughter industry structure, transport conditions, educational standards, legislation and tradition. Norway and Iceland are not part of the EU, in contrast to Sweden and Finland, but are closely connected through similarities in regulations and practices. For the same reasons, the risks identified in this study may differ from other countries where SS of sheep is applied.

Conclusions

From risk assessment based on expert opinion, we conclude that overnight lairage at the slaughter plant is associated with the strongest negative welfare effects at both small- and large-scale sheep slaughter in Norway, Iceland, Sweden and Finland. We also conclude that prolonged insufficient feeding and watering during lairage potentially are the largest threats to animal welfare, depending on their occurrence. Small-scale slaughter appears to have a potential for better animal welfare than large-scale slaughter. For most factors relevant to welfare, the risks are higher in large-scale than in small-scale slaughter, except for splitting of groups during lairage, separation of one sheep from the group during driving to stunning, and single sheep while waiting for stunning. In small-scale plants, a comparatively low line speed probably allows more consideration for the individual needs of animals being slaughtered.

Abbreviations

EFSA: European Food Safety Authority; IQR: interquartile range; LS: large-scale slaughter; ML: most likely; OIE: World Organisation for Animal Health; SS: small-scale slaughter.

Authors' contributions

JH and BA planned the study. JH chaired the risk assessment workshop, collected the data and carried out the statistical analysis. All authors participated in the workshop and contributed with expert opinion data. All authors read and approved the final manuscript.

Author details

[1] Department of Animal Environment and Health, Swedish University of Agricultural Sciences, P. O. Box 234, 53223 Skara, Sweden. [2] Department of Animal Environment and Health, Swedish University of Agricultural Sciences, P. O. Box 234, 53223 Skara, Sweden. [3] Department of Animal Environment and Health, Swedish University of Agricultural Sciences, P. O. Box 7068, 75007 Uppsala, Sweden. [4] Veterinary Public Health, Norwegian Veterinary Institute, P. O. Box 750, Sentrum, 0106 Oslo, Norway. [5] Vallnäsvägen 3, 70358 Örebro, Sweden. [6] Icelandic Food and Veterinary Authority, Austurvegur 64, 800 Selfoss, Iceland. [7] Swedish Board of Agriculture, 551 82 Jönköping,

Sweden. [8] Brahea Centre for Training and Development, University of Turku, 20014 Turku, Finland.

Acknowledgements
Financial support was provided by the Nordic Council of Ministers. The authors gratefully acknowledge experiences shared by Torill Malmstrøm, Mobilslakt AS.

Competing interests
The authors declare that they have no competing interests.

References
1. Liu HW, Zhong RZ, Zhou DW, Sun HX, Zhao CS. Effects of lairage time after road transport on some blood indicators of welfare and meat quality traits in sheep. J Anim Physiol Anim Nutr. 2012;96:1127–35.
2. Karlsson T, Cornell B. Nordiskt seminarium kring gårdsnära slakt inom småskalig livsmedelsförädling [Nordic seminar on farmbased slaughter in small-scale food processing]. Nordic Council of Ministers, Copenhagen, Report ANP 776; 2006.
3. Karlsson T. Slaughtering at farm in Nordic countries. Development by improvements in live animal inspection and slaughter waste treatment. Nordic Innovation, Oslo. 2011. http://eldrimner.com/core/files/technical_report_till_ni_ver2.pdf. Accessed 19 Apr 2016.
4. Food and Agriculture Organization of the United Nations. FAOSTAT. FAO, Rome. 2016. http://faostat.fao.org/. Accessed 19 Apr 2016.
5. Animalia. Kjøttets tilstand. Status i norsk kjøtt-og eggproduksjon [The state of meat. Status in Norwegian meat and egg production]. Animalia, Oslo. 2015. http://flashbook.no/animalia/kjottetstilstand15/index.html. Accessed 19 Apr 2016.
6. Lindow K, Lannhard Öberg Å. Marknadsrapport får- och lammkött juni 2015 [Market report sheep and lamb meat June 2015]. Swedish Board of Agriculture, Jönköping. 2015. http://www.faravelsforbundet.com/startsida/marknadsstatistik/1848-marknadsrapport-2015. Accessed 19 Apr 2016.
7. European Food Safety Authority. Scientific Opinion. Guidance on Risk Assessment for Animal Welfare. EFSA, Parma. EFSA J. 2012;10:2513. http://www.efsa.europa.eu/en/efsajournal/pub/2513. Accessed 19 Apr 2016.
8. Eriksson S. Riskbedömning av djurvälfärd inom småskalig fårslakt [Risk assessment of animal welfare in small-scale sheep slaughter]. Department of Animal Environment and Health, Swedish University of Agricultural Sciences, Uppsala. Graduation Report 2012:25; 2012.
9. Skog Eriksen M, Rødbotten R, Grøndahl AM, Friestad M, Andersen L, Mejdell CM. Mobile abattoir versus conventional slaughterhouse—impact on stress parameters and meat quality characteristics in Norwegian lambs. Appl Anim Behav Sci. 2013;149:21–9.
10. Fisher MW, Muir PD, Gregory NG, Thomson BC, Smith NB, Johnstone PD, Bicknell N. The effects of depriving feed to facilitate transport and slaughter in sheep—a case study of cull ewes held off pasture for different periods. N Z Vet J. 2015;63:260–4.
11. Silanikove N. The struggle to maintain hydration and osmoregulation in animals experiencing severe dehydration and rapid rehydration: the story of ruminants. Exp Physiol. 1994;79:281–300.
12. Jacob RH, Pethick DW, Clark P, D'Souza DN, Hopkins DL, White J. Quantifying the hydration status of lambs in relation to carcass characteristics. Aust J Exper Agric. 2006;46:429–37.
13. Occupational Safety & Health Service. Health and safety recommendations for fasting of sheep prior to shearing. OSH, Department of Labour, Wellington. 2003. http://www.business.govt.nz/worksafe/information-guidance/all-guidance-items/fasting-of-sheep-prior-to-shearing-health-and-safety-recommendations-for. Accessed 19 Apr 2016.
14. Hargreaves AL, Hutson GD. Changes in heart rate, plasma cortisol and hematocrit of sheep during a shearing procedure. Appl Anim Behav Sci. 1990;26:91–101.
15. Winfield CG, Syme GJ, Pearson AJ. Effect of familiarity with each other and breed on the spatial behaviour of sheep in an open field. Appl Anim Ethol. 1981;7:67–75.
16. Mounier L, Dubroeucq H, Andanson S, Veissier I. Variations in meat pH of beef bulls in relation to conditions of transfer to slaughter and previous history of the animals. J Anim Sci. 2006;84:1567–76.
17. Krawczel PD, Friend TH, Archer GS. Behavior of lambs in rest pens during long-distance transport. J Appl Anim Welf Sci. 2008;11:337–45.
18. Ferguson DM, Warner RD. Have we underestimated the impact of pre-slaughter stress on meat quality in ruminants? Meat Sci. 2008;80:12–9.
19. Algers A, Algers B, Franzén U, Lindencrona M, Moen M, Ohnell S, Waidringer J, Wiberg S. Logistik i samband med transport till slakt. Livsmedel och miljö—optimerade djurtransporter, En förstudie [Logistics at transport to slaughter. Food and environment—optimised animal transport]. Swedish University of Agricultural Sciences, Department of Animal Environment and Health, Skara, Report 10. 2006. https://people.ifm.liu.se/unwen/djurskydd/Rapport_10_logistik_skara.pdf. Accessed 19 Apr 2016.
20. Moen O, Algers B, Waidringer J. Planning, operations and control to assure good animal welfare in transportation to slaughter—Application of modern logistics in EU. Proc. XIV ISAH Congress, 19–23 July 2009, Vechta. p. 433–6.
21. Parrott RF, Misson BH, de la Riva CF. Differential stressor effects on the concentrations of cortisol, prolactin, and catecholamines in the blood of sheep. Res Vet Sci. 1994;56:234–9.
22. Cockram MS, Random M, Imlah P, Goddard PJ, Burrells C, Harkiss GD. The behavioural endocrine and immune responses of sheep to isolation. Anim Prod. 1994;58:389–99.
23. Baldock NM, Sibly RM. Effects of handling and transportation on the heart rate and behaviour of sheep. Appl Anim Behav Sci. 1990;28:15–39.
24. Yates DT, Otis AR, Warner CA, Yates LJ, Halalsheh RA, Horvath MB, Hallford DM, Ross TT. Effects of physical isolation on serum and salivary cortisol and components of complete blood counts in yearling ewes. Sheep Goat Res J. 2010;25:39–44.
25. Færevik G, Andersen IL, Bøe KE. Preferences of sheep for different types of pen flooring. Appl Anim Behav Sci. 2005;90:265–76.
26. Hall SJG, Kirkpatrick SM, Lloyd DM, Broom DM. Noise and vehicular motion as potential stressors during the transportation of sheep. Anim Sci. 1998;67:467–73.
27. Algers B, Anil H, Blokhuis H, Fuchs K, Hultgren J, Lambooij B, Nunes T, Paulsen P, Smulders F. Project to develop Animal Welfare Risk Assessment Guidelines on Stunning and Killing, EFSA proposal CFP/EFSA/AHAW/2007/01. Swedish University of Agricultural Sciences, Skara. 2009. http://www.efsa.europa.eu/en/supporting/pub/11e. Accessed 19 April 2016.
28. European Food Safety Authority. Opinion of the Scientific Panel on Animal Health and Welfare (AHAW) on a request from the Commission related to welfare aspects of the main systems of stunning and killing the main commercial species of animals. EFSA, Parma. EFSA J. 2004;45:1–29. http://www.efsa.europa.eu/en/efsajournal/pub/45. Accessed 19 Apr 2016.
29. Rushen J, de Passillé AMB. The scientific assessment of the impact of housing on animal welfare: a critical review. Can J Anim Sci. 1992;72:721–43.
30. Hemsworth PH, Coleman GJ. Human-livestock interactions: the stockperson and the productivity and welfare of intensively farmed animals. Wallingford: CABI; 1998.
31. Hutson GD, Grandin T. Behavioural principles of sheep handling. In: Grandin T, editor. Livestock Handling and Transport. 4th ed. Wallingford: CABI; 2014. p. 193–217.
32. Grandin T. Making slaughterhouses more humane for cattle, pigs, and sheep. Ann Rev Anim Biosci. 2013;1:491–512.
33. European Food Safety Authority. Scientific Opinion on the welfare risks related to the farming of sheep for wool, meat and milk production. EFSA, Parma. EFSA J. 2014;12:3933. http://www.efsa.europa.eu/en/efsajournal/pub/3933. Accessed 19 Apr 2016.
34. Probst JK, Spengler Neff A, Leiber F, Kreuzer M, Hillmann E. Gentle touching in early life reduces avoidance distance and slaughter stress in beef cattle. Appl Anim Behav Sci. 2012;139:42–9.

17

In vitro assessment of the antimicrobial activity of silver and zinc oxide nanoparticles against fish pathogens

Mohamed Ibrahim Shaalan[1,2], Magdy Mohamed El-Mahdy[2], Sarah Theiner[3], Mansour El-Matbouli[1*] and Mona Saleh[1]

Abstract

Background: Antibiotic resistance is a global issue that threatens public health. The excessive use of antibiotics contributes to this problem as the genes of antibiotic resistance can be transferred between the bacteria in humans, animals and aquatic organisms. Metallic nanoparticles could serve as future substitutes for some conventional antibiotics because of their antimicrobial activity. The aim of this study was to evaluate the antimicrobial effects of silver and zinc oxide nanoparticles against major fish pathogens and assess their safety in vitro. Silver nanoparticles were synthesized by chemical reduction and characterized with UV–Vis spectroscopy, transmission electron microscopy and zeta sizer. The concentrations of silver and zinc oxide nanoparticles were measured using inductively coupled plasma-mass spectrometry. Subsequently, silver and zinc oxide nanoparticles were tested for their antimicrobial activity against *Aeromonas hydrophila, Aeromonas salmonicida* subsp. *salmonicida, Edwardsiella ictaluri, Edwardsiella tarda, Francisella noatunensis* subsp. *orientalis, Yersinia ruckeri* and *Aphanomyces invadans* and the minimum inhibitory concentrations were determined. MTT assay was performed on eel kidney cell line (EK-1) to determine the cell viability after incubation with nanoparticles. The interaction between silver nanoparticles and *A. salmonicida* was investigated by transmission electron microscopy.

Results: The tested nanoparticles exhibited marked antimicrobial activity. Silver nanoparticles inhibited the growth of both *A. salmonicida* and *A. invadans* at a concentration of 17 μg/mL. Zinc oxide nanoparticles inhibited the growth of *A. salmonicida, Y. ruckeri* and *A. invadans* at concentrations of 15.75, 31.5 and 3.15 μg/mL respectively. Silver nanoparticles showed higher cell viability when compared to zinc oxide nanoparticles in the MTT assay. Transmission electron microscopy showed the attachment of silver nanoparticles to the bacterial membrane and disruption of its integrity.

Conclusions: This is the first study on inhibitory effects of silver and zinc oxide nanoparticles towards *A. salmonicida* and *A. invadans.* Moreover, zinc oxide nanoparticles inhibited the growth of *Y. ruckeri.* In low concentrations, silver nanoparticles were less cytotoxic than zinc oxide nanoparticles and represent an alternative antimicrobial compound against *A. hydrophila, A. salmonicida* and *A. invadans.*

Keywords: Antibacterial, Antifungal, Fish diseases, Silver nanoparticles, Zinc oxide nanoparticles

Background

Increases in global fish consumption have resulted in greater development and intensification of aquaculture worldwide [1, 2] which have led to a massive use of antibiotics for promoting growth and prophylaxis, especially in intensive aquaculture [2]. The EU has prohibited the use of antibiotics as growth promoters in animals since 2006 [3]. However, it is difficult to assess the quantity and identify the classes of antimicrobial agents in aquaculture [4]. Tuševljak et al. [5] conducted a survey of fish

*Correspondence: mansour.el-matbouli@vetmeduni.ac.at
[1] Clinical Division of Fish Medicine, University of Veterinary Medicine, Veterinärplatz 1, 1210 Vienna, Austria

farms in 25 countries in North America, South America, Europe, Africa and Asia, and found that tetracycline and quinolones are applied frequently, especially in salmon aquaculture. Nevertheless, detailed investigations about the types and the amounts of antibiotics in fish farms are still needed [4, 6]. The problem of antibiotic resistance has become a major concern in human and veterinary medicine [2, 3, 7]. The antibiotic resistance genes could be transferred between bacteria from different environments. Sharing of such genes occurs between bacteria which infect aquatic animals, terrestrial animals and humans, and thereby poses a hazard to animal and human health [7]. The closing statement of the joint science ministers meeting at the G8 summit in 2013 emphasized that antimicrobial resistance is one of the most important global health challenges in the 21st century. At the same time, bacterial, viral, mycotic and parasitic fish diseases constitute a massive threat to the aquaculture industry [8]. *Aeromonas hydrophila* is a major bacterial pathogen, which causes dermal ulceration and haemorrhagic septicemia in many fish species [9]. *Aeromonas salmonicida* was one of the first discovered causative agents of fish diseases, and is a widely-occurring pathogen of salmonids, which causes septicemia with high mortality rates [10, 11]. *Edwardsiella ictaluri* is responsible for enteric septicemia of channel catfish (*Ictalurus punctatus*), while *Edwardsiella tarda* is the causative agent of emphysematous putrefactive disease in the same species [12, 13]. *Francisella noatunensis* subsp. *orientalis* is an intracellular bacterial pathogen, which infects tilapia and produces a chronic granulomatous inflammation [14]. *Yersinia ruckeri* is the causative agent of enteric red mouth disease (ERM), which causes a wasting condition in fish and result in cumulative mortalities with high economic losses in fish farms [15, 16]. In spite of the production of a commercial vaccine against motile and non-motile strains of *Y. ruckeri*, field cases of vaccination failure have been reported [17]. Oomycete infections caused by *Aphanomyces invadans* induce skin ulcerations that extend deep into the underlying muscles leading to high morbidity and mortality in fish during outbreaks of epizootic ulcerative syndrome (EUS) [18].

Sørum [7] has reported the emergence of antibiotic resistant strains of *A. hydrophila, A. salmonicida*, and *Y. ruckeri* in fish farms. One of the recent strategies to combat microbes and multi-drug resistant bacteria is the application of metallic nanoparticles, which exhibit antimicrobial activities [19–22].

Antimicrobial effects on fish pathogens have been observed with silver and gold nanoparticles [21–28], and zinc oxide nanoparticles [29, 30].

Silver nanoparticles show antibacterial effects against *A. hydrophila, Aeromonas bestiarum, Pseudomonas flourescens, E. tarda, Vibrio harveyi, Proteus* spp. and *Flavobacterium* spp. [23–28, 30] and inhibit the growth of multiple drug resistant isolates of *Staphylococcus aureus, Micrococcus luteus* and *Klebsiella pneumonia* [31, 32]. One advantage of silver nanoparticles over conventional antibiotics is that their antimicrobial action arises through interference with multiple cellular processes of the bacteria, so the emergence of resistance is less likely [33]. Exact mechanisms that underlie the antibacterial actions of silver nanoparticles are not completely understood [34, 35]. However, modes of action have been suggested by different researchers [22, 33–36] and include the interaction of the silver nanoparticles with the bacterial cell wall, production of reactive oxygen species (ROS), interaction with DNA, and release of Ag^+ ions.

Similarly, zinc oxide nanoparticles exhibit potent antimicrobial activities [29, 30, 37], which are suspected of arising through complex mechanisms of action that include release of Zn^{2+} ions, production of ROS and interference with bacterial replication by inhibition of cellular processes like glycolysis, acid tolerance and transmembrane proton translocation [36, 38].

In this study, we investigated the antibacterial and antifungal activity of silver and zinc oxide nanoparticles against *A. hydrophila, A. salmonicida* subsp. *salmonicida, E. ictaluri, E. tarda, F. noatunensis* subsp. *orientalis, Y. ruckeri* and *A. invadans.* We also assessed cytotoxicity and host cell viability using an MTT assay after incubating nanoparticles with eel kidney-1 cells (EK-1).

Methods

Materials

Silver (≈100 nm) and zinc oxide (≈66 nm) nanoparticles were purchased from Sigma-Aldrich, Austria. Chemicals and reagents used for silver nanoparticles synthesis [silver nitrate, sodium citrate tribasic hydrate, sodium borohydride, polyvinyl pyrrolidone (PVP) and de-ionized water] were also purchased from Sigma.

Silver nanoparticles synthesis

All beakers and cylinders were thoroughly cleaned and autoclaved before use and deionized water was used for the synthesis. Silver nanoparticles synthesis was carried out by the chemical reduction method as previously described [39]. Briefly, silver nitrate was used as a source of silver, sodium borohydride solution was used as a reducing agent, and PVP acted as a stabilizing agent to prevent particles agglomeration [40]. Sodium citrate tribasic hydrate functions as both reducing and stabilizing agent at the same time, besides, the combination of PVP and sodium citrate increases the stability of the newly formed nanoparticles [41]. Silver nitrate was dissolved completely in de-ionized water then sodium citrate tribasic hydrate and PVP were added. After complete dissolving, sodium borohydride solution was added to the mixture and stirred for 30 min. The color of the solution changed from colorless to brown indicating the formation of silver nanopaticles.

As silver nanoparticles are sensitive to light, they were kept dark in a clean autoclaved bottle at 4 °C.

Characterization of silver nanoparticles

The absorption spectra were determined using a UV–Vis spectrophotometer (NanoDrop 2000®, Thermo Fischer Scientific, Massachusetts, USA) against the spectrum of deionized water as a blank. All measurements were performed at room temperature on 3 separate days.

Morphology of the synthesized nanoparticles was investigated using transmission electron microscopy (EM 900, Zeiss, Oberkochen, Germany) operating at an accelerating voltage of 80 kV. One drop of silver nanoparticle solution was deposited on the carbon-coated copper grid then left to evaporate at room temperature forming a monolayer. The mean size of the particles was calculated using (Image SP Viewer®) software to measure 100 randomly sampled nanoparticles.

Nanoparticles size distribution and zeta potential were measured based on the dynamic light scattering (DLS) using a Malvern zeta sizer Nano ZS® device. Three separate measurements on different days were performed at room temperature.

Determination of nanoparticles concentration

Elemental concentrations of the nanoparticle solutions were measured using inductively coupled plasma-mass spectrometry (ICP-MS). Milli-Q water and nitric acid were used in all samples, with elemental standards for ICP-MS measurements from CPI international (Amsterdam, The Netherlands). Samples were digested in nitric acid using a microwave discover SP-D system (CEM Microwave Technology, Germany) with parameters: temperature 200 °C; ramp time 4 min; hold time 6 min; maximum power 300 W. Digested samples were diluted with Milli-Q water to give nitric acid concentrations lower than 3% and zinc and silver concentrations lower than 20 ng/g.

ICP-MS measurements were performed according to Theiner et al. [42] using an ICP-quadrupole MS instrument Agilent 7500ce (Agilent Technologies, Waldbronn, Germany) equipped with a CETAC ASX-520 autosampler (Nebraska, USA) and a MicroMist nebulizer, at a sample uptake rate of approx. 0.25 mL/min. The instrument was tuned daily, and rhenium served as an internal standard for zinc and silver. The ICP-MS was equipped with nickel cones and operated at an RF power of 1550 W. Argon was used as plasma gas with a flow of 15 L/min and as a carrier gas with a flow of ~1.1 L/min. The dwell time was set to 0.3 s and replicates of 10 measurements were taken. Agilent MassHunter® (Workstation Software, Version B.01.01, 2012) was used for data processing.

Bacterial strains and growth conditions

Six bacterial strains were tested: *A. hydrophila* (252/13), *A. salmonicida* subsp. *salmonicida* (A-14390), *E. ictaluri* (93/146), *E. tarda* (30.1/14), *F. noatunensis* subsp. *orientalis, Y. ruckeri* biotype-2 (7959-11); all were obtained from our MikroBank in the clinical division of fish medicine, University of Veterinary Medicine, Vienna, Austria. *A. hydrophila* was isolated from naturally-infected common bream (*Abramis brama* L.), *A. salmonicida* subsp. *salmonicida* and *Y. ruckeri* were isolated from naturally-infected rainbow trout (*Oncorhynchus mykiss*). *E. ictaluri* and *E. tarda* were isolated from infected channel catfish (*I. punctatus*) and discus (*Symphysodon aequifasciatus*), respectively. *F. noatunensis* subsp. *orientalis* was isolated from Malawi cichlid (*Aulonocara stuartgranti*). A loop from each pure strain was streaked on Müller-Hinton (MH) agar plates (Sigma-Aldrich) except for *F. noatunensis,* which was inoculated firstly in cystine heart broth and incubated for 24 h then streaked on cystine heart agar supplemented with 2% horse blood. All cultured agar plates were incubated at 22 °C for 24 h except for *A. salmonicida* which was incubated at 15 °C for 48 h and *F. noatunensis* which requires 5 days incubation at 22 °C for colony growth.

Bacterial growth inhibition test

A single bacterial colony from each strain was inoculated in brain heart infusion (BHI) broth (Sigma-Aldrich) except for *F. noatunensis* which was inoculated in modified Müller-Hinton II cation-adjusted broth (Sigma-Aldrich) enriched with 2% IsoVitalex (Becton–Dickinson). After inoculation, all isolates were incubated in a shaking incubator (144 rpm) at 22 °C for 24 h, except for *A. salmonicida* which was incubated at 15 °C for 48 h. A spectrophotometer (Eppendorf BioPhotometer®, Eppendorf, Hamburg, Germany) was used to determine the optical density (OD_{600}). Bacterial cultures were diluted with BHI broth to adjust their concentration at 10^6 CFU/mL, which was confirmed by plate counting. Equal volumes of each nanoparticle solution and each bacterial strain were mixed to reach a final concentration of 5×10^5 CFU/mL. A negative control was prepared by mixing equal volumes of bacteria and deionized water. All samples were then incubated overnight in a shaking incubator at the same conditions as above. After that, 100 μL of each sample was streaked on Müller Hinton agar plate (Sigma Aldrich) or cystine heart agar supplemented with 2% horse blood and incubated in a static incubator to observe the bacterial growth, according to Bresee et al. [43]. The test was performed in triplicate.

Minimal inhibitory concentration (MIC)

Nanoparticles that inhibited bacterial growth were subjected to the minimal inhibitory concentration (MIC) assay in triplicate, according to Swain et al. [30] with some modifications. Double fold serial dilutions of nanoparticles were added to the cultures containing 10^6 CFU/mL of bacteria and incubated as before. Then 100 μL of each was streaked on Müller Hinton agar plates. The double fold serial dilutions were prepared for each nanoparticle solution up to five times to determine the MIC value at which no bacterial growth on the plate was observed.

The effect of silver and zinc oxide nanoparticles on bacterial growth kinetics in BHI broth was measured using Eppendorf ® spectrophotometer at 600 nm. The determined MICs of silver and zinc oxide nanoparticles were applied in this assay. Oxytetracycline (25 μg/mL) and bacterial cultures only were used as positive and negative controls, respectively. The absorbance values (OD 600) were recorded at 4, 8, 12, 16, and 24 h. The experiment was performed in triplicate.

Fungal growth inhibition test

Silver and zinc nanoparticles were tested for their inhibitory effects against *A. invadans*. The fungus was isolated from infected dwarf gourami (*Colisa lalia*). It was grown on glucose-peptone (GP) agar and incubated at 26 °C for 5 days [18]. An anti-fungal assay was conducted as described by Mori et al. [44] with some modifications. Mycelia from the periphery of the growing fungus (about 1 mm) were inoculated in 2 mL GP broth in 10 mL falcon tubes. Equal volumes (2 mL) of each tested nanoparticle solution were added to the broth. An equal volume (2 mL) of deionized water was added to one tube as a negative control. All tubes were incubated at 26 °C for 5 days. Then, 100 μL of broth from each tube was inoculated in the center of a GP agar plate and incubated again at 26 °C for 5 days to monitor fungal growth or inhibition. Nanoparticles that inhibited the fungal growth were further diluted in twofold serial dilutions to determine the MIC. The experiment was performed in triplicate.

Assessment of cytotoxicity via MTT assay

We assessed three concentrations of silver and zinc oxide nanoparticles for their cytotoxicity, to determine the safety of these concentrations as therapeutants in vitro. Nanoparticle concentrations were chosen based on our MIC data. Eel kidney cells (EK-1) were used in 96-well plates at approximately 1.5×10^4 cells per well in L-15 medium + GlutaMAX (Gibco) supplemented with 10% fetal bovine serum (FBS) and antibiotics (Penicillin100 IU/mL and streptomycin 100 μg/mL). After 24 h incubation at 26 °C, three concentrations of silver (8.5, 17, 25.5 μg/mL) and zinc oxide nanoparticles (7.88, 15.75, 23.63 μg/mL) were added to the EK-1 cells; cells with medium alone served as negative controls. The medium was then removed and wells were washed with phosphate buffered saline (PBS) twice to remove any residual nanoparticles. Subsequently, cell viability was assessed by incubating the triplicate wells of silver and zinc oxide nanoparticles, negative control cells and blank (medium only) with MTT (3-[4,5-dimethylthiazol-2-yl]-2,5-diphenyl tetrazolium bromide, Sigma-Aldrich). MTT assay was performed as described by Mosmann [45]. 10 μL of the MTT (5 mg mL^{-1} dissolved in PBS) per 100 μL media were added to each well and incubated for 3 h at the same temperatures as described above. After that, 100 μL of MTT solubilization solution (Sigma-Aldrich) was added into each well to solubilize formazan crystals, and mixed using a rotatory shaker. The absorbance values of each well were recorded at 570 nm using EnSpire® multimode plate reader. Triplicate tests were performed for each concentration and the control. After blank correction, the percentage of cell viability was calculated as the optical density values of nanoparticles-treated cells/the mean optical density of non-treated control cells ×100. Data were analyzed using one-way ANOVA test with SPSS® 16.0 software.

Ultrastructural interaction between silver nanoparticles and *A. salmonicida*

Aeromonas. salmonicida was incubated in BHI broth at 15 °C for 2 days, as described by Bresee et al. [43] with some modifications (Pellet was fixed with 5% glutaraldehyde in 0.1 M PBS for 4 h instead of overnight fixation with 2.5% glutaraldehyde in 0.1 M sodium cacodylate buffer). The culture was adjusted to 2.1×10^8 CFU/mL, then, 1 mL added to 1 mL of silver nanoparticles (34 μg/mL), and incubated for 1 h at room temperature. The mixture was centrifuged at 11,600×*g* for 15 min, then the pellet was re-suspended in 1 mL PBS. Centrifugation was repeated with the same conditions. The pellet was fixed with 500 μL of glutaraldehyde (5% in 0.1 M PBS) at 4 °C for 4 h. Glutaraldehyde was removed and the pellet washed twice with 0.1 M PBS and incubated overnight at 4 °C. The pellet was post-fixed in 1% osmium tetroxide for 2 h at 4 °C and washed twice with PBS. Samples were dehydrated using graded alcohol series (70, 96 and 100%) before a 1:1 mixture of glycidyl ether and propylene oxide was added for 45 min then incubated overnight with a 3:1 mixture of glycidyl ether and propylene oxide. Samples were embedded in gelatin capsules then ultrathin sections were prepared using an ultramicrotome. For transmission electron microscopy (TEM) imaging, we used an

EM 900 (Zeiss®, Oberkochen, Germany) and Image SP Viewer® software.

Results

Characterization of silver nanoparticles

UV–Vis analysis of the synthesized silver nanoparticles showed a sharp absorption peak (0.806) at 395 nm (Fig. 1a). TEM images of the synthesized silver nanoparticles showed they were spherical (Fig. 1b), with a mean diameter of 21 nm (range of sizes 11–39 nm). DLS showed two peaks: a smaller peak at 8.3 nm and a larger peak at 44.5 nm (Fig. 1c), which indicated the presence of two populations of silver nanoparticles, zeta potential value was -30.7 ± 0.45 mV.

Determination of nanoparticles concentration

ICP-MS measurements revealed a silver concentration of 34 µg/mL in the synthesized silver nanoparticles and 16 µg/mL in the commercial silver nanoparticles. The concentration of zinc in zinc oxide nanoparticles was 63 µg/mL. Sizes and concentrations of nanoparticles are summarized in Table 1.

Bacterial growth inhibition test

The synthesized silver nanoparticles and the commercial zinc oxide nanoparticles exhibited antibacterial activity against *A. hydrophila*, *A. salmonicida* and *Y. ruckeri*. However, they were not able to inhibit the growth of *E. ictaluri*, *E. tarda* and *F. noatunensis*. Commercial silver nanoparticles did not inhibit bacterial growth of the strains in this study (Table 2).

Minimal inhibitory concentration (MIC)

The growth of both *A. hydrophila* and *A. salmonicida* was inhibited completely after incubation with the synthesized silver nanoparticles at 17 µg/mL or zinc oxide nanoparticles at 15.75 µg/mL. This was confirmed by the absence of bacterial growth on Müller Hinton agar

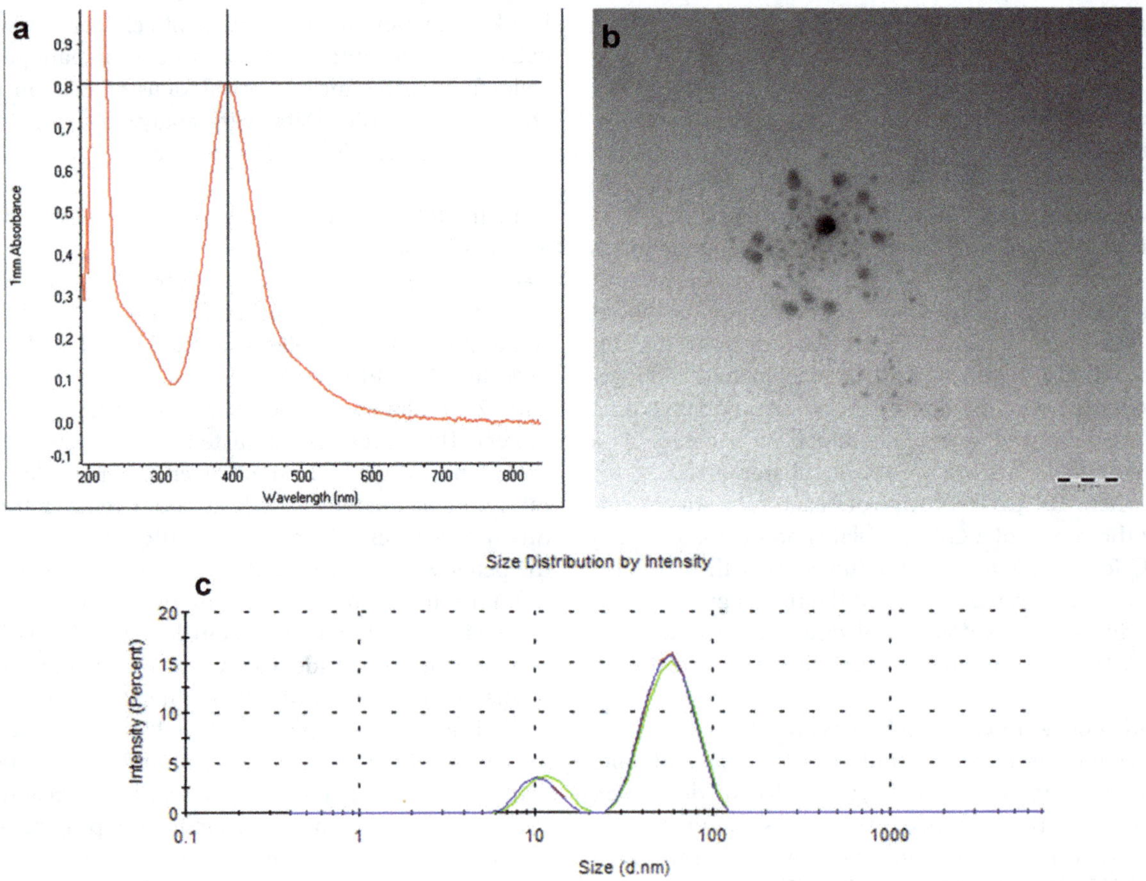

Fig. 1 Characterization of silver nanoparticles. **a** UV–Vis analysis of silver nanoparticles showed peak absorption (0.806) at 395 nm, which matches with the surface plasmon resonance of silver nanoparticles, **b** TEM micrograph showing the morphology of silver nanoparticles: they are *spherical* with a mean size of 21 nm. (*scale bar* = 50 nm), **c** particle size distribution of the synthesized silver nanoparticles, showing two peaks: a smaller peak at 8.3 nm and a larger peak at 44.5 nm, which indicate presence of two particle size populations

Table 1 The properties of the tested nanoparticles (sizes and concentrations)

Type of nanoparticles	Size by TEM (nm)	Size by DLS (nm)	Concentration (μg/mL)
Silver nanoparticles (synthesized)	21	Two sizes: 8.3 and 44.5	34
Silver nanoparticles (commercial)	100	96	16
Zinc oxide nanoparticles (commercial)	–	66	63

Table 2 Antimicrobial effects of the tested metallic nanoparticles and their minimum inhibitory concentrations (MICs) in μg/mL

Pathogen	Silver nanoparticles (synthesized) (μg/mL)	Silver nanoparticles (commercial) (μg/mL)	Zinc oxide nanoparticles (commercial) (μg/mL)
A. hydrophila	17	–	15.75
A. salmonicida	17	–	15.75
E. ictaluri	–	–	–
E. tarda	–	–	–
F. noatunensis	–	–	–
Y. ruckeri	–	–	31.5
A. invadans	17	–	3.15

(–) = MIC was not reached

plates (Figs. 2, 3), and the complete inhibition of bacterial growth in BHI as observed by a spectrophotometer (Fig. 4a, b). The growth of *Y. ruckeri* was inhibited after incubation with zinc oxide nanoparticles at 31.5 μg/mL (Table 2). That was confirmed by OD 600 measurements, which indicated complete inhibition of bacterial growth after incubation with zinc oxide nanoparticles at 24 h. In contrast, oxytetracycline (25 μg/mL) failed to reach complete inhibition of *Y. ruckeri* at the same time point (Fig. 4c).

Fungal growth inhibition test

Silver and zinc oxide nanoparticles inhibited *A. invadans* growth in both GP broth and agar. After double fold serial dilutions, the MIC values were 17 and 3.15 μg/mL for synthesized silver and zinc oxide nanoparticles, respectively (Table 2).

Assessment of cytotoxicity via MTT assay

Viability of EK-1 cells varied widely between silver and zinc oxide nanoparticles. The cells viability after addition 8.5 μg/mL of synthesized silver nanoparticles showed no significant difference ($P \leq 0.05$) when compared with non-treated control cells. After incubation of the cells with 17 and 25.5 μg/mL of silver nanoparticles the cell viability measured 69.1 and 63% respectively (Table 3). For zinc oxide nanoparticles, all concentrations resulted in 100% cell death.

Ultrastructural interaction between silver nanoparticles and *A. salmonicida*

Silver nanoparticles were observed attached to the outer membrane of *A. salmonicida* (Fig. 5a). At two-times higher magnification, we observed that silver nanoparticles induced widening of periplasmic space (arrowhead), and caused diffuse intra-cytoplasmic edema (arrow) (Fig. 5b). Smaller nanoparticles (8 nm) were observed inside the bacterial cytoplasm (arrow) (Fig. 5c). Finally, silver nanoparticles disrupted the bacterial cell membrane, leading to complete cell lysis and leakage of intracellular content (Fig. 5d).

Discussion

Infectious diseases caused by parasites, bacteria, fungi and viruses constitute major threats to cultured fish [8]. Concurrently, there is a need to minimize use of antibiotics in farming, to combat antibiotic resistance [3, 4]. Thus, there is a growing need for alternative antimicrobial therapeutics, and metal and metal oxide nanoparticles are being widely investigated for their potential medical applications, including their use in fish medicine [22].

In this study, we investigated the antibacterial and antifungal effects of commercially obtained zinc oxide and silver nanoparticles, and synthesized silver nanoparticles in-house. For this synthesis, we used PVP as a capping agent, to stabilize the nanoparticles and prevent them from aggregating [46], with the direct benefit that

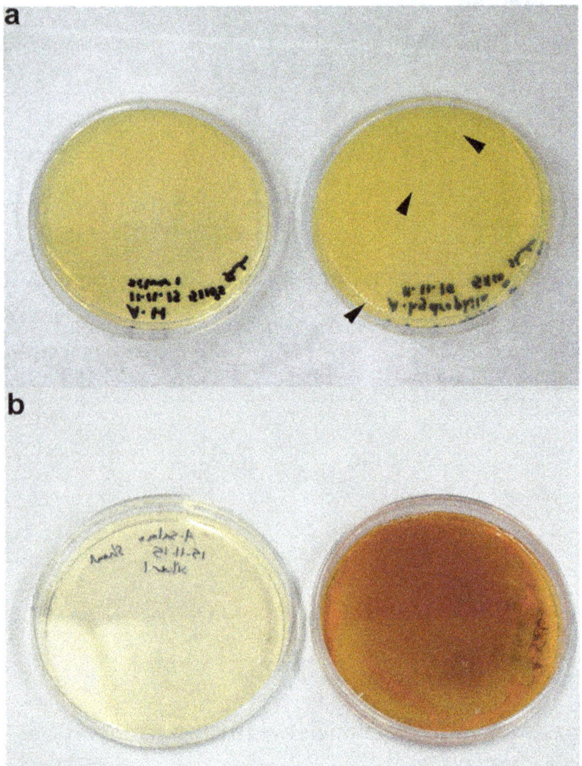

Fig. 2 Minimum inhibitory concentration determination for silver nanoparticles. **a** Note the formation of small pinpoint colonies (*arrowheads*) of *A. hydrophila* on the control plate (*on the right*), while no bacterial growth was observed after incubation with 17 µg/mL silver nanoparticles (*on the left*), **b** growth of *A. salmonicida* with production of brown pigments on the control plate (*on the right*), while neither bacterial growth nor pigment production was observed after incubation with 17 µg/mL silver nanoparticles (*on the left*)

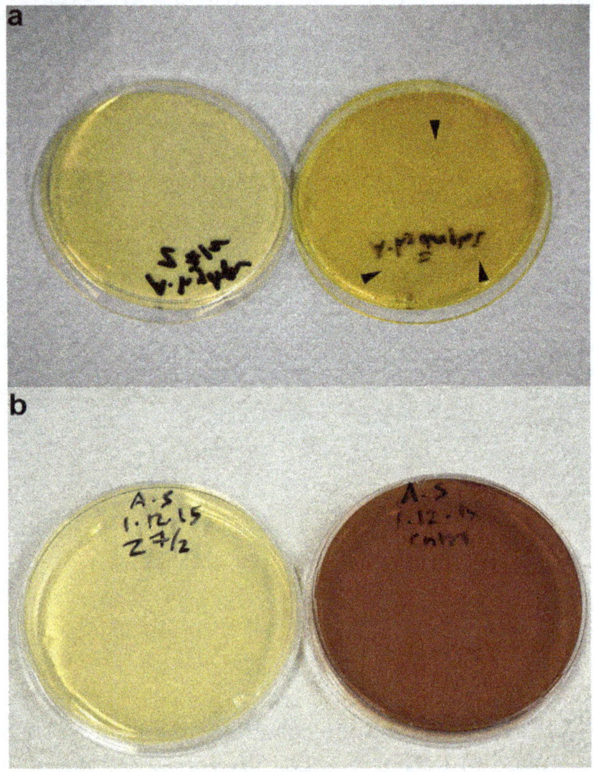

Fig. 3 Minimum inhibitory concentration determination for zinc oxide nanoparticles. **a** Note the formation of small pinpoint colonies (*arrowheads*) of *A. hydrophila* on the control plate (*on the right*), while no bacterial growth was observed after incubation with 15.75 µg/mL zinc oxide nanoparticles (*on the left*), **b** growth of *A. salmonicida* with production of brown pigments on the control plate (*on the right*), while neither bacterial growth nor pigment production was observed after incubation with 15.75 µg/mL zinc oxide nanoparticles (*on the left*)

PVP-capped nanoparticles are an ideal form for administration in water for fish.

UV–Vis analysis of the synthesized silver nanoparticles showed absorbance peak at 395 nm which lies in the spectrum range of silver nanoparticles and confirms the successful synthesis [47, 48]. The analysis of the size distribution of silver nanoparticles using zeta sizer revealed the presence of two peaks, one peak at 8.3 nm and a larger peak at 44.5 nm, which indicates the presence of two populations of silver nanoparticles where the majority of particles were located under the larger peak with mean size of 44.5 nm. TEM images confirmed that silver nanoparticles were spherical in shape, with an average particle size of 21 nm. While TEM provides the morphology and the mean size of the nanoparticles, zeta sizer indicates the real size distribution.

In our study, silver nanoparticles showed antibacterial activity against *A. hydrophila* which agreed with the results from previous studies [23, 25, 30]. Also, zinc oxide nanoparticles exhibited antibacterial activity against *A. hydrophila* which corresponded with Swain et al. [30]. However, in our study the MIC was measured at 15.75 µg/mL which is lower than their results which ranged from 250 to 2500 µg/mL. This difference is mostly due to the variation in the size of the nanoparticles used when comparing these two studies. The particle size along with the concentration plays a crucial role in the antibacterial properties of the nanoparticles. Smaller-sized nanoparticles have a higher surface area which increases their antibacterial activity [38].

To the best of our knowledge, this is the first study to demonstrate the inhibitory effects of silver and zinc oxide nanoparticles against *A. salmonicida* and *A. invadans,* in addition to the inhibitory effect of zinc oxide nanoparticles against *Y. ruckeri* [49].

Synthesized silver nanoparticles at a concentration of 17 µg/mL were capable of complete inhibition of the growth of both *A. salmonicida* and *A. invadans*. In comparison, oxytetracycline (25 µg/mL) required longer

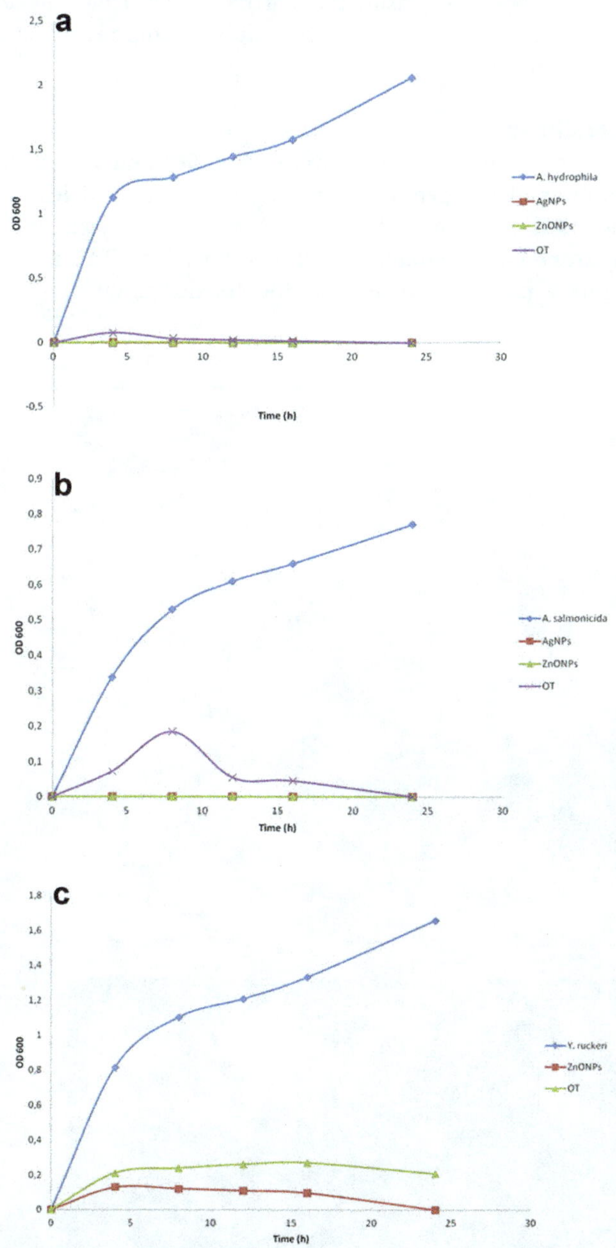

Fig. 4 Absorbance values (OD 600) measurements for the bacterial cultures only and after incubation with silver nanoparticles, zinc oxide nanoparticles or oxytetracycline, **a** OD 600 values for *A. hydrophila*, **b** OD 600 values for *A. salmonicida*, **c** OD 600 values for *Y. ruckeri*. *AgNPs* silver nanoparticles (17 μg/mL), *ZnONPs* zinc oxide nanoparticles for *A. hydrophila* and *A. salmonicida* (15.75 μg/mL) and for *Y. ruckeri* (31.5 μg/mL), *OT* oxytetracycline (25 μg/mL)

time to inhibit the growth of *A. salmonicida* as shown in Fig. 4b.

Using MTT assay, there was no significant difference between the lowest concentration of silver nanoparticles (8.5 μg/mL) and the control group. Silver nanoparticles were less cytotoxic to EK-1 cells when compared with zinc oxide nanoparticles. However, higher concentrations of silver nanoparticles were reported as cytotoxic and genotoxic to the fish cell lines and zebrafish [50].

Commercial silver nanoparticles failed to inhibit the bacterial growth of the tested pathogens in this study, possibly due to their lower concentration and bigger particle size in comparison with the synthesized silver nanoparticles.

Residual silver nanoparticles in the aqueous environment bind to organic and inorganic sulfur in sea or fresh water. Sulfidation of silver nanoparticles leads to significant decrease of their toxicity due to the lower solubility of the resulting silver sulfide and thus cause low detrimental impact on the environment [51].

Zinc oxide nanoparticles inhibited the growth of *A. hydrophila* and *A. salmonicida* at a concentration of 15.75 μg/mL, which is near to the MICs of silver nanoparticles.

Zinc oxide nanoparticles (31.5 μg/mL) inhibited the growth of *Y. ruckeri*, while oxytetracycline could not completely inhibit the growth of *Y. ruckeri* after 24 h (Fig. 4c).

Moreover, zinc oxide nanoparticles showed a strong antifungal activity against *A. invadans* at concentration of only 3.15 μg/mL, which was much lower than the MIC of silver nanoparticles against the same fungus. Unfortunately, the zinc oxide nanoparticles were highly toxic against the EK-1 cell line at all concentrations (7.88, 15.75, 23.63 μg/mL). These results are in accordance with Fernández et al. [52] who report high sensitivity of RTG-2, RTH-149 and RTL-W1 fish cell lines to zinc oxide nanoparticles. The observed cytotoxicity may be attributed to release of free Zn^{+2} ions [53, 54].

When zinc oxide nanoparticles are released into the aquatic environment, their behavior is controlled by water environment such as oxygen level, pH, ionic strength and amount of organic matter. Due to the high ionic strength in sea water, the zinc oxide nanoparticles tend to aggregate and become less mobile [55], while in fresh water they tend to dissolve rapidly which increases the risk of acute toxicity for aquatic organisms [56].

We investigated the interaction between silver nanoparticles and *A. salmonicida* on the ultrastructural level. TEM showed larger nanoparticles (>20 nm) bound to the bacterial cell membrane (Fig. 4), thereby presumably interfering with its integrity and function. Smaller particles (8 nm) were observed inside the bacterial cytoplasm (Fig. 4c). These observations were in concordance with previous reports [35, 57]. Presence of nanoparticles in the cytoplasm suggests that the small-sized nanoparticles could pass through the S-layer pores, which range from 2 to 8 nm in diameter as described in *A. salmonicida*

Table 3 Effect of different silver nanoparticles concentrations (0, 8.5, 17, 25.5 μg/mL) on EK-1 cells viability

Concentrations μg/mL	Viability %
0.0	100.3 ± 18.6^a
8.5	92.8 ± 12.1^a
17	69.1 ± 37.0^b
25.5	63.0 ± 14.3^b

The values are expressed as mean ± SD. Different letters (a, b) in the same column means that they are significantly different ($P \leq 0.05$)

[58]. In the cytoplasm, the particles would be able to react directly with the intracellular components and mechanisms.

Conclusions

Due to their high antimicrobial activity and low environmental and cytotoxic effects, silver nanoparticles can be used as an effective antimicrobial agent against *A. hydrophila*, *A. salmonicida* and *A. invadans*. This represents a proof-of-concept for the consideration of silver

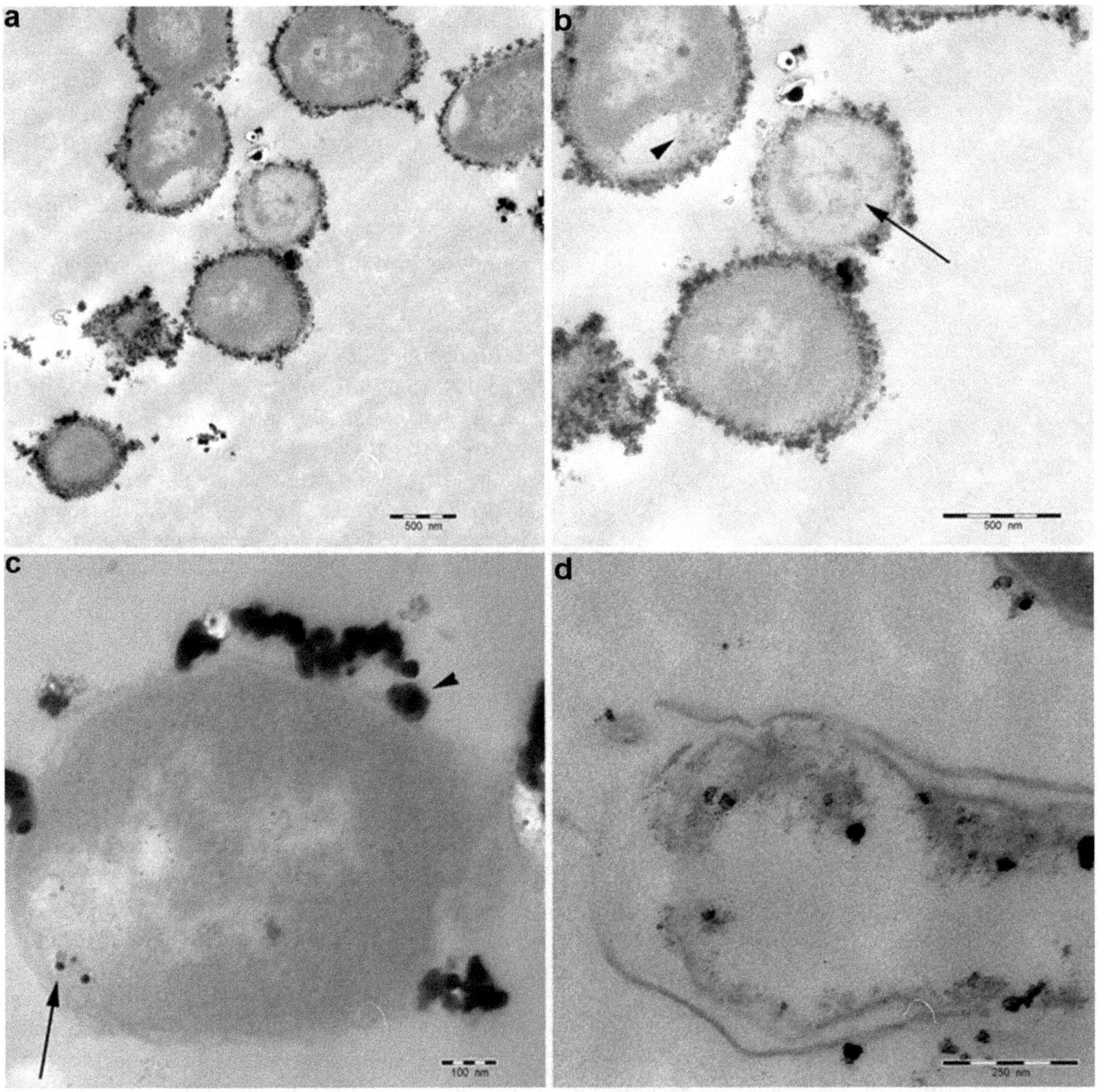

Fig. 5 Transmission electron microscopy microphotograph showing the interaction between silver nanoparticles and *A. salmonicida*, **a** electron-dense silver nanoparticles attached to the outer membrane of *A. salmonicida* (*bar* = 500 nm). **b** Widening of periplasmic space, presence of silver nanoparticles inside the periplasm (*arrowhead*), and marked intra-cytoplasmic edema which appears electron lucent (*arrow*) (*bar* = 500 nm). **c** Silver nanoparticles attached to the outer membrane (*arrowhead*) of *A. salmonicida*, with some particles inside the bacterial cytoplasm (*arrow*) (*bar* = 100 nm). **d** Complete lysis of *A. salmonicida* by silver nanoparticles (*bar* = 250 nm)

nanoparticles in novel therapeutics development and disease management in aquaculture. Additional in vivo studies are needed to investigate the efficacy and safety of the silver nanoparticles in the living fish.

Authors' contributions

MIS, MS and MEL designed the study. MIS performed the experiment and drafted the manuscript. MS, MEL and MME revised the manuscript. ST performed the ICP-MS analysis. All authors read and approved the final manuscript.

Author details

[1] Clinical Division of Fish Medicine, University of Veterinary Medicine, Veterinärplatz 1, 1210 Vienna, Austria. [2] Department of Pathology, Faculty of Veterinary Medicine, Cairo University, Giza 12211, Egypt. [3] Institute of Analytical Chemistry, University of Vienna, Währinger Straße 38, 1090 Vienna, Austria.

Acknowledgements

We would like to thank the FWF for funding the research work (Project No. P 23850-B17), Dr. Andrea Dressler for her help with the bacteriology, Mag. Nora Dinhopl for the electron microscopy imaging and Dr. Olga Jovanovic for her help in zetasizer measurements.

Competing interests

The authors declare that they have no competing interests.

Funding

This work was funded by the Austrian Science Fund (FWF), Project No. P 23850-B17.

References

1. Goldburg R, Naylor R. Future seascapes, fishing, and fish farming. Front Ecol Environ. 2005;3:21–8.
2. Cabello FC. Heavy use of prophylactic antibiotics in aquaculture: a growing problem for human and animal health and for the environment. Environ Microbiol. 2008;8:1137–44.
3. Menanteau-Ledouble S, Krauss I, Santos G, Fibi S, Weber B, El-Matbouli M. Effect of a phytogenic feed additive on the susceptibility of *Onchorhynchus mykiss* to *Aeromonas salmonicida*. Dis Aquat Org. 2015;115:57–66.
4. Cabello FC, Godfrey HP, Tomova A, Ivanova L, Dölz H, Millanao A, Buschmann AH. Antimicrobial use in aquaculture re-examined: its relevance to antimicrobial resistance and to animal and human health. Environ Microbiol. 2013;15:1917–42.
5. Tuševljak N, Dutil L, Rajić A, Uhland FC, Mcclure C, St-Hilaire S, Reid-Smith RJ, McEwen SA. Antimicrobial use and resistance in aquaculture: findings of a globally administered survey of aquaculture-allied professionals. Zoonoses Public Health. 2013;60:426–36.
6. Sapkota A, Sapkota AR, Kucharski M, Burke J, Mckenzie S, Walker P, Lawrence R. Aquaculture practices and potential human health risks: current knowledge and future priorities. Environ Int. 2008;34:1215–26.
7. Sørum H. Antibiotic resistance associated with veterinary drug use in fish farms. In: Lie Ø, editor. Improving farmed fish quality and safety. Cambridge: Woodhead Publishing; 2008. p. 157–82.
8. Meyer FP. Aquaculture disease and health management. J Anim Sci. 1991;69:4201–8.
9. Cipriano RC, Bullock GL, Pyle SW. *Aeromonas hydrophila* and motile aeromonad septicemias of fish. Fish disease leaflet 68. Washington, DC: United States Department of the Interior, Fish and Wildlife Service, Division of Fishery Research; 1984. p. 23.
10. Austin B, Austin DA. *Aeromonadaceae* representative (*Aeromonas salmonicida*). In: Austin B, Austin DA, editors. Bacterial fish pathogens. 6th ed. Switzerland: Springer International Publishing; 2016. p. 215–321.
11. Menanteau-Ledouble S, Kumar G, Saleh M, El-Matbouli M. *Aeromonas salmonicida*: updates on an old acquaintance. Dis Aquat Org. 2016;120:49–68.
12. Hawke JP, Mcwhorter AC, Steigerwalt AG, Brenner DJ. *Edwardsiella ictaluri* sp. nov., the causative agent of enteric septicemia of catfish. Int J Sys Evol Microbiol. 1981;31:396–400.
13. Meyer FP, Bullock GL. *Edwardsiella tarda*, a new pathogen of channel catfish (*Ictalurus punctatus*). Appl Microbiol. 1973;25:155–6.
14. Birkbeck TH, Feist SW, Verner-Jeffreys DW. Francisella infections in fish and shellfish. J Fish Dis. 2011;34:173–87.
15. Furones MD, Rodgers CJ, Munn CB. *Yersinia ruckeri*, the causal agent of enteric redmouth disease (ERM) in fish. Annu Rev Fish Dis. 1993;3:105–25.
16. Kumar G, Menanteau-Ledouble S, Saleh M, El-Matbouli M. *Yersinia ruckeri*, the causative agent of enteric redmouth disease in fish. Vet Res. 2015;46:103.
17. Huang Y, Jung A, Schäfer WJ, Mock D, Michael GB, Runge M, Schwarz S, Steinhagen D. Analysis of *Yersinia ruckeri* strains isolated from trout farms in northwest Germany. Dis Aquat Org. 2015;116:243–9.
18. Roberts RJ, Willoughby LG, Chinabut S. Mycotic aspects of epizootic ulcerative syndrome (EUS) of Asian fishes. J Fish Dis. 1993;16:169–83.
19. Huh AJ, Kwon YJ. "Nanoantibiotics": a new paradigm for treating infectious diseases using nanomaterials in the antibiotics resistant era. J Control Release. 2011;156:128–45.
20. Pelgrift RY, Friedman AJ. Nanotechnology as a therapeutic tool to combat microbial resistance. Adv Drug Deliv Rev. 2013;65:1803–15.
21. Saleh M, Kumar G, Abdel-Baki A, Al-Quraishy S, El-Matbouli M. In vitro antimicrosporidial activity of gold nanoparticles against *Heterosporis saurida*. BMC Vet Res. 2016;12:44.
22. Shaalan M, Saleh M, El-Mahdy M, El-Matbouli M. Recent progress in applications of nanoparticles in fish medicine: a review. Nanomedicine. 2016;12:701–10.
23. Antony JJ, Nivedheetha M, Siva D, Pradeepha G, Kokilavani P, Kalaiselvi S, Sankarganesha A, Balasundaramb A, Masilamani V, Achiraman S. Antimicrobial activity of *Leucas aspera* engineered silver nanoparticles against *Aeromonas hydrophila* in infected *Catla catla*. Colloids Surf B Biointerfaces. 2013;109:20–4.
24. Mahanty A, Mishra S, Bosu R, Maurya UK, Netam SP, Sarkar B. Phytoextracts-synthesized silver nanoparticles inhibit bacterial fish pathogen *Aeromonas hydrophila*. Indian J Microbiol. 2013;4:438–46.
25. Soltani M, Ghodratnema M, Ahari H, Ebrahimzadeh Mousavi HA, Atee M, Dastmalchi F, Rahmanya J. The inhibitory effect of silver nanoparticles on the bacterial fish pathogens. *Streptococcus iniae*, *Lactococcus garvieae*, *Yersinia ruckeri* and *Aeromonas hydrophila*. Int J Vet Res. 2009;3:137–42.
26. Umashankari J, Inbakandan D, Ajithkumar TT, Balasubramanian T. Mangrove plant, *Rhizophora mucronata* (Lamk, 1804) mediated one pot green synthesis of silver nanoparticles and its antibacterial activity against aquatic pathogens. Aquat Biosyst. 2012;8:11.
27. Vaseeharan B, Ramasamy P, Chen JC. Antibacterial activity of silver nanoparticles (AgNps) synthesized by tea leaf extracts against pathogenic *Vibrio harveyi* and its protective efficacy on juvenile *Feneropenaeus indicus*. Lett Appl Microbiol. 2010;50:352–6.
28. Velmurugan P, Iydroose M, Lee SM, Cho M, Park JH, Balachandar V, Oh BT. Synthesis of silver and gold nanoparticles using cashew nut shell liquid and its antibacterial activity against fish pathogens. Indian J Microbiol. 2014;54:196–202.
29. Ramamoorthy S, Kannaiyan P, Moturi M, Devadas T, Muthuramalingam J, Natarajan L, Arunachalam N, Ponniah AG. Antibacterial activity of zinc oxide nanoparticles against *Vibrio harveyi*. Indian J Fish. 2013;60:107–12.
30. Swain P, Nayak SK, Sasmal A, Behera T, Barik SK, Swain SK, Mishra SS, Sen AK, Das JK, Jayasankar P. Antimicrobial activity of metal based nanoparticles against microbes associated with diseases in aquaculture. World J Microbiol Biotechnol. 2014;30:2491–502.

31. Ayala-Núñez NV, Lara HH, Turrent LDCI, Padilla CR. Silver nanoparticles toxicity and bactericidal effect against methicillin resistant *Staphylococcus aureus*: nanoscale does matter. Nanobiotechnol. 2009;5:2–9.
32. Prakash P, Gnanaprakasam P, Emmanuel R, Arokiyaraj S, Saravanan M. Green synthesis of silver nanoparticles from leaf extract of *Mimusops elengi*, Linn. for enhanced antibacterial activity against multi drug resistant clinical isolates. Colloids Surf B Biointerfaces. 2013;108:255–9.
33. Knetsch ML, Koole LH. New strategies in the development of antimicrobial coatings: the example of increasing usage of silver and silver nanoparticles. Polymers. 2011;3:340–66.
34. Durán N, Durán M, De Jesus MB, Seabra AB, Fávaro WJ, Nakazato G. Silver nanoparticles: a new view on mechanistic aspects on antimicrobial activity. Nanomedicine. 2016;12:789–99.
35. Mosselhy DA, El-Aziz MA, Hanna M, Ahmed MA, Husien MM, Feng Q. Comparative synthesis and antimicrobial action of silver nanoparticles and silver nitrate. J Nanopart Res. 2015;17:1–10.
36. Seil JT, Webster TJ. Antimicrobial applications of nanotechnology: methods and literature. Int J Nanomed. 2012;7:2767–81.
37. Gunalan S, Sivaraj R, Rajendran V. Green synthesized ZnO nanoparticles against bacterial and fungal pathogens. Prog Nat Sci Mater Int. 2012;22:693–700.
38. Sirelkhatim A, Mahmud S, Seeni A, Kaus NHM, Ann LC, Bakhori SKM, Hasan H, Mohamad D. Review on zinc oxide nanoparticles: antibacterial activity and toxicity mechanism. Nano-Micro Lett. 2015;7:219–42.
39. El Mahdy MM, Eldin TAS, Aly HS, Mohammed FF, Shaalan MI. Evaluation of hepatotoxic and genotoxic potential of silver nanoparticles in albino rats. Exp Toxicol Pathol. 2015;67:21–9.
40. Wang H, Qiao X, Chen J, Wang X, Ding S. Mechanisms of PVP in the preparation of silver nanoparticles. Mater Chem Phys. 2005;94:449–53.
41. Cao VD, Tran NQ, Nguyen TPP. Synergistic effect of citrate dispersant and capping polymers on controlling size growth of ultrafine copper nanoparticles. J Exp Nanosci. 2015;10:576–87.
42. Theiner S, Varbanov H, Galanski M, Egger AE, Berger W, Heffeter P, Keppler BK. Comparative in vitro and in vivo pharmacological investigation of platinum(IV) complexes as novel anticancer drug candidates for oral application. J Biol Inorg Chem. 2014;20:89–99.
43. Bresee J, Bond CM, Worthington RJ, Smith CA, Gifford JC, Simpson CA, Carter CJ, Wang G, Hartman J, Osbaugh NA, Shoemaker RK, Melander C, Feldheim DL. Nanoscale structure-activity relationships, mode of action, and biocompatibility of gold nanoparticle antibiotics. J Am Chem Soc. 2014;136:5295–300.
44. Mori T, Hirose H, Hanjavanit C, Hatai K. Antifungal activities of plant extracts against some aquatic fungi. Biocontrol Sci. 2002;7:187–91.
45. Mosmann T. Rapid colorimetric assay for cellular growth and survival: application to proliferation and cytotoxicity assays. J Immunol Methods. 1983;65:55–63.
46. El Badawy AME, Luxton TP, Silva RG, Scheckel KG, Suidan MT, Tolaymat TM. Impact of environmental conditions (pH, ionic strength, and electrolyte type) on the surface charge and aggregation of silver nanoparticles suspensions. Environ Sci Technol. 2010;44:1260–6.
47. Bijanzadeh AR, Vakili MR, Khordad R. A study of the surface plasmon absorption band for nanoparticles. Int J Phys Sci. 2012;7:1943–8.
48. Slistan-Grijalva A, Herrera-Urbina R, Rivas-Silva JF, Ávalos-Borja M, Castillón-Barraza FF, Posada-Amarillas A. Classical theoretical characterization of the surface plasmon absorption band for silver spherical nanoparticles suspended in water and ethylene glycol. Physica E Low Dimens Syst Nanostruct. 2005;27:104–12.
49. Shaalan M, El-Mahdy M, El-Matbouli M, Saleh M. Zinc oxide nanoparticles as a novel tool to combat *Yersinia ruckeri* and *Aphanomyces invadans*. J Comp Pathol. 2017;1:74.
50. Kim S, Ryu DY. Silver nanoparticle-induced oxidative stress, genotoxicity and apoptosis in cultured cells and animal tissues. J Appl Toxicol. 2013;33:78–89.
51. Levard C, Hotze EM, Lowry GV, Brown GE Jr. Environmental transformations of silver nanoparticles: impact on stability and toxicity. Environ Sci Technol. 2012;46:6900–14.
52. Fernández D, García-Gómez C, Babín M. In vitro evaluation of cellular responses induced by ZnO nanoparticles, zinc ions and bulk ZnO in fish cells. Sci Total Environ. 2013;452:262–74.
53. Brunner TJ, Wick P, Manser P, Spohn P, Grass RN, Limbach LK, Bruinink A, Stark WJ. In vitro cytotoxicity of oxide nanoparticles: comparison to asbestos, silica, and the effect of particle solubility. Environ Sci Technol. 2006;40:4374–81.
54. Kahru A, Dubourguier HC, Blinova I, Ivask A, Kasemets K. Biotests and biosensors for ecotoxicology of metal oxide nanoparticles: a minireview. Sensors. 2008;8:5153–70.
55. Yung MMN, Mouneyrac C, Leung KMY. Ecotoxicity of zinc oxide nanoparticles in the marine environment. Encycl Nanotechnol. 2014. doi:10.1007/978-94-007-6178-0_100970-1.
56. Franklin NM, Rogers NJ, Apte SC, Batley GE, Gadd GE, Casey PS. Comparative toxicity of nanoparticulate ZnO, bulk ZnO, and $ZnCl_2$ to a freshwater microalga (*Pseudokirchneriella subcapitata*): the importance of particle solubility. Environ Sci Technol. 2007;41:8484–90.
57. Feng QL, Wu J, Chen GQ, Cui FZ, Kim TN, Kim JO. A mechanistic study of the antibacterial effect of silver ions on *Escherichia coli* and *Staphylococcus aureus*. J Biomed Mater Res. 2000;52:662–8.
58. Tomás JM. The main *Aeromonas* pathogenic factors. ISRN Microbiol. 2012;2012:1–22. doi:10.5402/2012/256261.

18

Mink (*Neovison vison*) kits with pre-weaning diarrhea have elevated serum amyloid A levels and intestinal pathomorphological similarities with New Neonatal Porcine Diarrhea Syndrome

Ronja Mathiesen[1,2*], Julie Melsted Birch[3], Mariann Chriél[4], Henrik Elvang Jensen[3], Jens Frederik Agger[3], Peter Mikael Helweg Heegaard[1,2] and Tina Struve[5]

Abstract

Background: Pre-weaning diarrhea (PWD) is a syndrome affecting farm-raised neonatal mink kits. Apart from diarrhea it causes greasy skin exudation, dehydration, and distressed behavior and can ultimately lead to death. No specific causative agents have been identified and the syndrome is regarded as multifactorial. The aim of the present study was to investigate a possible inflammatory state in mink kits with PWD, as indicated by raised serum concentrations of the acute phase protein serum amyloid A (SAA) and by changes in intestinal pathomorphology and intestinal contents of bacteria. Samples collected from 20 diarrheic mink kits with PWD and 20 age-matched non-diarrheic control mink kits from two commercial Danish farms during the pre-weaning period (April–May) in 2016 were analyzed.

Results: Concentrations of SAA in serum samples from mink kits with PWD were significantly higher (up to 1000-fold) compared to non-diarrheic control mink kits. Significant features of enterocytic vacuolization, atrophy and fusion of villi in jejunum and mucosal atrophy of the colon of kits with PWD were found. Moreover, attachment of coccoid bacteria to enterocytes was more often found in kits suffering from PWD, while intra-cytoplasmic eosinophil bodies were more frequently observed in control kits. Cellular infiltrations with mononuclear and neutrophil leukocytes were not associated with disease status. Bacteria from the *Staphylococcus intermedius* group, such as *Staphylococcus delphini*, were more frequently cultivated from control mink kits, whereas *Enterococcus* spp. dominated in mink kits with PWD. *Escherichia coli* was cultivated from both control and mink kits with PWD, but with a higher frequency from mink kits with PWD.

Conclusion: A significant increase in circulating concentrations of SAA was found in PWD affected mink kits from 6 to 23 days old compared to controls. The histopathological changes in PWD mink kits suggest that the type of diarrhea is secretory. Attachment of coccoid bacteria, therefore, might be responsible for an enterotoxic effect causing a loss of balance in movements of ions and water leading to the vacuolization and swelling of the enterocytes. The slight to moderate infiltrations of neutrophils irrespectively of diarrheic status and the attachment of coccoid bacteria to enterocytes are comparable to observations found in piglets suffering from New Neonatal Porcine Diarrhea

*Correspondence: romat@dtu.dk
[1] Innate Immunology Group, National Veterinary Institute, Technical University of Denmark, Kemitorvet, Building 204, 2800 Kgs. Lyngby, Denmark
Full list of author information is available at the end of the article

Syndrome. Mechanisms behind the correlation between increased SAA levels and the observed pathological intestinal features remain obscure.

Keywords: Bacteriology, Histology, Mink kits, (*Neovison vison*), Pre-weaning diarrhea, Serum amyloid A

Background

The pre-weaning diarrhea syndrome (PWD) in mink (*Neovison vison*) kits is a major cause of concern in the mink industry due to both economic losses and decreased animal welfare. It may affect more than 30% of the litters [1, 2] and has been observed in farm-raised neonatal mink for several decades worldwide [3]. Mink kits affected by PWD display diarrhea with concomitant excessive secretions from the cervical apocrine glands, and exudate on the skin surface, the tail, and the claws. Moreover, dehydration may ultimately lead to the death of the affected kits [4, 5]. The onset of clinical signs generally occurs in the whole litter during the pre-weaning period, at 5–20 days of age, with a morbidity rate varying from 0 to more than 30% of the litters, and a mortality of typically one or two kits per litter [6, own findings, 2017]. The PWD syndrome is considered multifactorial, and there is a lack of consistency in isolated bacteria and viruses in kits with PWD. Studies have aimed to define the causality of the syndrome and mink astrovirus (MiAstV) isolated from mink kits with PWD indicate involvement in the syndrome [7–11]. However, all of the proposed putative pathogens including also *Campylobacter jejuni*, rota-, calici-, and mink coronavirus, *Escherichia coli*, and *Staphylococcus delphini* have also been isolated from clinically healthy kits, so their role in PWD remains elusive [10–13]. Apart from having a multifactorial infectious origin, other factors including management factors have been associated with an increased risk of developing PWD. For example, litters from 1-year old females and in females with low energy supply in the late gestation period are at increased risk of being affected by PWD [2, 14]. Moreover, the presence of dogs on the farm area as well as the size of the farm (total number of females) have also been associated with high morbidity of PWD [2]. Regarding the intestinal pathomorphology accompanying PWD, only a few studies have been published [15, 16]. Moreover, intestinal lesions in mink kits suffering from PWD have not been classified, according to the standard pathomorphological paradigm, as either non-inflammatory/secretory, inflammatory or invasive [17]. A possible biomarker to assess infection or inflammation in mink kits suffering from PWD is serum amyloid A (SAA). SAA is an acute phase protein found in low concentrations in healthy animals and is released following inflammation, infection, or tissue injury in both mink [18–20] and many other species, including humans [21, 22]. It is synthesized predominantly by the liver in response to the cytokine interleukin 1, however, other organs such as the intestine, have also been shown to produce it [19]. The aim of the present study was to examine if the levels of SAA could be a biomarker for PWD in mink kits and to characterize and compare the intestinal pathomorphology, and the bacterial intestinal contents between healthy controls and mink kits suffering from PWD.

Methods

Animals

In total, 20 mink (*Neovison vison*) kits with PWD and 20 age-matched healthy kits (controls), between 6 and 23 days old, were obtained during the pre-weaning period (April–May) from two (A and B) commercial Danish mink farms with outbreaks of PWD. Sick mink kits were selected based on the liquid consistency of the feces and the following clinical manifestations: sticky cutaneous exudation, red swollen anus and perineal soiling (own findings, 2017). Mink female and their kits were housed in separate cages with conventional nest boxes, females were fed conventional feed and had unlimited access to water. Mink kits were euthanized with CO or CO_2, bled, and the intestine was removed aseptically immediately thereafter.

Serum amyloid A ELISA

Un-stabilized blood samples from the kits were obtained at the time of euthanasia. Blood was allowed to clot and serum was obtained as the supernatant after centrifugation at 4000*g* for 15 min at 4 °C. Serum was stored at −20 °C until analysis. A commercially available multispecies sandwich ELISA (Phase SAA assay, Tridelta Development Ltd., Kildare, Ireland, #TP 802) was used to quantify SAA concentrations in the serum samples. This assay is a quantitative sandwich ELISA using rat anti–human monoclonal antibodies [23]. Mink kit serum samples were diluted 500 times according to the manufacturer's instructions for canine SAA. The lower limit of quantification was 6.25 μg/mL (canine SAA units) as given by the lowest concentration of the standard dilution series included on each plate. Readings below the lower limit of quantification were assigned the value 6.3 μg/mL. Data was transferred to GraphPad Prism version 7 (GraphPad Software, San Diego, California, USA, https://www.graphpad.com) for graphic representation and for statistical analysis. Significant difference in SAA concentrations in circulation between PWD kits and control kits were identified using the Mann–Whitney test in Prism. P values < 0.05 were considered significant.

Histology

Duodenal, mid-intestinal (jejunum) and aboral colon sections from each kit were fixed with needles on a piece of styrene foam and placed in 10% neutral buffered formalin in a CellStor Pot (CellPath, Newtown, Powys, UK). Two pieces from each of the three gut sections were embedded in paraffin and sections of 4–5 μm were prepared and stained with hematoxylin and eosin (HE). Selected sections were stained with Periodic acid–Schiff (PAS), Gram, and Warthin–Starry (WS). Each of the three sections was histologically examined and graded blindly according to the following manifestations (Table 1).

For each of the included animals a score for duodenum + jejunum and colon sections was established, respectively. Thus, for the dichotomous variables the summary score was "absent" (−), if absent in all gut sections and "present" (+), if present in any of the gut sections. For the assessment of vacuolization a cumulated score was established and categorized as absent (−) if the cumulated score was 0, or present (+) if the cumulated score was > 0. For the assessment of infiltration with neutrophils in the villi a cumulated score was established, and categorized based on the mean score as high or low i.e. ≥ 2/< 2 for duodenum + jejunum sections. Associations between disease status of the kit and each variable was tested with the SAS Enterprise Guide 7.1 using Chi square and where relevant Fisher's exact test (expected < 5). A cumulated number of mitosis in enterocytes of duodenum and jejunum from PWD and control mink kits were tested with Students t-test. P values < 0.05 were considered significant.

Bacteriology

Post mortem, the intestine was removed from the abdomen as previously described [24]. The aboral part of the colon was aseptically opened with a sterile scalpel and swabbed for bacterial cultivation (Transport Swabs, VWR, Radnor, PA, USA). The total of 17 pooled swab control samples were generated by pooling swabs from two healthy kits from the same litter, on the same day, from 17 litters age-matched to the kits affected by PWD. The age-matching of the mink kits unfortunately resulted in some of the kits being pooled into the same tube. This left only 17 pooled samples, instead of 20, from

Table 1 Histological criteria for assessing sections from duodenum, jejunum and aboral colon of mink kits

Histological examinations	Assessment	Score
Degree of vacuolization of the enterocytes	Loss of staining of the cytoplasm in a group of enterocytes seen together with elongation and hypertrophy due to micro-vacuolization	Absent (0) Mild: present focally (1) Severe: present multifocal or disseminated (2)
Coccoid bacteria and rod-shaped bacteria (duodenum and jejunum)	Attached to enterocytes on the villi	Absent (−) Present (+)
Semi-quantified degree of infiltration of neutrophils (duodenum and jejunum)	Neutrophils in villi	≤ 5 neutrophils/villi (0) Several villi contained 5–10 neutrophils (1) Several villi contained > 10 neutrophils (2)
Infiltrations of mononuclear cells	Distinguished from Peyer's patches as diffuse, disorderly infiltrations of mononuclear cells in the lamina propria	Absent (−) Present (+)
Intra-cytoplasmic eosinophil bodies of the enterocytes	Circular elements often located adjacent to the nuclei [15, 16]	Absent (−) Present (+)
Atrophy and fusion of the villi (duodenum and jejunum)	Reduction of the height of villi and the spaces between them [15]	Absent (−) Present (+)
Amount of enterocytic proliferation (duodenum and jejunum)	Number of mitosis in enterocytes	Number
Atrophy of mucosal lining (colon)	Reduction of mucosal height and normal architecture	Absent (−) Present (+)

kits without PWD. From the diarrheic kits, the samples were cultured individually. The swabs were stored at 5 °C until analysis by blinded cultivation. The swabs were inoculated on blood agar plates enriched with 5% bovine blood (blood agar base, Oxoid, Thermo Scientific, Watham, MA, USA) and incubated at 37 °C aerobically for 1–2 days. The two most frequently occurring bacterial colonies were then sub-cultivated before they were identified by Matrix-Assisted Laser Desorption Ionization Time-Of-Flight mass spectrometry (MALDI–TOF–MS) using a VITEK MS MALDI-TOF (BioMérieux, Marcy-l'Etoile, France) as previously described [25]. If two bacterial species were equally frequent next to a single more frequent species both were sub-cultivated, and hence three isolates were identified.

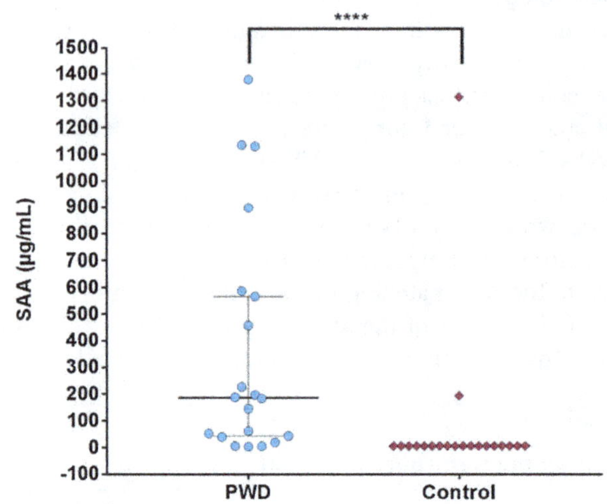

Fig. 1 Serum concentration of serum amyloid A (SAA) protein in PWD and healthy control mink kits as determined by SAA ELISA. Median of the serum SAA concentrations with 95% confidence interval is depicted (n = 20). The Mann–Whitney test showed a statistically significant higher concentration of serum SAA in PWD kits than in control kits (****P < 0.0001)

Results

Serum SAA concentrations

The difference in serum SAA concentration between PWD kits and control kits was highly statistically significant (Mann–Whitney test, P < 0.0001) (Fig. 1). Only 2/20 (10%) control mink kits had SAA concentrations higher than the lower limit of quantification of 6.3 µg/mL, while 17/20 (85%) kits with PWD had SAA concentrations higher than 6.3 µg/mL.

Histology

The results of the histologic evaluations are presented in Table 2. Compared to normal kits (Fig. 2a) PWD mink kits expressed significant features of enterocytic hydropic vacuolization (PAS negative) in the jejunum and colon (Fig. 2b, c). Atrophy and fusion of villi in the small intestine and atrophy of the mucosa lining in the colon were also associated with presence of the disease, and were most prominent in jejunum and colon (Fig. 2d, e). The association between attachment of coccoid bacteria to enterocytes and disease status was highly significant in duodenum + jejunum and colon (P < 0.0001 and P = 0.001, respectively), and was equally present in all parts of the intestine (Fig. 2b). Selected Gram stained sections revealed that the coccoid bacteria were Gram positive. Rod-shaped bacteria were also significantly observed more frequently in intestines from PWD kits,

Table 2 Histopathological findings in duodenum ± jejunum and colon from control to PWD mink kits, respectively

Histopathologic features	PWD (n = 20)	Control (n = 20)	P-value
Duodenum + jejunum			
Vacuolization (hydropic degeneration) of enterocytes (+/−)	8/12	1/19	0.02
Coccoid bacteria attached to enterocytes (+/−)	16/4	1/19	< 0.0001
Rod-shaped bacteria attached to enterocytes (+/−)	4/16	0/20	0.11
Infiltration of neutrophils in villi (high/low)	9/11	14/6	0.11
Infiltration of mononuclear cells (+/−)	0/20	0/20	-
Eosinophilic bodies in enterocytes (+/−)	2/18	12/8	0.001
Atrophy of villi (+/−)	4/16	0/20	0.11
Fusion of villi (+/−)	5/15	0/20	0.05
Number of mitosis [mean, (standard deviation)]	66.3 (30.3)	39.8 (20.9)	0.003
Colon			
Vacuolization (hydropic degeneration) of enterocytes (+/−)	11/9	1/19	0.001
Infiltration of mononuclear cells (+/−)	3/17	1/19	0.61
Eosinophilic bodies in enterocytes (+/−)	2/18	4/16	0.66
Atrophy of the mucosa (+/−)	9/11	1/19	0.01

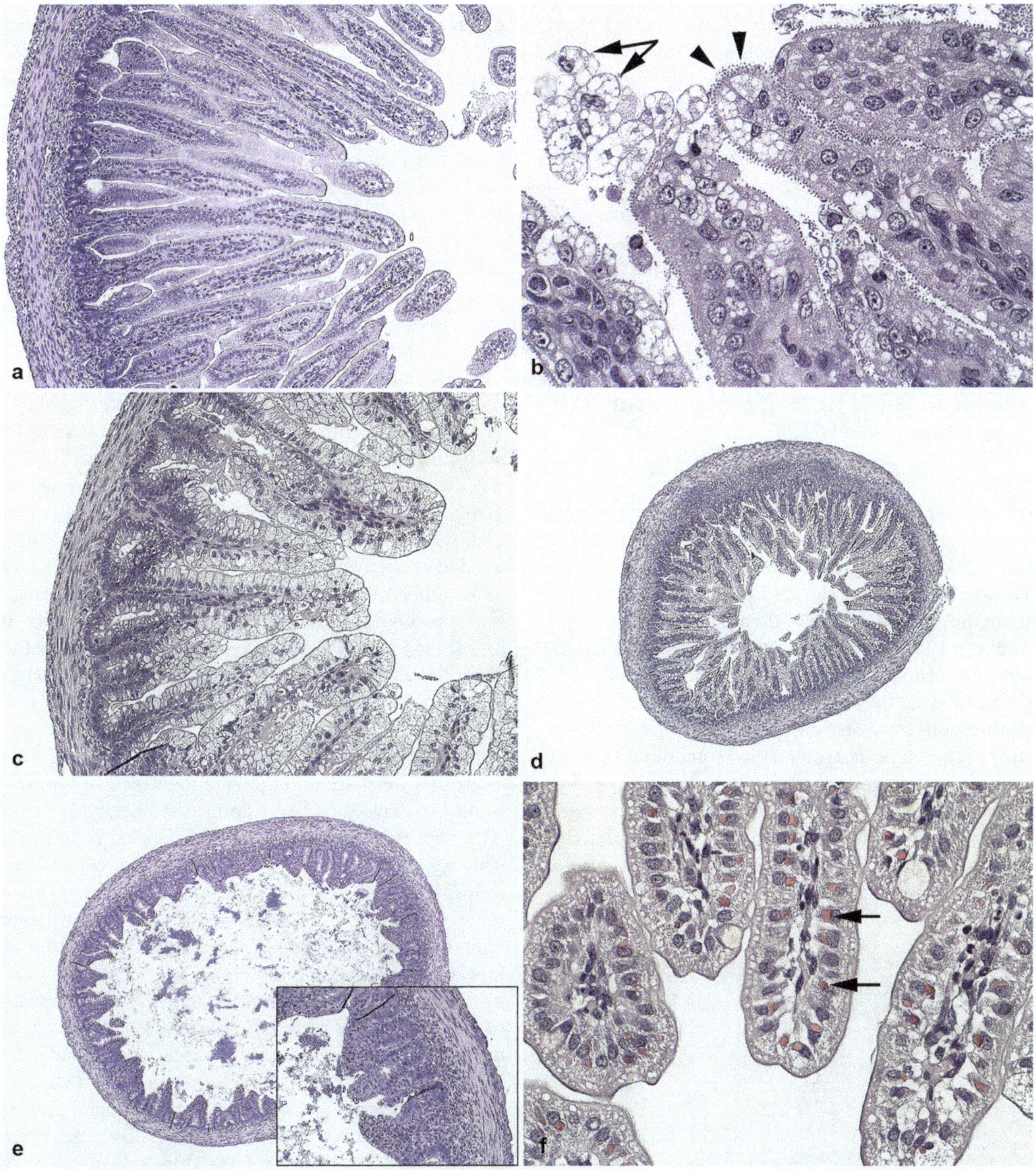

Fig. 2 Photomicrographs of representative examples of intestines from mink kits. **a** Jejunum from healthy mink kit. **b** Vacuolization on the tip of the villi (arrows) and pronounced attachment of coccoid bacteria (arrow heads) to the enterocytes in jejunum of a mink kit with PWD. **c** Severe vacuolization and hypertrophied enterocytes in the colon of a mink kits with PWD. **d** Colon from a healthy mink kit. **e** Atrophy of the mucosa of the colon from a mink kit with PWD. Inset: higher magnification of the mucosal atrophy. **f** Eosinophilic bodies in the enterocytes from jejunum in a healthy mink kit (arrows)

but the attachment to villi was sporadic and in combination with coccoid bacteria. Intra-cytoplasmic eosinophilic bodies (PAS positively stained vacuoles) were significantly more frequent in control kits compared to PWD kits, and most often in jejunum (Fig. 2f). Infiltrations with mononuclear and neutrophil leucocytes were not associated with disease status. Moreover, the mitotic activity of enterocytes in the small intestine were significantly higher in PWD kits compared to control kits (P = 0.003).

Bacteriology

The number of bacterial isolates obtained from healthy mink kits and kits with PWD is shown in Table 3. The dominating species cultivated from healthy control mink kits was from the *Staphylococcus intermedius* group, whereas *Enterococcus* spp. was the main species found in mink kits with PWD. On Farm B, *E. coli* was cultivated more frequently from mink kits with PWD (58.8% of the isolates) than from control kits (41.7% of isolates). On farm A, *E. coli* was not isolated from any of the control kits, but accounted for 28.6% of the isolates from the mink kits suffering from PWD.

Discussion

We report for the first time that PWD in mink kits between 6 and 23 days old is associated with a significant increase in circulating concentrations of SAA. Two of the control kits showed elevated concentrations of SAA in serum, however only one of them (1315 μg/mL; Fig. 1) showed signs of cholangitis, which could explain the elevated concentration of SAA (data not shown). SAA have been shown by Bruun et al. [20] to be elevated in mink after subcutaneous injection with lipopolysaccharide from *E. coli*. The gastrointestinal tract of mink is very short and the passage of feed through the entire gastrointestinal tract takes approximately 2–3 h [26]. Previous studies have shown the difficulty in culturing bacteria from the small intestine in mink [27] and therefore we decided to use swabs from the colon, where the density of bacteria is relatively high. Furthermore, the decision to only cultivate the bacteria aerobically was based on the fact that only aerobic bacteria have so far been isolated from PWD-affected mink, whereas anaerobic bacteria have not [11, 28, 29]. We isolated *E. coli* most frequently from kits suffering from PWD, which corresponds well with previous findings that *E. coli* is commonly isolated from PWD mink kits [11, 16, 30, 31]. A quantitative study of healthy mink kits showed that the intestinal counts of *E. coli* were highest when kits were around 4 weeks of age [30], but in the present study *E. coli* was isolated from younger kits suffering from PWD. However, *E. coli* has also been identified as part of the normal mink kit intestinal microflora [11, 16, 30, 32]. Moreover, analysis of virulence factors of *E. coli* has revealed that the population of *E. coli* in mink consists of several serogroups with no apparent association to outbreaks of PWD [11, 32]. In general, enterococci are not regarded as pathogenic in mink, but *Enterococcus hirae* has been associated with diarrhea in 4–7 week old mink kits submitted for diagnostic testing (Chriél, pers. comm., 2017), as well as in other neonatal animals such as suckling rats, kittens and piglets [33–35]. Gut sections from PWD mink kits showed clear disease associated changes, including vacuolization of enterocytes and pronounced attachment of coccoid bacteria, both of which have been observed in other studies [7, 15, 16]. The intracytoplasmic eosinophilic bodies (PAS positive vacuoles) within the enterocytes that most frequently were identified in the healthy mink kits have also been described previously [15, 16]. Although their role has not been clarified in mink, their staining properties and localization is comparable to the absorptive, intra-cytoplasmic vacuoles found in neonates of pigs and ruminants [36]. Therefore, the presence of these vacuoles in enterocytes of healthy mink kits is not surprising and may be related to the intestinal uptake of maternal milk antibodies [37], taking place up to 4–5 weeks after birth in mink kits [37]. Although more pronounced changes of the gut architecture like atrophy and fusion of villi were present in the PWD kits, no significant difference in the degree of neutrophil and mononuclear leucocyte infiltration were observed between controls and PWD mink kits. This lack of histopathological signs of inflammation indicates that PWD in the mink kits represents a secretory type of diarrhea. The observed attachment of coccoid bacteria may be responsible for an enterotoxic effect causing a loss of balance of movements of ions and water leading to the vacuolization and swelling of the enterocytes. Interestingly, the attachment of enterococci and *E. coli* to enterocytes and the slight to moderate infiltrations of neutrophils irrespective of diarrheic status has recently been found in

Table 3 Number and percentages of bacterial isolates from control and PWD mink kits

Bacterial isolates	Farm A		Farm B	
	Control[a]	PWD[b]	Control[a]	PWD[b]
Number of samples	9	10	8	10
Escherichia coli	–	4 (28.6%)	5 (41.7%)	10 (58.8%)
Staphylococcus intermedius group	7 (58.3%)	2 (14.3%)	6 (50%)	1 (5.9%)
Staphylococcus schleiferi	2 (16.7%)	–	–	–
Enterococcus faecalis	1 (8.3%)	–	–	–
Enterococcus faecium	2 (16.7%)	8 (57.1%)	–	–
Enterococcus durans	–	–	1 (8.3%)	–
Enterococcus hirae	–	–	–	6 (35.3%)
Total number of isolates	12	14	12	17

[a] The samples from the control kits from each farm were pooled samples (two kits from the same litter, sampled on the same day, constituted the samples)

[b] The samples from the PWD kits were not pooled

piglets suffering from New Neonatal Porcine Diarrhea Syndrome (NNPDS) [38–40], suggesting similarities in mechanisms between diarrhea in the pre-weaning period of mink kits and piglets. Elevated levels of SAA and adhesion of bacteria to the intestinal wall has been seen for segmented filamentous bacteria (SFB), which adhere to the enterocytes, inducing epithelial SAA production [41, 42]. Atarashi et al. [43] colonized rats and germ-free mice with SFB from 20 strains of bacteria isolated from feces from patients suffering from ulcerating colitis and from *E. coli* and found that they all promote the induction of Th17 cells, which in turn could lead to an increased SAA production in enterocytes. Research on local expression of SAA in the intestine is needed to elucidate if circulating SAA levels are increased as a consequence of local production of SAA by epithelial intestinal cells in mink kits affected by PWD. In rodent models, a local induction of SAA in enteric epithelial cells in response to an altered microbiota in the absence of inflammation has indeed been demonstrated [43], however the impact on circulating SAA concentrations has not been reported. Although more pronounced changes of the gut architecture, like atrophy and fusion of villi were present in the PWD kits, no significant difference in the degree of neutrophil and mononuclear leucocyte infiltration were observed between controls and PWD mink kits. Thus, the possibility of an association between increased SAA levels and an unidentified inflammatory state in mink kits suffering from PWD should be investigated in more detail.

The most frequent bacterial isolate from control mink kits belonged to the *S. intermedius* group, which in mink has been shown to be *S. delphini* [44]. This finding is in line with previous studies of the normal intestinal microflora of mink kits [12, 30]. Although mink are natural hosts of *S. delphini* this bacterial species was suggested to be responsible for an outbreak of PWD through enterotoxin production, which again leads to the question if *S. delphini* could be an opportunistic bacterium after a primary infection during an episode of PWD [29]. In contrast, MiAstV, mink coronavirus, mink enteritis virus, and rotavirus A were not found by PCR [45] in any of the kits analyzed (data not shown), suggesting a low presence of virus.

Conclusions

We identified a significant increase in circulating concentrations of SAA and attachment of coccoid bacteria in kits affected by PWD. The slight to moderate infiltrations of neutrophils irrespectively of diarrheic status and the attachment of coccoid bacteria to enterocytes show similarities with observations found in piglets suffering from NNPDS, and suggest that PWD in mink is a secretory type of diarrhea.

Authors' contributions

RM and JMB conceived the study. RM and JMB planned the sampling, performed the experiments and drafted the manuscript with contributions from PMHH, HEJ, MC, JFA and TS. RM, JMB and TS did the necropsies. RM analyzed the SAA concentration. JMB and HEJ evaluated all histological sections and described the histopathological lesions. JMB did the bacteriology. TS participated in the collection of blood and samples. All authors read and approved the final manuscript.

Author details

[1] Innate Immunology Group, National Veterinary Institute, Technical University of Denmark, Kemitorvet, Building 204, 2800 Kgs. Lyngby, Denmark. [2] Present Address: Innate Immunology Group, Department of Biotechnology and Biomedicine, Technical University of Denmark, Kemitorvet, Building 204, 2800 Kgs. Lyngby, Denmark. [3] Department of Veterinary and Animals Sciences, Faculty of Health and Medical Sciences, University of Copenhagen, Ridebanevej 3, 1870 Frederiksberg C, Denmark. [4] Diagnostics & Scientific Advice, National Veterinary Institute, Technical University of Denmark, Kemitorvet, Building 204, 2800 Kgs. Lyngby, Denmark. [5] Kopenhagen Fur, Langagervej 60, 2600 Glostrup, Denmark.

Acknowledgements

Farmers K. J. Hansen and J. Jensen who helped with the sampling for the project are greatly acknowledged. The technical assistance and invaluable help from Henriette Vorsholt, Marion Baltzer Petersen, Mette Sif Hansen, Dennis Brok, and Annie Ravn Pedersen are also greatly acknowledged.

Competing interests

The authors declare that they have no competing interests.

Funding

The project was co-funded by Pelsdyrafgiftsfonden (The Danish production levy fund for mink), Pelsdyrenes Forskningsfond, the Innovation Fund Denmark, and the Technical University of Denmark.

References

1. Chriél M. Greasy kits-an efficient effort limits losses. Dansk Pelsdyravl. 1994;4:180–1 **(in Danish)**.
2. Birch JM, Agger JF, Dahlin C, Jensen VF, Hammer AS, Struve T, et al. Risk factors associated with diarrhea in Danish commercial mink (*Neovison vison*) during the pre-weaning period. Acta Vet Scand. 2017;59:43.
3. Svennekjær NC. Mink diseases and current problems in mink farming. Dansk Pelsdyravl. 1954;12:384–404 **(in Danish)**.

4. Hyldgaard-Jensen C. "Greasy kits" in mink. Observations over a three year period. Dansk Veterinærtidskrift. 1989;72:566–71 **(in Danish)**.
5. Clausen TN, Dietz HH. Greasy kits. Annual Report, Kopenhagen Research. Kopenhagen Fur. 2004; p. 209–14 **(in Danish)**.
6. Olesen CR, Hansen M, Clausen TN. Sticky kits-risk factors and causality. Dansk Pelsdyravl. 1992;4:170–2 **(in Danish)**.
7. Englund L, Chriél M, Dietz HH, Hedlund KO. Astrovirus epidemiologically linked to pre-weaning diarrhoea in mink. Vet Microbiol. 2002;85:1–11.
8. Ullman K, Hammer AS, Hedlund KO, Thorén P, Czifra G. Prevalence of mink astrovirus (MiAstV) in faecal samples in mink kits during the pre-weaning period. Annual Report, Kopenhagen Research. Kopenhagen Fur. 2007. p. 159–64 **(in Danish)**.
9. Hammer AS, Ullman K, Czifra G. Astrovirus infections in mink kits-virological and pathological findings in mink kits with pre-weaning diarrhea submitted for diagnostic investigation. Annual Report, Kopenhagen Research. Kopenhagen Fur. 2007. p. 165–70 **(in Danish)**.
10. Hansen S, Krarup LJ, Agger JF, Ullman K, Hedlund KO, Klingström J, et al. Investigation of parvo-, corona-, and astrovirus as causative agents in outbreaks of diarrhea in Danish mink kits in the nursing and growth period 2013—Preliminary results. Annual Report, Kopenhagen Research. Kopenhagen Fur. 2014. p. 131–8 **(In Danish)**.
11. Jørgensen M, Scheutz F, Strandbygaard B. *Escherichia Coli* and virus isolated from "Sticky Kits". Acta Vet Scand. 1996;37:163–9.
12. Guardabassi L, Schmidt KR, Petersen TS, Espinosa-Gongora C, Moodley A, Agersø Y, Olsen JE. Mustelidae are natural hosts of *Staphylococcus delphini* group A. Vet Microbiol. 2012;159:351–3.
13. Bell JA, Manning DD. Prevalence of *Campylobacter jejuni* in ranch mink at pelting: cultural, serological, and histological evidence of infection. Can Vet J. 1990;31:367–71.
14. Møller SH, Chriél M. Health effects of feeding strategies in the pre mating and gestation periods of mink. Scientifur. 2000;24:37–41.
15. Järplid B, Mejerland T. Villous atrophy in the small intestine of mink kits with diarrhea. Scientifur. 1998;22:157–60.
16. Dietz HH, Rattenborg E. Histopatological and bacteriological investigation of healthy and greasy mink kits. Annual Report, Kopenhagen Research. Kopenhagen Fur. 1996. p. 135–8 **(in Danish)**.
17. Gelberg HB. Alimentary system and the peritoneum, omentum, mesentery and peritoneal cavity. In: Zachary JF, editor. Pathol basis Vet Dis. St. Louis: Elsevier; 2016. p. 324–411.
18. Jespersen A, Jensen HE, Agger JF, Heegaard PMH, Damborg P, Aalbæk B, et al. The effect of color type on early wound healing in farmed mink (*Neovison vison*). BMC Vet Res. 2017;13:135.
19. Rygg M, Nordstoga K, Husby G, Marhaug G. Expression of serum amyloid A genes in mink during induction of inflammation and amyloidosis. Biochim Biophys Acta. 1993;1216:402–8.
20. Bruun CF, Rygg M, Nordstoga K, Sletten K, Marhaug G. Serum amyloid A protein in mink during endotoxin induced inflammation and amyloidogenesis. Scand J Immunol. 1994;40:337–44.
21. Petersen HH, Nielsen JP, Heegaard PMH. Application of acute phase protein measurements in veterinary clinical chemistry. Vet Res. 2004;35:164–87.
22. De Buck M, Gouwy M, Wang JM, Van Snick J, Opdenakker G, Struyf S, et al. Structure and expression of different serum amyloid A (SAA) variants and their concentration-dependent functions during host insults. Curr Med Chem. 2016;23:1725–55.
23. McDonald TL, Weber A, Smith JW. A monoclonal antibody sandwich immunoassay for serum amyloid A (SAA) protein. J Immunol Methods. 1991;144:149–55.
24. Hammer ASV, Dietz HH. Necropsy of the mink. In: Jensen HE, editor. Necropsy A Handb Atlas. 1st ed. Frederiksberg C: Biofolia; 2011. p. 231–50.
25. Fang H, Ohlsson AK, Ullberg M, Özenci V. Evaluation of species-specific PCR, Bruker MS, VITEK MS and the VITEK 2 system for the identification of clinical *Enterococcus* isolates. Eur J Clin Microbiol Infect Dis. 2012;31:3073–7.
26. Gugołek A, Zalewski D, Strychalski J, Konstantynowicz M. Food transit time, nutrient digestibility and nitrogen retention in farmed and feral American mink (*Neovison vison*) - a comparative analysis. J Anim Physiol Anim Nutr. 2013;97:1030–5.
27. Pedersen K, Jørgensen M. Lactic acid bacteria for mink. Colonization and persistence of *Enterococcus faecium* Cernelle 68 in the digestive tract of mink. Acta Vet Scand. 1992;33:95–103.
28. Jørgensen M. *E. coli*-bacteria frequent guests in wet kits. Dansk Pelsdyravl. 1994;12:546–51 **(in Danish)**.
29. Sledge DG, Danieu PK, Bolin CA, Bolin SR, Lim A, Anderson BC, et al. Outbreak of neonatal diarrhea in farmed mink kits (*Mustella vison*) associated with enterotoxigenic *Staphylococcus delphini*. Vet Pathol. 2010;47:751–7.
30. Vulfson L, Pedersen K, Chriél M, Andersen TH, Dietz HH. Assessment of the aerobic faecal microflora in mink (*Mustela vison* Schreiber) with emphasis on *Escherichia coli* and *Staphylococcus intermedius*. Vet Microbiol. 2003;93:235–45.
31. Hammer AS, Rasmussen LB, Hansen S, Krarup L, Damgaard PP, Aalbek B. Bacterial etiology of diarrhea in mink kits. In: NJF Semin Proc; 2014. p. 170–2.
32. Vulfson L, Pedersen K, Chriél M, Frydendahl K, Andersen TH, Madsen M, et al. Serogroups and antimicrobial susceptibility among *Escherichia coli* isolated from farmed mink (*Mustela vison* Schreiber) in Denmark. Vet Microbiol. 2001;79:143–53.
33. Etheridge ME, Yolken RH, Vonderfecht SL. *Enterococcus hirae* implicated as a cause of diarrhea in suckling rats. J Clin Microbiol. 1988;26:1741–4.
34. Nicklas JL, Moisan P, Stone MR, Gookin JL. In situ molecular diagnosis and histopathological characterization of enteroadherent *Enterococcus hirae* infection in pre-weaning-age kittens. J Clin Microbiol. 2010;48:2814–20.
35. Larsson J, Lindberg R, Aspán A, Grandon R, Westergren E, Jacobson M. Neonatal piglet diarrhoea associated with enteroadherent *Enterococcus hirae*. J Comp Pathol. 2014;151:137–47.
36. Uzal FA, Plattner BL, Hostetter JM. Intestine. Normal form and function. In: Maxie MG, editor. Pathol Domest Anim. 6th ed. Philadelphia: Saunders Elsevier; 2016. p. 60–3.
37. Coe JE, Race RE. Ontogeny of Mink IgG, IgA, and IgM (40039). Proc Soc Exp Biol Med. 1978;157:289–92.
38. Kongsted H, Jonach B, Haugegaard S, Angen Ø, Jorsal S, Kokotovic B, et al. Microbiological, pathological and histological findings in four Danish pig herds affected by a new neonatal diarrhoea syndrome. BMC Vet Res. 2013;9:206.
39. Jonach B, Boye M, Stockmarr A, Jensen TK. Fluorescence in situ hybridization investigation of potentially pathogenic bacteria involved in neonatal porcine diarrhea. BMC Vet Res. 2014;10:68.
40. Hedegaard CJ, Strube ML, Hansen MB, Lindved BK, Lihme A, Boye M, et al. Natural pig plasma immunoglobulins have anti-bacterial effects: potential for use as feed supplement for treatment of intestinal infections in pigs. PLoS ONE. 2016;11:1–14.
41. Sano T, Huang W, Hall JA, Yang Y, Chen A, Gavzy SJ, et al. An IL-23R/IL-22 Circuit regulates epithelial serum amyloid A to promote local effector Th17 responses. Cell. 2015;163:381–93.
42. Bel S, Hooper LV. A bacterial nudge to T-cell function. Nature. 2015;526:328–30.
43. Atarashi K, Tanoue T, Ando M, Kamada N, Nagano Y, Narushima S, et al. Th17 Cell induction by adhesion of microbes to intestinal epithelial cells. Cell. 2015;163:367–80.
44. Larsen C. Hemolytic Staphylococci in mink. Veterinary Master Thesis. University of Copenhagen; 2014 **(in Danish)**.
45. Hartby CM, Andersen MR, Kvistgaard LK, Chriél M, Larsen LE, Hjulsager CK. Pooling of faecal samples for quantitative virus diagnostics by real-time PCR. In: Mäki-Tanila A, Valaja J, Mononen J, Sironen T, Vapalahti O, editors. Proceenings XIth Int Sci Congr Fur Anim Prod. Helsinki: Libris Oy; 2016. p. 27–30.

19

Effect of a live attenuated vaccine against *Lawsonia intracellularis* in weaned and finishing pig settings

Kati Susanna Peiponen[1,3*], Birger Taneli Tirkkonen[2,3], Jouni Juho Tapio Junnila[4] and Mari Leena Heinonen[3]

Abstract

Background: The intracellular bacterium *Lawsonia intracellularis* is an important pathogen in modern swine production. The aim of this study was to investigate the effect of a live attenuated *L. intracellularis* vaccine (Enterisol Ileitis®) on the health and production parameters of weaned and finishing pigs in a commercial Finnish 850-sow farm with diagnosed *L. intracellularis* infection. The herd was free from enzootic pneumonia, swine dysentery, progressive atrophic rhinitis, sarcoptic mange and salmonellosis. Four weekly groups of approximately 500 piglets were included in the study for a total of approximately 2000 piglets. Half of these piglets were vaccinated at 3 weeks of age and the other half served as controls. The study piglets were ear-tagged with individual numbers and colour-coded and were individually weighed at weaning (4 weeks), delivery to the finishing farm (12–14 weeks) and at slaughter. Mortality, symptoms of diseases and medications of the study piglets were registered in the nursery and finishing unit. Feed conversion rate was calculated for the finishing period and lean meat percentage was measured at slaughter.

Results: Vaccinated piglets had a higher live weight than unvaccinated piglets at delivery to the finishing unit (+ 1.18 kg, $P = 0.002$) and at slaughter (+ 3.57 kg, $P < 0.001$). The daily weight gain of vaccinated piglets was better than unvaccinated piglets in the nursery (+ 14.8 g/d, $P = 0.013$) and in the finishing unit (+ 30.9 g/d, $P < 0.001$). Vaccination had no effect on feed conversion rate or lean meat percentage ($P = 0.102$). Altogether, 3.9 and 4.6% of the pigs were medicated for different reasons in the vaccinated and control groups, respectively. The return on investment for the vaccination was calculated to be 0.41.

Conclusions: Immunisation of piglets with a live attenuated *L. intracellularis* vaccine resulted in higher meat yield in pig production via significantly higher live weight and average daily weight gain in a Finnish specific pathogen-free setting.

Keywords: Average daily weight gain, *Lawsonia intracellularis*, Live attenuated vaccine, Pig, Vaccination

Background

The intracellular bacterium *Lawsonia intracellularis* is an important pathogen in modern commercial swine production. A disease with suspected infectious aetiology later known to be caused by *L. intracellularis* was first described in pigs in 1931 [1]. The disease is now recognised to have an economic impact via performance decrease in piglets, which in 2006 resulted in losses of approximately 1.5–3.0 USD per animal in the weaning period [2]. The costs arise from increased mortality, reduced daily weight gain and need for medications.

Lawsonia intracellularis is easily transmitted and is widespread in many countries, including the Nordic countries. The prevalence of *L. intracellularis* is 48% of piglet-producing herds in Sweden [3] and 93.7% of such herds in Denmark [4]. No reports have been published regarding the prevalence of *L. intracellularis* in Finland. There is anecdotal evidence that *L. intracellularis* is also a common pathogen causing enteric disease in Finnish pig herds [5].

*Correspondence: susanna.peiponen@vetcare.fi
[1] Vetcare Finland Ltd, Hiomotie 3 A, 00380 Helsinki, Finland
Full list of author information is available at the end of the article

Lawsonia intracellularis causes the condition known as proliferative enteropathy. This condition may lead to various symptoms, such as diarrhoea and wasting in growing pigs to acute intestinal haemorrhage in adult pigs naive to the pathogen [6]. Diagnosis is made via laboratory identification of antibodies against *L. intracellularis* from blood samples, direct identification of bacteria or bacterial DNA from faecal samples or by identification of typical morphological changes for *L. intracellularis* infection at necropsy. Many antimicrobial agents can be used for the treatment of proliferative enteropathy. In Finland, the Finnish Food Safety Authority Evira recommends tylosin or other macrolides (first-line treatment) or tiamulin or tetracycline (second-line treatment) [7]. Although antimicrobial use in Finnish pork production is among the lowest worldwide [8], Finland is aiming to decrease this use further. One way to lower medication use for intestinal infections is to identify alternative means to control *L. intracellularis* in pig farms. Vaccination is investigated as one possible measure and is also mentioned in the national recommendations.

Vaccination against *L. intracellularis* has been previously reported in some successful field studies in Denmark [9], Australia [10], Korea [11], Switzerland [12] and Hungary [13]. These studies reported increased weight gain, decreased mortality and lower antimicrobial use. Some studies have shown that vaccination increased the immunity of piglets against *L. intracellularis* and decreased intestinal lesions and bacterial shedding [14–17]. In Finland, the pathogen load of herds is different from those mentioned above; most of the herds belong to the health classification system Sikava that requires absence of enzootic pneumonia, swine dysentery, salmonella, progressive atrophic rhinitis and sarcoptic mange [18]. The results of *L. intracellularis* vaccine use have not been reported in herds with a similar specific pathogen-free (SPF) system.

This study aimed to investigate the effect of a live attenuated *L. intracellularis* vaccine in a Finnish sow farm with diagnosed *L. intracellularis* infection. The goal of the study was to measure the effect of the vaccine when used in a Finnish SPF setting. Our first hypothesis was that *L. intracellularis* vaccination would have a positive effect on production, namely better weight gain, lower mortality and morbidity, smaller variation in slaughter weight, better feed conversion rate and financially better return on investment. We also hypothesised that *L. intracellularis* vaccination use is associated with lower antimicrobial use.

Methods

Procedures in the study herds

The study was performed in a piglet-producing farm with 850 sows and in a finishing herd with room for 1632 finishing pigs. Both herds were free from *Salmonella* sp., *Mycoplasma hyopneumoniae, Brachyspira hyodysenteriae,* sarcoptic mange and progressive atrophic rhinitis. The sow farm had a history of persistent diarrhoea typical of *L. intracellularis* in nursery pigs 2–3 weeks after weaning. The herd was diagnosed with a *L. intracellularis* infection in March 2014. Four piglets with typical diarrhoea were euthanised and sent for necropsy at Finnish Food Safety Authority Evira. One of the piglets was diagnosed with *L. intracellularis* with macroscopic and histologic lesions typical of proliferative enteropathy and identification of *L. intracellularis*-like organisms in Warthin–Starry stained tissue sections. Blood samples were obtained from six (age 6 weeks) and 11 (age 12 weeks) piglets; one (17%) and 11 (100%), respectively, were serologically positive in an ELISA test for *L. intracellularis.* Two finishing pigs from a farm receiving piglets only from the study sow farm were also investigated at Evira. Necropsy findings revealed *L. intracellularis*-infection in both of the finishers. The diagnosis was confirmed by examination of Warthin–Starry stained sections (one case) and by PCR (EVIRA6307 PCR for *Lawsonia intracellularis*) (one case). The farm had started to treat the pigs prophylactically with oral tylvalosin, 4.25 mg/kg (Aivlosin®, ECO Animal Health Limited) for 10 days from 3 days after weaning.

The sow farm weaned approximately 500 piglets every week in one of their all-in-all-out nursery departments. At weaning, the piglets were on average 28 days old. About 15% of the piglets were too small to be weaned at 4 weeks; their weaning was postponed until they were 5 weeks old. Litters from most sows were mixed at weaning, but the vaccine and control groups were raised in their own pens.

The nursery pen floor consisted of one-third concrete slats and two-thirds of solid concrete floor with floor heating. Every pen had a liquid feeding system with long troughs and two water nipples. Altogether, 23–26 piglets were placed in every pen, providing them with approximately 0.35 m^2 of floor space per piglet.

After a rearing time of approximately 7 weeks in the nursery, piglets in the trial group were delivered to a finishing farm, where also their feed consumption could be followed. The finishing period of the piglets moved to two other farms were not included in the study.

Piglets were delivered to the finishing farm in 4 weekly groups of 408 piglets; half of were vaccinated and half served as controls (total 1632 piglets). All 408 pigs of the same batch were in one compartment and no other pigs were kept in the same compartments. Vaccinated and control pigs were kept in separate pens throughout the study and they were not mixed with pigs not included in this study.

The finishing farm had four compartments with 34 pens per compartment and 12 pigs per pen, providing about 0.9 m^2 for each pig. Two pens shared one feed distribution valve. The pigs were fed five times a day with a liquid feeding system with approximately 32 cm of trough per pig.

All pigs in one trial group (originally 408 pigs) were sent to slaughter on the same day even if all of them had not reached the optimum slaughter weight. Due to higher than normal stocking density in the pens, eight pigs had to be culled before slaughter and were excluded from the study. Under normal production circumstances, the farmer would have sent these pigs to slaughter in two or three batches as they reached the optimal slaughter weight, thus lowering the stocking density for the last days of final production phase. The delivery date to slaughter was fixed by batches in the study so that the pigs could be followed at the slaughterhouse. The pigs in this study were sent to slaughter 79–86 days after arrival in the finishing farm. They were tattooed on their backs the day before transport to slaughterhouse. The tattoo included the following information: farm identity number, compartment number and treatment group (V=vaccinated and C=control group). Most of the slaughter pigs also had their individual identification ear tags intact at the time of transport to slaughter.

Vaccination and control groups

Four weekly weaning groups were followed in the study. One group consisted of approximately 500 piglets, of which half were vaccinated with *L. intracellularis* vaccine at the age of 3 weeks about 7 days before weaning (V=vaccine group). The other half of non-vaccinated piglets served as controls (C=control). The litters were chosen randomly and all piglets in a litter were either vaccinated or served as controls. One vaccine group piglet at a time was lifted from the ground and administered 2 mL of *L. intracellularis* vaccine (Enterisol Ileitis®, Boehringer Ingelheim Vetmedica GmbH) directly into the mouth with a drench and injected intramuscularly 1 mL of circovirus vaccine (Ingelvac CircoFLEX®, Boehringer Ingelheim Vetmedica GmbH) behind its ear. The control group piglets were lifted similarly but only received the circovirus vaccine. Vaccinated piglets were marked with an individually numbered red ear tag in their right ear. Similarly, control piglets received a numbered yellow ear tag in their left ear.

Follow up of weight and weight gain

All study piglets were weighed individually at weaning (weaning weight) and within a week prior to delivery to the finishing farm (delivery weight). At that time, they were roughly 30 kg live weight and 12–14 weeks of age.

The slaughterhouse provided the individual carcass weight of each pig. Live weight at slaughter was calculated from the carcass weight by conversion from 74.5% slaughter yield. Unfortunately, the ear tags for roughly half of the pigs (n=807) were lost during the scalding of the carcasses. This was likely due to the 'widening' of the ear tag hole during the growth of the pinnae, which caused the tag to fall off easily. Therefore, we could obtain a partial data set with individual parameters from some of the pigs and the data with parameters with group-level accuracy from the pigs that lost their ear tag.

Medications and treatments of the pigs

Routine or group treatment antimicrobials were not used for the trial groups. Because of the use of a live vaccine, we advised the farmer not to give any antimicrobial medications to piglets for 3 days before and after vaccination. Piglets that required medication with antimicrobials during these restriction days were excluded from the trial.

The animals were medicated due to sickness or injury according to the normal treatment routine advised by the herd veterinarian. The farmer recorded all medications for the piglets both in the nursery and in the finishing units individually, including date, indication or symptoms and medicine used.

Mortality

The farmers both in the nursery and in the finishing unit registered individually the dates of death and euthanasia.

Feed conversion rate

Feed consumption was registered at the pen level by the finishing farmer for different study groups in a table planned for this purpose. As vaccination and control piglets were kept in separate pens, feed consumption could be then traced at the vaccination versus control level.

Lean meat percentage

The slaughterhouse provided the information of the lean meat percentage for each pig individually at slaughter; this was measured with the AutoFom system (Carometec A/S, Denmark).

Return of investment

The return on investment (ROI) for the vaccine was calculated as

$$(\textit{increased revenues}(\textit{increased meat from the slaughterhouse}) - \textit{increased costs}(\textit{price of vaccine} + \textit{price of labour} + \textit{increased feed intake for increased live weight})) \div \textit{increased costs}.$$

Statistical methods

Weight at weaning was considered as the baseline measurement. The difference between treatment groups in change from baseline in weight was analysed with repeated measures analysis of covariance model (RM-ANCOVA). The model included vaccination group, timepoint and the interaction between treatment group and baseline measurement as fixed terms, the baseline measurement as covariate and the pig as a random term. The difference between the treatments overall and at delivery and slaughter was estimated from the model using contrasts. A similar RM-ANCOVA model was fitted for the response of daily growth (g). Daily growth was defined in two different ways. First, the daily growth was calculated from the previous measurement. Second, the daily growth was calculated from the baseline measurement, regardless of the timepoint as a sensitivity analysis.

Weight was also analysed using the actual values (instead of change from baseline) by applying a linear mixed model for repeated measures. The model included treatment, timepoint and their interaction as fixed terms and the pig as a random term.

For the pigs missing their ear tags at scalding, daily growth could not be calculated (as the values of the baseline and delivery measurement were unknown). To analyse the full data at slaughter weighing, the following data imputations were performed. The baseline (weaning) date was imputed as the first date of the two possible weighing dates within the group. The first date was selected as a vast majority of the pigs (80–90%) were weighed on the first date. The delivery date was imputed as the date of delivery weighing of the corresponding group. The baseline/delivery weight of the pigs with missing ID at slaughter was imputed as the mean weight of the corresponding group and treatment.

Using the imputed data, an analysis of covariance (ANCOVA) model was fitted for the daily growth at slaughter. The model included the treatment group and the baseline-weight covariate as fixed terms.

The incidence of deaths between the treatment groups separately at both delivery and slaughter was compared with Fisher's exact tests.

The meat percentage between the treatment groups at slaughter was analysed with independent samples t-test.

The feed consumption was reported by pen in the original data (without pig identifications) and all calculations were made at the pen level. To calculate the feed conversion ratio, the following decisions on calculations and data derivations were made to make the values as unbiased as possible:

- The total feed consumption of the pen was calculated as:

$$\textit{feed consumption}(\textit{energy}) \times \textit{number of pigs in the pen}.$$

Deceased and euthanised pigs were removed from the total number of pigs in the pen.

- To calculate the overall weights at delivery and slaughter, the weight data was modified as follows: pigs reported as deceased or euthanised were deleted from the data. Using this dataset, the total weight at delivery and slaughter by treatment and trial group were calculated.
- The feed conversion ratio at the pen level was calculated with the following formula:

$$\text{feed consumption} \div (\text{weight at slaughter} - \text{weight at delivery}).$$

All statistical analyses were performed at 4Pharma Ltd using SAS® System for Windows, version 9.3 (SAS Institute Inc., Cary, NC, USA).

Results

Weight and daily weight gain

Vaccinated pigs were significantly heavier than control pigs at time of delivery to the finishing unit and at slaughter. Daily weight gain was better in vaccinated pigs than that in control pigs. Detailed results of the weights and average daily weight gains are presented in Tables 1 and 2. Live pig weight data was obtained from the individual weighings of identified pigs. The weight data from the slaughtering process was identified only at the treatment group level (vaccine vs control).

Mortality

In the nursery, 64 vaccinated (6.5%) and 55 control piglets (5.6%) died or were euthanised ($P = 0.451$). In the finishing farm, nine pigs (1.2%) in both groups were found dead or were euthanised due to sickness. There was no statistical difference between the groups.

Medications and clinical symptoms

At the time of the study, the nursery farmer decided not to use any medications in the nursery; the researchers had no influence on this decision. Instead, the farmer

Table 1 Weight of the study pigs at different timepoints during the study

Timepoint	Vaccinated pigs		Control pigs		Mean difference, kg (SE)*	P-value*
	n	Weight in kg, average (SD)#	n	Weight in kg, average (SD)#		
Weaning	962	7.1 (1.2)	960	6.9 (1.2)	0.1 (0.4)	0.697
Delivery to finishing unit	861	24.1 (7.0)	923	22.9 (6.9)	1.2 (0.4)	0.002
Slaughter	800	103.9 (13.8)	800	100.3 (12.3)	3.6 (0.4)	< 0.001

Vaccinated piglets received an oral dose of *L. intracellularis* vaccine at the age of 3 weeks; control pigs were untreated

n number of pigs

Descriptive data, * based on the linear mixed model for weight

Table 2 The average daily weight gain of the study pigs at different timepoints during the study

Timepoint	Vaccine		Control		Mean difference (SE)*	P-value*
	n	Average daily weight gain g/day (SD)	n	Average daily weight gain g/day (SD)		
Weaning-delivery	842	325.1 (123.1)#	905	306.0 (123.3)#	14.8 (6.0)	0.013
Delivery-slaughter	800	938.6§	800	907.7§	30.9 (7.4)§	< 0.001

Vaccinated piglets received an oral dose of *L. intracellularis* vaccine at the age of 2 weeks; control pigs were untreated

n number of pigs

Descriptive data, * based on the statistical models, § imputed data

decided to euthanise all piglets in need of treatment for economic reasons. These piglets are included in the mortality figures described above.

The medications used in the finishing farm were minimal and the medications consisted of 68 individually treated pigs. A total of 3.9 and 4.6% of the vaccinated and control pigs were medicated during finishing, respectively. Treatments included injectable and peroral antimicrobials, nonsteroidal anti-inflammatory agents or trace minerals. The clinical symptoms recorded with medications that could be linked to *L. intracellularis* were diarrhoea (4 and 6 pigs in the vaccination and control groups, respectively), rectal prolapse (2 pigs in the vaccination group) and anorexia (0 in the vaccination group, 1 in control group). Altogether, 55 pigs were treated in the finishing unit due to symptoms unlikely to be related to intestinal disorders (lameness and inability to stand up, arthritis, abscesses, tail biting, and runts).

Feed conversion ratio

The mean feed conversion ratio (FCR) in the finishing unit was 2.63 FE/kg (vaccination group) and 2.65 FE/kg (control group).

Lean meat percentage

For lean meat percentage, a total of 1600 pigs were included in the analysis (800 vaccinated pigs and 800 control pigs). The mean lean meat percentage for vaccinated pigs was 59.3% (SD 3.3) and 59.6% (SD 3.8) for control pigs. There was no statistical difference between the groups (P = 0.102).

Return on investment

During the study, the price per kilogram of meat paid to the farmer from the slaughterhouse was 1.40 EUR. As the difference between vaccination and control group in live weight was 3.6 kg at slaughter, the estimated difference in kg meat was 2.7 kg (3.6 * 0.745). The increased revenue was thus 3.78 EUR per pig. The costs were estimated to be 0.70 EUR per piglet in the Finnish setting, including the costs of the vaccine and labour. The cost of increased feed intake was also included in the calculation and was estimated to be 1.99 EUR (2.63 FE/kg * 3.6 kg * 0.21 EUR/FE).

Return of investment was calculated to be with these estimates 0.41.

Discussion

Our results indicate that oral vaccination with live attenuated *L. intracellularis* resulted in both a significantly higher live weight and a significantly higher average daily weight gain (ADWG) than that of the control group. This is consistent with other results from vaccination field trials [11]. This indicates that *L. intracellularis* is an important pathogen in a Finnish SPF setting at the herd level and can limit optimal performance throughout the chain. There was a need to evaluate the effect of the vaccine in an environment where the pathogen load is low compared to other similar trials.

The FCR was similar in treatment and control groups as seen in other published field trials [10]. The results might have been different if more accurate data regarding feed consumption was available. As the vaccine is reported to increase ADWG and decrease the formation of intestinal lesions in pigs [14], we can assume that this would also influence the FCR favourably.

There was no statistical difference in lean meat percentage between the groups. This indicates that vaccination leads via significantly higher slaughter weight to better gain in the amount of lean meat (kg) per slaughtered animal and is therefore a possible tool to increase the efficacy of pork production at the farm level. To the authors' knowledge, this is the first time that the effect of *L. intracellularis* vaccination on lean meat percentage has been investigated in a field trial. In the study of McOrist et al. [10], back fat depth was reduced in vaccinated pigs, indicating 'leaner' growth patterns during the growing phase.

A decrease in antimicrobial usage after immunisation against *L. intracellularis* has been demonstrated in previous studies [9] and was also the hypothesis of our study. We could not confirm this difference. A possible explanation could be our more restrictive approach to oral group antimicrobial treatments and our relatively small sample size compared to the previous study by Bak and Rathkjen [9], where the sample size was altogether 15,656 pigs. Minimal antimicrobial use was attempted in our study herds, in accordance with the National Recommendations for the Use of Antimicrobials Against the Most Important Infectious Diseases of Animal [7]. Therefore, the starting level of antimicrobial use was already low, and a decrease was difficult to achieve. The obvious advantage with this study was that the farm could stop using the in-feed antimicrobial agents against *L. intracellularis* required for the weaned piglets before the vaccination trial started. We hypothesised that we would record more clinical symptoms typical of *L. intracellularis* in the control group, but this was not observed during the study. The disease of younger pigs has typically low mortality and most of the affected animals recover and thereafter grow normally [6]. It is possible that the overall reduced infection pressure and good management kept the clinical symptoms at a manageable level. However, as the significant difference in growth between the vaccinated and control pigs shows, infection in the control pigs had some effect even if the symptoms were subclinical.

The mortality during the nursery phase was much higher than that in other Finnish SPF farms. Statistics from the National Finnish Porcine Healthcare reports (2015 and 2016) reported national nursery mortality to be at the level of 1.6% and euthanised 0.7% of the piglets [19]. The owner decided to euthanise all sick animals in lieu of medication use. This was an unusual decision and we did not have access to data on the percentages of euthanised and dead pigs. This data would have provided a better understanding of the situation at farm level. In the finishing unit, the mortality was about the same as in most similar herds. Other *L. intracellularis* vaccination studies report similar mortalities in the vaccination and control groups [10, 11] or a lower mortality in the vaccination group [10, 12]. The effect of the vaccine can be different at the farm level as shown in McOrist et al. [10], which refers to the variable expression of the infection on different farms.

A positive ROI for the use of the vaccine was expected in this study, as it is demonstrated in previous studies [11, 12]. For example, Park et al. [11] estimated in their cost–benefit analysis a 4.2:1 ROI. However, the assumptions and circumstances (meat and feed price, pig health status) varied between the studies and generalisations on expected revenues between farms should be viewed with caution. As the mortality during finishing was low and similar between treatment groups and there were no differences in medication demand between groups, the ROI was based solely on increased revenues from increased meat production. The ROI is expected to be better in farms where mortality is more commonly observed due to *L. intracellularis* infection and where medications are needed.

There were some limitations to the study. It was challenging to follow all animals in a field setting and some of them were lost during the study period. The loss of ear tags during scalding also decreased the number of animals with individual numbering throughout the study. For future studies, it is advisable to plan the feed consumption measurements to a more precise level, as the method used in this study did not yield data that could be used in statistical calculations. As the study was conducted only on one sow farm and one finishing farm, the results should be interpreted with caution and may not be valid for the entire Finnish swine industry.

Conclusions

Immunisation of piglets with live attenuated *L. intracellularis* vaccine resulted in a higher meat yield in pig production via significantly higher live weight and average daily weight gain in a Finnish SPF farm. Immunisation ultimately led to better financial results. Vaccination is a tool to improve production in farms diagnosed with *L. intracellularis* infection.

Authors' contributions

SP wrote the draft of the manuscript. SP and TT conducted the herd visits and manual data collection from the slaughterhouse. JJ conducted the statistical analyses. SP, TT and MH were actively involved in planning the study. All authors read and approved the final manuscript.

Author details
[1] Vetcare Finland Ltd, Hiomotie 3 A, 00380 Helsinki, Finland. [2] Atria Pork/A-Farmers Ltd, Po. Box 910, 60061 Atria, Finland. [3] Department of Production Animal Medicine, Faculty of Veterinary Medicine, University of Helsinki, Paroninkuja 20, 04920 Saarentaus, Finland. [4] 4Pharma Ltd, Arkadiankatu 7, 00100 Helsinki, Finland.

Acknowledgements
We wish to thank the farmers who permitted our herd visits and assisted in data collection.

Competing interests
TT, JJ and MH declare that they have no competing interests. SP has worked in the University of Helsinki while specialising in production animal medicine and running this field study as part of her specialisation studies. SP is an employee of Vetcare Finland Ltd.

Funding
This work received funding from Atria Pork/A-Farmers Ltd, Boehringer Ingelheim Vetmedica Inc. and Vetcare Ltd. The funding bodies had no influence on study design, collection, analysis, data interpretation or the manuscript.

References

1. Biester HE, Schwarte LH. Intestinal adenoma in swine. Am J Pathol. 1931;7:175–85.
2. Jensen HM. Health management with reduced antibiotic use—experiences of a Danish pig vet. Anim Biotechnol. 2006;17:189–94.
3. Jacobson M, Gerth Lofstedt M, Holmgren N, Lundeheim N, Fellstrom C. The prevalences of *Brachyspira* spp. and *Lawsonia intracellularis* in Swedish piglet producing herds and wild boar population. J Vet Med B Infect Dis Vet Public Health. 2005;52:386–91.
4. Stege H, Jensen TK, Moller K, Baekbo P, Jorsal SE. Prevalence of intestinal pathogens in Danish finishing pig herds. Prev Vet Med. 2000;46:279–92.
5. Finnish Food Safety Authority website. 2016. https://www.evira.fi/elaimet/elainten-terveys-ja-elaintaudit/elaintaudit/siat/suolistotulehdukset/. Accessed 29 Dec 2016.
6. Lawson GH, Gebhart CJ. Proliferative enteropathy. J Comp Pathol. 2000;122:77–100.
7. Finnish Food Safety Authority Evira. Recommendations for the use of antimicrobials against the most important infectious diseases of animal. 2016. https://www.evira.fi/tietoa-evirasta/julkaisut/elaimet/oppaat/mikrobilaakkeiden-kayttosuositukset-elainten-tarkeimpiin-tulehdus–ja-tartuntatauteihin/. Accessed 31 Aug 2017.
8. European Medicines Agency. Sales of veterinary antimicrobial agents in 29 European countries in 2014 Trends from 2011 to 2014 Sixth ESVAC report. 2017. http://www.ema.europa.eu/docs/en_GB/document_library/Report/2016/10/WC500214217.pdf. Accessed 31 Aug 2017.
9. Bak H, Rathkjen PH. Reduced use of antimicrobials after vaccination of pigs against porcine proliferative enteropathy in a Danish SPF herd. Acta Vet Scand. 2009;51:1. https://doi.org/10.1186/1751-0147-51-1.
10. McOrist S, Smits RJ. Field evaluation of an oral attenuated *Lawsonia intracellularis* vaccine for porcine proliferative enteropathy (ileitis). Vet Rec. 2007;161:26–8.
11. Park S, Lee JB, Kim KJ, Oh YS, Kim MO, Oh YR, et al. Efficacy of a commercial live attenuated *Lawsonia intracellularis* vaccine in a large scale field trial in Korea. Clin Exp Vaccine Res. 2013;2:135–9.
12. Weibel H, Sydler T, Brugnera E, Voets H, Grosse Liesner B, Sidler X. Efficacy of simultaneous vaccination with Enterisol(R) Ileitis and Ingelvac(R) CircoFLEXTM in a Swiss breeding farm. Schweiz Arch Tierheilkd. 2012;154:445–50.
13. Almond PK, Bilkei G. Effects of oral vaccination against *Lawsonia intracellularis* on growing-finishing pig's performance in a pig production unit with endemic porcine proliferative enteropathy (PPE). Dtsch Tierarztl Wochenschr. 2006;113:232–5.
14. Kroll JJ, Roof MB, McOrist S. Evaluation of protective immunity in pigs following oral administration of an avirulent live vaccine of *Lawsonia intracellularis*. Am J Vet Res. 2004;65:559–65.
15. Guedes RM, Gebhart CJ. Onset and duration of fecal shedding, cell-mediated and humoral immune responses in pigs after challenge with a pathogenic isolate or attenuated vaccine strain *of Lawsonia intracellularis*. Vet Microbiol. 2003;91:135–45.
16. Riber U, Heegaard PM, Cordes H, Stahl M, Jensen TK, Jungersen G. Vaccination of pigs with attenuated *Lawsonia intracellularis* induced acute phase protein responses and primed cell-mediated immunity without reduction in bacterial shedding after challenge. Vaccine. 2015;33:156–62.
17. Nogueira MG, Collins AM, Dunlop RH, Emery D. Effect of the route of administration on the mucosal and systemic immune responses to *Lawsonia intracellularis* vaccine in pigs. Aust Vet J. 2015;93:124–6.
18. Kortesniemi, P, Nikunen S. Online register with health classification—an efficient tool to control swine diseases. In: Proceedings of European symposium of porcine health management; May 7.9.2014. p. 184.
19. Annual healthcare reports 2015 and 2016, Sikava. 2017. https://www.sikava.fi/. Accessed 24 Aug 2017.

20

Canine breeds associated with gastric carcinoma, metaplasia and dysplasia diagnosed by histopathology of endoscopic biopsy samples

Marcus Vinicius Candido[1*], Pernilla Syrjä[2], Susanne Kilpinen[1] and Thomas Spillmann[1]

Abstract

Background: Gastric carcinoma (GC) is a rather rare pathological finding in dogs, with the exception of some breeds which seem predisposed. The etiopathogenesis is largely unknown in dogs, whereas in humans GC often develops from gastric mucosal metaplasia and dysplasia. This study investigates whether dogs of certain breeds are more often subject to gastroduodenoscopy (GDS), and diagnosed with GC, mucosal metaplasia or dysplasia. A retrospective clinical database search was performed at the Veterinary Teaching Hospital at the University of Helsinki, Finland. The following inclusion criteria were applied to estimate relative risk for metaplasia/dysplasia and GC: dogs from pure breeds with at least five individuals subject to GDS with histopathology of gastric biopsies.

Results: Between 2006 and 2016, from a total of 54945 canine patients presented, 423 dogs underwent GDS. Inclusion criteria were met in 180 dogs of 20 different pure breeds. Eight dogs had GCs (mean age $= 9.8 \pm 1.7$ years): Belgian Tervuren (n = 4), Collie (n = 2), Golden Retriever (n = 1) and Jack Russel Terrier (n = 1). Fourteen dogs of eight breeds had gastric mucosal metaplasia or dysplasia. A log-binomial statistical model revealed that dogs in the following breeds had a significantly higher probability to undergo GDS than the others in the study population: Australian Terrier, Belgian Tervuren, Cairn Terrier, Collie and Siberian Husky. Belgian Tervuren was found at higher risk to be diagnosed with GC [RR = 19 (5.7–63.9; $P < 0.0001$)], as well as mucosal metaplasia/dysplasia [RR (7.6; 2.95–19.58; $P < 0.0001$)], as compared to the other breeds included. Shetland Sheepdog had an increased RR (5.83; 1.75–19.45; $P = 0.0041$) for metaplasia.

Conclusions: The results indicate a very low incidence of GC in dogs. The Belgian Tervuren, however, appears as predisposed. The histopathologic descriptions of mucosal changes such as metaplasia and dysplasia were also rare, but were more frequent in the Belgian Tervuren. Previous reports of these changes in dogs are very scarce, but they might be presumably related to GC in dogs, as they are in humans. Future research should investigate the possible role of metaplasia and dysplasia in the development of GC in dogs, especially those of predisposed breeds.

Keywords: Breed predisposition, Cancer, Dog, Dysplasia, Endoscopy, Gastric carcinoma, Gastroduodenoscopy, Metaplasia

*Correspondence: marcus.candido@helsinki.fi

[1] Department of Equine and Small Animal Medicine, Faculty of Veterinary Medicine, University of Helsinki, P.O. Box 57, 00014 Helsinki, Finland

Full list of author information is available at the end of the article

Background

Gastric carcinoma (GC) is a rare pathologic finding in dogs, as it corresponds to less than one percent of all neoplastic changes identified in dogs [1, 2]. The most common type of gastric neoplasm in dogs is adenocarcinoma, which is diagnosed at around 10 years of age, with initial clinical signs similar to those of other chronic gastrointestinal disorders [2–5]. Most gastrointestinal carcinomas in humans are known to evolve from superficial, flat changes classified as metaplastic or dysplastic according to their degree of cellular differentiation [6, 7]. GC is the fifth most common type of cancer in people worldwide, and endoscopic biopsy is essential for diagnostic and staging [8]. Visual enhancement techniques such as chromoendoscopy and narrow band imaging are often applied for cancer screening and surveillance, as they can help improve the diagnostic yield of discrete mucosal changes [9]. The pathogenesis in humans is complex and not fully understood, but in approximately 90% of the cases it involves a multistep, multifactorial process. The progression from normal mucosa to chronic gastritis, further evolving to atrophic gastritis, intestinal metaplasia, dysplasia and adenocarcinoma, occurs over several years [10]. However, challenging this classic histogenetic pathway in which metaplasia and dysplasia are well-recognized pre-neoplastic changes, human GC can also develop from otherwise normal gastric mucosa. Diffuse gastric cancer, for example, is rare and often develops in a hereditary setting from foci of superficial signet ring carcinoma in situ [11]. Gastric infection with *Helicobacter pylori* plays a major role among environmental factors contributing to an increased risk of gastric cancer in humans [12], along with dietary factors including high intake of salt and preserved or smoked food (especially meat products), and low consumption of fresh fruit and vegetables [13].

The etiology of GC in dogs is still unknown, and it is suspected to be as complex as in humans [14]. The cardinal histological changes in canine gastric carcinogenesis remain undetermined, and the correlation between gastric polyps, *Helicobacter* spp. and GC has not yet been demonstrated [5, 15, 16]. A study on 14 Norwegian Lundehund dogs describes findings of mucous metaplasia in association with varying degrees of atrophic gastritis and intestinal lymphangiectasia. Additionally, four of those dogs had gastric neoplasia, which suggests that the changes represent a single pathological process [17]. In a further study with a total of eight Lundehunds with gastric neoplasia, it seems that such tumors are rather of neuroendocrine origin (derived from enterochromaffin-like-cells), possibly secondary to gastric atrophy and hypergastrinemia [18]. However, canine GC is not always associated with atrophic gastritis and comprehensive studies demonstrating the progression of atrophy towards metaplasia, dysplasia and gastric cancer in dogs are still lacking.

Previous retrospective studies based on data from canine cancer registry, records from specialists, pathology laboratories and breeders have shown breed predisposition to GC in the Belgian Tervuren, Bouvier des Flandres, Groenendael, Collie, Chow–Chow, Poodle, Norwegian Elkhound and a few other breeds, which implies a genetic background for the disease [1, 3, 4, 19, 20]. In Finland, information about breed association to gastric cancer has been missing.

The present study was conducted to investigate which pure breeds are most commonly subject to gastroduodenoscopy (GDS) at the Veterinary Teaching Hospital of the University of Helsinki, a national referral center. The most important objective was to determine the probability of dogs in different breeds undergoing endoscopy with mucosal biopsy for histology to be diagnosed with gastric carcinoma, metaplasia or dysplasia, as a possible evidence of breed predisposition also in Finland. The overall aim of this study was to gather information about gastric cancer and metaplastic or dysplastic changes as recognizable features in canine patients undergoing endoscopy with gastric mucosal biopsy for histology. This study relies on the hypothesis that, in the clinical setting of an endoscopic unit, certain breeds can be found affected with GC and mucosal metaplasia/dysplasia more commonly than others. The study therefore aims at investigating a possible association between individual breed, submission to GDS, and diagnosis of gastric carcinoma and metaplastic or dysplastic mucosal changes in histopathology.

Methods

The study was designed as a retrospective cohort on the diagnosis of GC, metaplasia and dysplasia in dogs subjected to GDS. The source population of this study comprises all dogs presented at the Veterinary Teaching Hospital between January 2006 and December 2016. A computerized database search was performed on the records throughout this period. The study population included dogs which belong to a pure breed having a minimum of five dogs subject to GDS with complete histopathological report based on gastric biopsies. The Belgian Tervuren is herein regarded as a breed on its own. The breed Collie includes both rough and smooth haircoat varieties (Border Collie and Shetland Shepherd being separate pure breeds).

The endoscopic biopsy samples were collected in a standardized fashion: at least eight gastric mucosal fragments were taken onto wood chips and then immediately immersed (upside down) in 10% neutral buffered formalin. After 24 h fixation, the biopsies were processed, paraffine-embedded, sectioned at 4 microns and stained with hematoxylin and eosin (HE). Special staining such as periodic acid-Schiff (PAS) or Warthin–Starry (WS) were applied when indicated.

The endoscopic mucosal biopsy samples were examined at the University of Helsinki by veterinary pathologists adhering to a standardized assessment protocol since 2006. The standard reporting template included the following parameters as main criteria for histopathological evaluation of the stomach: number of biopsy samples examined, epithelial surface characterization, amount of intraepithelial lymphocytes, presence of *Helicobacter*-like organisms, characterization and amount of mononuclear and granulocyte infiltration in lamina propria, presence of lymphoid follicles, characterization of fundic glands, and whether pepsinogen and HCl-producing cells are identified regularly, or else substituted by mucous cells (metaplasia) [21]. Gland structure was also evaluated regarding presence of fibrosis, glandular nesting and structural changes which could be related to dysplasia. The World Small Animal Veterinary Association standards and guidelines were applied from 2008 onwards and the template was updated accordingly, regarding grading of inflammatory changes (0–3: normal, mild, moderate, severe) [22, 23]. The diagnoses were given under the supervision of, and in consensus with, a board-certified pathologist (PS).

The complete histopathological record of endoscopic biopsies from each patient of the study population was revisited for findings consistent with either gastric carcinoma (GC), dysplasia or metaplasia, in addition to other features [21–23]. Histologic sections from the patients presenting these specific lesions were re-examined by a board-certified pathologist (PS) for verification of the diagnosis and consistency of the results.

Statistical methods

All of the outcomes tested were binary, because the presence or absence of GDS, GC or metaplasia/dysplasia was considered for each case studied. A log-binomial model was applied for each outcome variable, and the probability of presence was modelled with 95% confidence intervals (CI). The models were re-run separately for each breed in the analysis population comparing the breed of interest to other breeds. Relative probability to undergo GDS (numerically equivalent to relative risk) was calculated for each selected breed in comparison to all other canine patients visiting the hospital in the period (source population). The individual histopathological diagnosis from dogs of breeds meeting the inclusion criteria (study population) was considered for the calculation of relative risk (RR) to be diagnosed with gastric metaplasia/dysplasia, or carcinoma, and computed for each breed in comparison to the other breeds included. P-values < 0.05 were considered significant. All analyses were done using SAS® System for Windows, version 9.3 (SAS Institute Inc., Cary, NC, USA).

Results

Pure breeds undergoing gastroduodenoscopy (GDS)

Between 2006 and 2016, the source population included a grand total of 54,945 canine patients being presented at the hospital. The study population was recruited out of 423 dogs which underwent GDS for diagnostic reasons, 30 of which being mixed-breed dogs. The inclusion criteria mentioned above were met by 180 dogs representing 20 different pure breeds. The study population consisted of 75 intact males, 26 castrated males, 46 intact females

Table 1 Study population: breeds with at least five dogs undergoing gastroduodenoscopy (GDS) and histopathological examination of biopsy samples, selected for inclusion from the source population of all dogs presented between 01.01.2006 and 31.12.2016

Breed	Total dogs presented	Dogs undergoing GDS
Australian Terrier	245	5
Belgian Tervuren	196	9
Border Collie	430	5
Cairn Terrier	522	11
Chihuahua	1729	5
Collie	673	27
Dachshund	1609	7
French bulldog	845	7
German Shepherd	2110	18
Golden Retriever	1216	15
Hovawart	328	5
Jack Russell Terrier	1149	7
Labrador retriever	2124	14
Miniature Schnauzer	1003	7
Parson Russell Terrier	496	6
Rottweiler	794	10
Shetland Sheepdog	734	5
Siberian Husky	219	5
Staffordshire Bull Terrier	592	6
West Highland White Terrier	690	6
Dogs in the breeds above	17,704	***180***
Other breeds/mixed (not included)	37,241	243[a]
All dogs in the period	*54,945*	423[b]

Study population is indicated in bolditalic

Source population is indicated in italic

[a] Includes individual dogs from the selected breeds which were excluded from the study due to lack of histopathological diagnosis (foreign body retrieval, no biopsy taken or biopsy lost to follow-up)

[b] Total number of GDS patients in the period

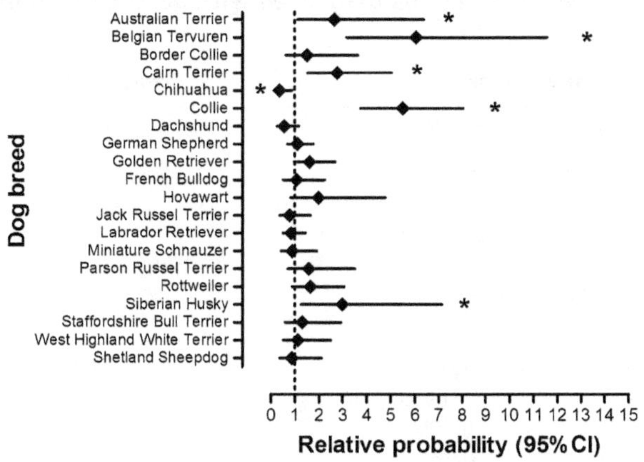

Fig. 1 Relative probability to undergo GDS for dogs of the selected breeds in comparison to all other dogs in the source population. *The difference is statistically significant ($P<0.05$)

Table 2 Number of dogs in each breed undergoing gastroduodenoscopy (GDS), and diagnosed with gastric carcinoma (GC), dysplasia or metaplasia from endoscopic biopsy samples taken from 01.01.2006 to 31.12.2016

Breed	GDS	GC	Dysplasia or metaplasia
Belgian Tervuren	9	4	4
Collie	27	2	2
Dachshund	7	–	1
Golden Retriever	15	1	2
Hovawart	5	–	1
Jack Russell Terrier	7	1	–
Shetland Sheepdog	5	–	2
Siberian Husky	5	–	1
Staffordshire Bull Terrier	6	–	1
Total in these breeds	86	8	14

and 33 sterilized females, which underwent GDS at the mean age of 5.3 ± 3.4 years (n = 180). These dogs correspond to 43% of all GDS patients in the period (Table 1). Twelve other individual dogs of the breeds included had already been excluded from the study either because histopathological information was lost (n = 3) or no biopsies were taken during GDS (n = 9). Six of those nine dogs had gastric foreign bodies removed (plastic; wood; needles; stone) and one presented biliary tract changes and underwent endoscopic retrograde cholangiopancreatography followed by surgical removal of the gallbladder.

When comparing the study population with the source population, a log-binomial model revealed significantly higher relative probability to undergo GDS in the following breeds as compared to dogs of other breeds (RR; 95% CI lower–higher; *P* value): Australian Terrier (2.67; 1.12–6.39; $P=0.0274$), Belgian Tervuren (6.07; 3.18–11.58; $P<0.0001$), Cairn Terrier (2.78; 1.54–5.03; $P=0.0007$), Collie (5.5; 3.75–8.06; $P<0.0001$) and Siberian Husky (2.99; 1.25–7.15; $P=0.0138$). Chihuahuas underwent GDS significantly less often than dogs of other breeds (0.37; 0.15–0.89; $P=0.0261$) (Fig. 1).

Gastric carcinoma

Eight of the dogs included in the study were diagnosed with gastric adenocarcinomas, which was the only type of gastric neoplasm seen in the study population. Affected dogs belonged to the following breeds: Belgian Tervuren (n = 4, including one signet-cell carcinoma), Collie (n = 2), Golden Retriever and Jack Russel Terrier (Table 2). Five of them were female and three were male. Concerning age at diagnosis of GC, the youngest patient was 7.8 years old when the examination was performed (mean age $= 9.8 \pm 1.7$ years; see also Table 3). The Belgian Tervuren was found at much greater relative risk for being diagnosed with GC from histopathological examination of endoscopically obtained gastric biopsies (33.4; 6.43–173.36; $P<0.0001$) in comparison to other breeds (Fig. 2).

Metaplasia and dysplasia in gastric mucosa

Changes histologically described as metaplastic or dysplastic were seen in 14 dogs in the following breeds: Belgian Tervuren (n = 4), Collie (n = 2), Golden Retriever (n = 2), Shetland Sheepdog (n = 2), Dachshund (n = 1), Hovawart (n = 1), Siberian Husky (n = 1) and Staffordshire Bull Terrier (n = 1). The mean age when these patients underwent GDS was 7.9 ± 2.6 years. Significant statistical differences were found for the diagnosis of either metaplasia or dysplasia in Belgian Tervuren compared to other breeds: RR (7.6; 2.95–19.58; $P<0.0001$). The Shetland Sheepdog was found at significantly increased RR (5.83; 1.75–19.45; $P=0.0041$) for metaplasia (dysplasia was not seen in this breed) compared to dogs of other breeds (Fig. 3).

Endoscopic and histopathological diagnosis

The final diagnosis considered for all of the analyses was achieved by endoscopic examination and sampling, followed by histopathological confirmation. All dogs presenting the changes of concern were also found with concomitant inflammatory changes (Table 3). Each set of sample images shown in this article correspond to a single patient, respectively diagnosed as carcinoma (Figs. 4, 5), metaplasia (Fig. 6) or dysplasia (Fig. 7). Chromoendoscopy and narrow band imaging were applied in one Belgian Tervuren presented with chronic vomiting, whose brother from the same litter had been euthanized

Table 3 Breed, age (years), sex and concomitant changes found in each of the dogs diagnosed with gastric carcinoma (GC)

Breed	Age	Sex	Inflammatory change	Structural change
Belgian Tervuren (n = 4)	7.8	F	Moderate chronic LP G	Glandular dysplasia
	9.7	F	Moderate chronic LP G	–
	9.2	M	Moderate chronic LP G with neutrophilic component and severe gland hyperplasia	Glandular dysplasia, epithelial dysplasia and atypia
	11.0	M	Severe chronic LP G	–
Collie (n = 2)	8.6	F	Moderate chronic LP G	–
	8.5	Fs	Moderate chronic atrophic G	Mucinous metaplasia
Golden Retriever	10.8	F	Severe chronic LP G with neutrophilic component and ulcerative mycotic G	–
Jack Russell Terrier	12.9	Mc	Severe gland hyperplasia, mild LP G	–

LP lymphoplasmacytic, *G* gastritis, *Fs* sterilized female, *Mc* castrated male

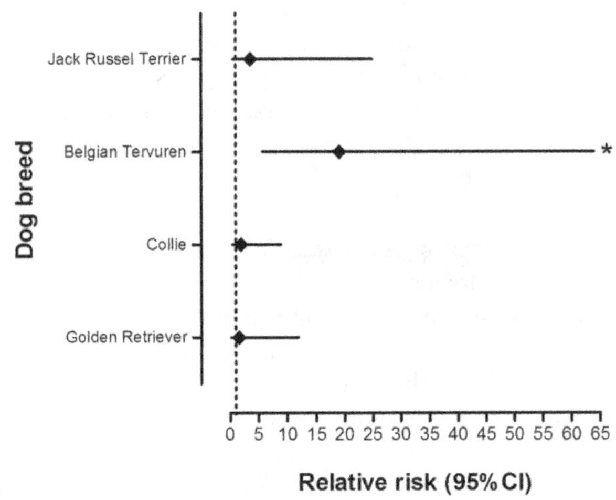

Fig. 2 Relative risk to be diagnosed with gastric carcinoma for selected breeds in comparison to the other breeds in the study population. *The difference is statistically significant ($P < 0.0001$)

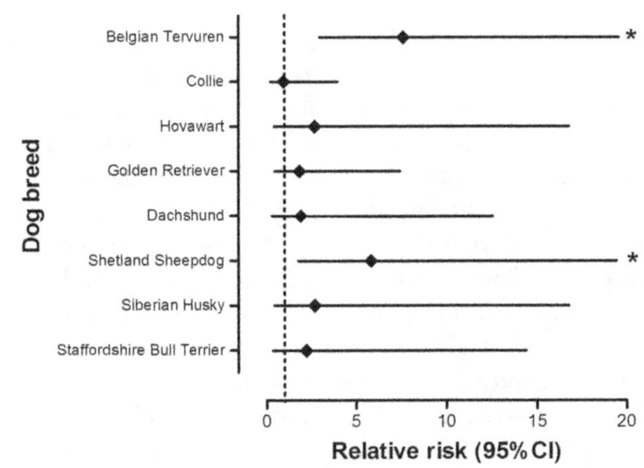

Fig. 3 Relative risk to be diagnosed with gastric mucosal metaplasia or dysplasia for selected breeds in comparison to the other breeds in the study population. *The difference is statistically significant ($P < 0.005$)

due to a massive GC. The most prominent endoscopic and respective histopathological changes found in this patient are in Fig. 7.

Discussion

Some dog breeds (namely Australian Terrier, Belgian Tervuren, Cairn Terrier, Collie and Siberian Husky) underwent GDS significantly more often as compared to the other breeds in this study. Chihuahua was scoped significantly less often than others; this breed with a relatively small body size is rather common in the source population. These findings remain largely unexplained, however breed distribution (Table 1) and relatively low overall frequency of GDS (low sample sizes) may have influenced the results. It is not clear whether it was the severity of gastrointestinal signs alone, or any other issues that might have influenced the probability for certain breeds to undergo GDS. It would be reasonable to speculate that an expected breed predisposition to GC, as previously reported for the Belgian Tervuren [1, 3, 19], might potentially bias the approach of clinicians and owners towards submitting patients of this breed to endoscopy earlier, or more often. The fact that dogs of certain breeds undergo GDS more often might as well indicate a higher prevalence of gastrointestinal disorders in general, which may warrant more extensive studies in such breeds.

The Belgian Tervurens that underwent GDS in this study were consistently found at much higher risk of being diagnosed with GC than dogs of any other breed. This finding is in accordance with previous studies that used pathological records and cancer registry data of

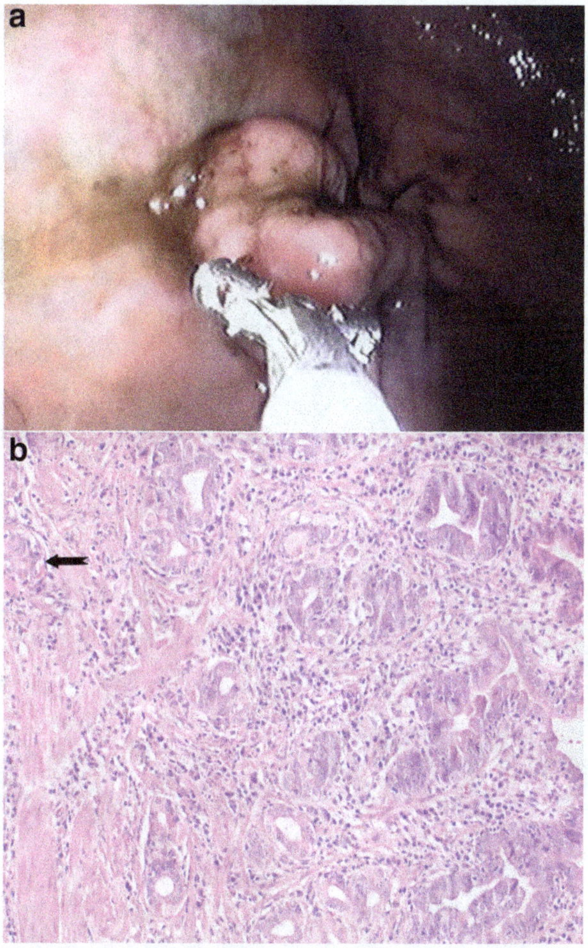

Fig. 4 Endoscopic and corresponding histologic images of an 8-year-old female Belgian Tervuren showing gastric adenocarcinoma. **a** White light endoscopic image of a gastric adenocarcinoma. Histology: **b** Well differentiated gastric adenocarcinoma with invasion of the *muscularis mucosae* (arrow). HE stain, Obj. 20×

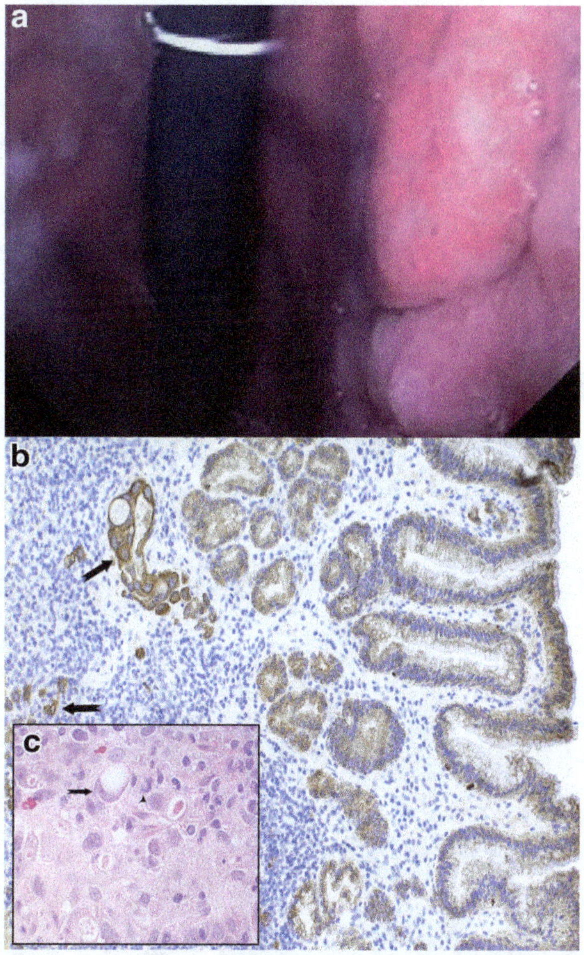

Fig. 5 Endoscopic and corresponding histologic images of a 10-year old female Belgian Tervuren representing gastric adenocarcinoma. **a** White light endoscopic image of a diffuse mass in the stomach. Histology: **b** Invasive gastric adenocarcinoma, with atypical tubular structures (arrow) and single cell invasion of deeper layers of the gastric wall (arrow), and **c** classical signet ring cells (arrow). **b** IHC cytokeratin stain, Obj. 20×. **c** HE stain, Obj. 40×

other countries such as Italy, Netherlands or Norway, in which the Belgian Tervuren were also considered to be highly predisposed to GC [1, 3, 19].

Gastric metaplasia or dysplasia were almost as rarely seen as GC, with significantly higher relative risks found for the Belgian Tervuren and Shetland Sheepdog. Although statistical significance could not be confirmed for every breed, both types of changes were found in Belgian Tervuren, Collie and Golden Retriever, sometimes in the same patient. Nonetheless, metaplasia and dysplasia can present as discrete, flat changes that are easily overlooked and possibly underdiagnosed [24], especially when considering the limitations of current white light endoscopy modalities available and non-directed sampling procedures in veterinary medicine. Visual enhancement techniques such as chromoendoscopy and narrow band imaging (Fig. 7) may help improve the diagnostic yield of discrete mucosal changes [9].

One of the major challenges in veterinary gastroenterology is that the extension and severity of macroscopic changes seen during endoscopy are not always consistent with the respective histopathological findings from endoscopic biopsy [25]. Cognitive aspects including specific knowledge, endoscopist experience and training, standardized grading systems, image quality and meticulous examination techniques are fundamental for the detection of subtle lesions [26]. In this study, the biopsies and histologic sections were prepared and then examined according to a uniform in-house standard. Such protocols help to control the risk of inaccuracy related to lack

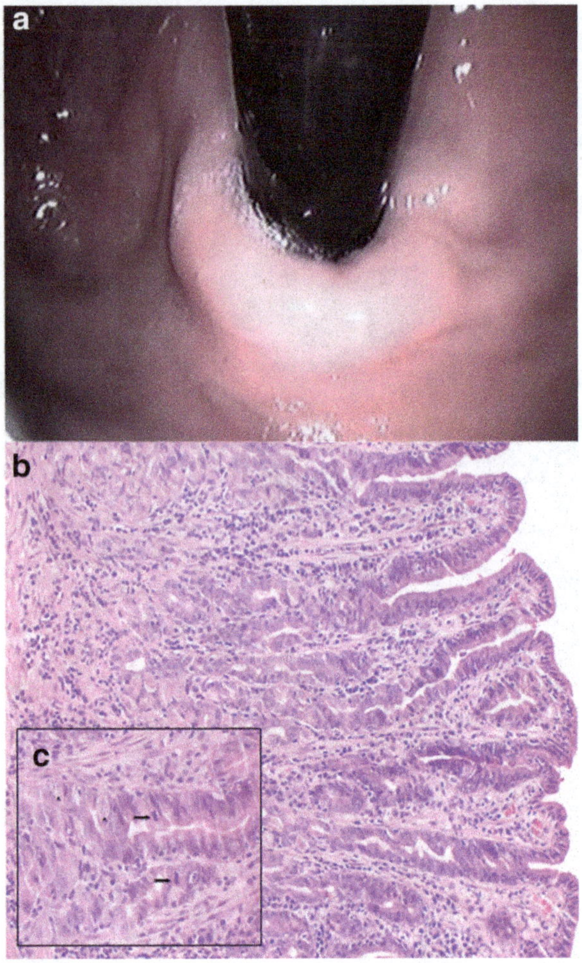

Fig. 6 Endoscopic and corresponding histologic images of a 9-year-old castrated male Dachshund representing metaplasia. **a** White light endoscopic image of gastric fundus with discrete mucosal changes. Histology: **b** Mucous/intestinal metaplasia within the gastric fundus; elongated hyperplastic mucous neck regions of fundic glands and diffuse moderate lymphoplasmacytic gastritis. **c** Increased mitotic figures within the hyperplastic mucous cells of the glandular neck area (arrow). Scattered parietal cells are visible (arrowhead) within the basal area of the glands. HE stain, **b** Obj. 20×, **c** Obj. 40×

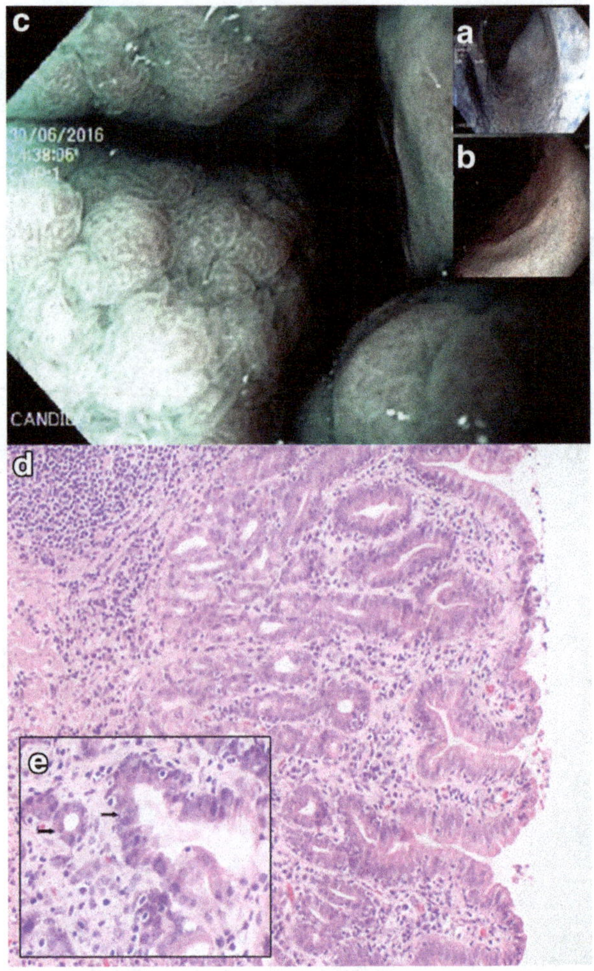

Fig. 7 Endoscopic and corresponding histologic images of a 9-year-old female Belgian Tervuren showing dysplasia. Endoscopic images (**a**, **b**, **c**) show diffuse mucosal texture irregularity along gastric fundus and body: **a** chromoendoscopy (CE), **b** narrow band imaging (NBI), **c** CE and NBI combined. Histology: **d** dysplasia of the fundic glands, with glandular dilatation and distortion. **e** Cellular dysplasia with flattening of the glandular cells and loss of cellular polarity (arrows). HE stain, **d** Obj. 20×, **e** Obj. 40×

of uniformity on sample quality and to interobserver variation in histopathological evaluation. Such issues have been reported as potentially detrimental when histologic material or reports originated from several different institutions are utilized [27, 28].

The diagnosis of metaplastic or dysplastic changes in breeds with predispositions to GC might indicate a stepwise progression in dogs, comparable to the better known pathway towards GC in humans [10]. Studies in Lundehund dogs with GC ponder on a similar pathogenesis [17, 18]. This might be the case especially for the Belgian Tervuren with its significantly higher relative risk for the suspected pre-neoplastic changes, along with its marked predisposition for GC. This hypothesis might be further explored by staging suspected lesions and screening dogs selected from predisposed breeds. Research should aim at applying more advanced endoscopic approaches such as chromoendoscopy or narrow band imaging, which are proven modalities in humans for improving the targeted sampling of lesions [29] that might be easily overlooked when using white light endoscopy alone. Metaplasia and dysplasia have not been consistently studied in canine gastroenterology and their potentially relevant role in the pathogenesis of canine GC must be further investigated, whereas in humans well-established staging protocols and advanced therapeutic approaches are routinely applied [30]. While standard guidelines for histopathology evaluation remain fluid in veterinary medicine, novel immune staining techniques and genetic examination of biopsy samples may provide valuable opportunities for both research and diagnosis in the near future [31].

The retrospective nature of the study and the sole inclusion of dogs that had undergone GDS led to some limitations that possibly influenced the interpretation of our results. This study did not include GC diagnosed after necropsy or full-thickness biopsy but rather focused on the findings of endoscopic biopsy samples. This approach resulted in a small case load, as endoscopy is typically performed in a relatively small proportion of dogs in the clinical population, thus it relies on specific indications and also the owner's compliance. A possible bias of indication for endoscopic procedures by different clinicians (e.g. awareness of certain breed predispositions), over such an extended time period, cannot be ruled out.

It is also worth mentioning that even in this selected population of canine patients with clinical signs of gastrointestinal disease, GCs were seen only in few individuals (8/180 = 4.4%), which further corroborates the rarity of the condition. The frequency of disease in this study cannot be directly compared with previous studies that used different approaches. However, the low frequency of diagnosis and the advanced age at diagnosis of GC in dogs found in this setting are in agreement with previous reports [1–4, 14].

Gaining knowledge about the actual prevalence of metaplasia and dysplasia in dogs may help to determine their possible role as pre-neoplastic changes. Furthermore, patient follow-up after the diagnosis of metaplastic and dysplastic changes might contribute to the knowledge about canine gastric carcinogenesis. Multi-center, prospective studies that utilize standardized approaches could help overcome the limitations related to reduced sample sizes in veterinary research, especially with regard to uncommon disease conditions like the ones reported in this study.

Conclusions

Belgian Tervurens, Collies, Siberian Huskies, Cairn Terriers and Australian Terriers underwent GDS more often than dogs of other breeds in our study population. The Belgian Tervurens were found to be at much higher risk (19-fold) of being diagnosed with GC than dogs of other breeds, which further corroborates predisposition for GC in this breed. Metaplastic or dysplastic changes were slightly more frequent than GC. Although no causal relationship could be established thus far, the presence of lesions of all three types in breeds such as the Collie, the Golden Retriever, and chiefly the Belgian Tervuren, even in the face of these low case numbers, might be a sign of associated pathogenesis requiring further investigation.

Authors' contributions

MVC applied the inclusion criteria to the database, revised the histopathological record of the individual patients included, prepared the data for statistical analysis, selected and prepared images, tables and graphics, and was the main responsible for the manuscript. PS acted as a co-author and consultant in pathology, and provided the photomicrographs and respective histopathological highlights, also participating as an active reviewer when drafting the manuscript. SK performed part of the endoscopies and acted as co-supervisor involved in drafting the manuscript. TS was the research director. He performed part of the endoscopies, the baseline search in the hospital database, co-authored and reviewed the manuscript on all steps. All authors read and approved the final manuscript.

Author details

[1] Department of Equine and Small Animal Medicine, Faculty of Veterinary Medicine, University of Helsinki, P.O. Box 57, 00014 Helsinki, Finland. [2] Department of Veterinary Biosciences, Faculty of Veterinary Medicine, University of Helsinki, P.O. Box 66, 00014 Helsinki, Finland.

Acknowledgements

Thanks go to Sofia Männikkö of '4Pharma' for her statistical analyses and technical assistance.

Competing interests

The authors declare that they have no competing interests.

Funding

This study was partly supported by a grant from the Brazilian Council for Science and Technology Development (CNPq). We also thank the Finnish Veterinary Foundation, the Finnish Foundation of Veterinary Research, and the Doctoral Program in Clinical Veterinary Medicine, for financial support.

References

1. Seim-Wikse T, Jörundsson E, Nødtvedt A, Grotmol T, Bjornvad CR, Kristensen AT, et al. Breed predisposition to canine gastric carcinoma-a study based on the Norwegian canine cancer register. Acta Vet Scand. 2013;55:25.
2. Terragni R, Vignoli M, van Bree HJ, Gaschen L, Saunders JH. Diagnostic imaging and endoscopic finding in dogs and cats with gastric tumors: a review. Schweiz Arch Tierh. 2014;156:569–76.
3. Lubbes D, Mandigers PJ, Heuven HC, Teske E. Incidence of gastric carcinoma in Dutch Tervueren shepherd dogs born between 1991 and 2002. Tijdschr Diergeneesk. 2009;134:606–10.
4. Von Babo V, Eberle N, Mischke R, Meyer-Lindenberg A, Hewicker-Trautwein M, Nolte I, et al. Canine non-hematopoietic gastric neoplasia. Tierarztl Prax Ausg K Kleintiere Heimtiere. 2012;40:243–9.
5. Taulescu MA, Valentine BA, Amorim I, Gärtner F, Dumitraşcu DL, Gal AF, et al. Histopathological features of canine spontaneous non-neoplastic

gastric polyps-a retrospective study of 15 cases. Histol Histopathol. 2014;29:65–75.

6. Park YH, Kim N. Review of atrophic gastritis and intestinal metaplasia as a premalignant lesion of gastric cancer. J Cancer Prev. 2015;20:25.
7. Schlemper RJ, Riddell RH, Kato YE, Borchard F, Cooper HS, Dawsey SM, et al. The Vienna classification of gastrointestinal epithelial neoplasia. Gut. 2000;47:251–5.
8. Carneiro F. Stomach cancer. In: Stewart B, Wild CP, editors. International agency for research on cancer. Lyon: WHO; 2014. p. 383–91.
9. Trivedi PJ, Braden B. Indications, stains and techniques in chromoendoscopy. QJM. 2013;106:117–31.
10. Correa P. Human gastric carcinogenesis: a multistep and multifactorial process—first American Cancer Society award lecture on cancer epidemiology and prevention. Cancer Res. 1992;52:6735–40.
11. Carneiro F, Huntsman DG, Smyrk TC, Owen DA, Seruca R, Pharoah P, et al. Model of the early development of diffuse gastric cancer in E-cadherin mutation carriers and its implications for patient screening. J Pathol. 2004;203:681–7.
12. Forman D, Newell DG, Fullerton F, Yarnell JW, Stacey AR, Wald N, Sitas F. Association between infection with Helicobacter pylori and risk of gastric cancer: evidence from a prospective investigation. BMJ. 1991;302:1302–5.
13. World Cancer Research Fund/American Institute for Cancer Research. Food, nutrition, physical activity, and the prevention of cancer: a global perspective. Washington DC: AICR; 2007. p. 265-6.
14. Hugen S, Thomas RE, German AJ, Burgener IA, Mandigers PJ. Gastric carcinoma in canines and humans, a review. Vet Comp Oncol. 2017;15:692–705.
15. Neiger R, Simpson KW. Helicobacter infection in dogs and cats: facts and fiction. J Vet Intern Med. 2000;14:125–33.
16. Amorim I, Taulescu MA, Ferreira A, Rêma A, Reis CA, Faustino AM, et al. An immunohistochemical study of canine spontaneous gastric polyps. Diagn Pathol. 2014;9:166.
17. Kolbjørnsen Ø, Press CM, Landsverk T. Gastropathies in the Lundehund. APMIS. 1994;102:647–61.
18. Qvigstad G, Kolbjørnsen Ø, Skancke E, Waldum HL. Gastric neuroendocrine carcinoma associated with atrophic gastritis in the Norwegian Lundehund. J Comp Pathol. 2008;139:194–201.
19. Scanziani E, Giusti AM, Gualtieri M, Fonda D. Gastric carcinoma in the Belgian shepherd dog. J Small Anim Pract. 1991;32:465–9.
20. Bilek A, Hirt RA. Breed-associated increased occurrence of gastric carcinoma in Chow-Chows. Wien Tierarztl Monatsschr. 2007;94:71–9.
21. Plattner B, Hostetter JM, Uzal FA. Alimentary system and peritoneum. In: Maxie MG, editor. Jubb, Kennedy and Palmer's pathology of domestic animals, vol. 2. St. Louis: Elsevier; 2016. p. 47.
22. Day MJ, Bilzer T, Mansell J, Wilcock B, Hall EJ, Jergens A, et al. International standards for the histopathological diagnosis of gastrointestinal inflammation in the dog and cat: a report from the World Small Animal Veterinary Association Gastrointestinal Standardization Group. J Comp Pathol. 2008;138:1–43.
23. Washabau RJ, Day MJ, Willard MD, Hall EJ, Jergens AE, Mansell J, et al. Endoscopic, biopsy, and histopathologic guidelines for the evaluation of gastrointestinal inflammation in companion animals. J Vet Intern Med. 2010;24:10–26.
24. Evans JA, Chandrasekhara V, Chathadi KV, Decker GA, Early DS, Fisher DA, et al. The role of endoscopy in the management of premalignant and malignant conditions of the stomach. Gastrointest Endosc. 2015;82:1–8.
25. Willard M, Mansell J. Correlating clinical activity and histopathologic assessment of gastrointestinal lesion severity: current challenges. Vet Clin North Am Small Anim Pract. 2011;41:457–63.
26. Tamura W, Fukami N. Early gastric cancer and dysplasia. Gastrointest Endosc Clin N Am. 2013;23:77–94.
27. Willard MD, Moore GE, Denton BD, Day MJ, Mansell J, Bilzer T, et al. Effect of tissue processing on assessment of endoscopic intestinal biopsies in dogs and cats. J Vet Intern Med. 2010;24:84–9.
28. Willard MD, Mansell J, Fosgate GT, Gualtieri M, Olivero D, Lecoindre P, et al. Effect of sample quality on the sensitivity of endoscopic biopsy for detecting gastric and duodenal lesions in dogs and cats. J Vet Intern Med. 2008;22:1084–9.
29. Subramanian V, Mannath J, Ragunath K, Hawkey CJ. Meta-analysis: the diagnostic yield of chromoendoscopy for detecting dysplasia in patients with colonic inflammatory bowel disease. Aliment Pharmacol Ther. 2011;33:304–12.
30. Rugge M, Fassan M, Pizzi M, Farinati F, Sturniolo GC, Plebani M, et al. Operative link for gastritis assessment vs operative link on intestinal metaplasia assessment. World J Gastroenterol. 2011;17:4596.
31. Jergens AE, Willard MD, Allenspach K. Maximizing the diagnostic utility of endoscopic biopsy in dogs and cats with gastrointestinal disease. Vet J. 2016;214:50–60.

21

Hock lesions in dairy cows in freestall herds

Lisa Ekman[1,2*], Ann-Kristin Nyman[3], Håkan Landin[3] and Karin Persson Waller[1,2]

Abstract

Background: Hock lesions (HL) in dairy cows are a common animal welfare problem in modern dairy production with freestall housing systems, but there are no large-scale studies addressing its epidemiology in Sweden. The aims of this cross-sectional study were to investigate the prevalence of HL of different severity in 100 Swedish freestall dairy herds, and to identify cow- and herd-related risk factors. Associations between HL and mastitis as well as culling were also investigated.

Results: In total, 3217 cows from 99 herds were included in the statistical analyses. The overall cow prevalence of hair loss on the hock (mild HL) was 68% and the prevalence of ulceration or evident swelling of the hock, with or without hair loss, (severe HL) was 6%. The within-herd prevalence varied among herds, between 23 and 100% for mild HL, and between 0 and 32% for severe ones. Breed (higher risk for Swedish Holstein than for Swedish Red) and days in milk (higher risk at 181–305 days than at 0–90 days) were cow-related risk factors associated with both types of lesions, whereas higher parity and cleaner cows were associated only with increased risk of severe HL. A reduced risk for mild HL was seen in cows housed on mattresses compared to rubber mats, and in cows housed on peat compared to other bedding materials. Also, cows in herds with a high proportion of not yet inseminated heifers older than 17 months had a lower risk of mild HL than cows in herds with a low proportion. Risk for severe HL was lower when cubicles were of recommended width compared to under recommendation, for organic production compared to conventional, and when teat dip or no treatment after milking was used, compared to teat spray. For both mild and severe HL, herringbone milking parlors were associated with higher risk than tandem parlors. We found no significant associations between HL and mastitis or culling.

Conclusions: The prevalence of HL is high in Swedish dairy herds, although most lesions are mild. Several cow- and herd-related risk factors were identified and the results can be used to improve recommendations for the prevention of HL in Swedish freestall dairy herds.

Keywords: Dairy cow, Epidemiology, Hock damage, Injury, Pressure ulcer, Skin lesion, Sweden

Background

During recent decades, the dairy industry in the Scandinavian countries has undergone marked structural rationalization resulting in increased milk production, larger herds and an increasing proportion of freestall housing systems [1, 2]. Freestalls facilitate natural behavior and several Nordic countries legislate such housing systems to improve animal welfare [3, 4]. However, the introduction of new housing systems is a challenge for dairy producers, as inadequate management or freestall design may lead to welfare problems such as lameness and skin lesions [5–7]. Hock lesions (HL) are a common problem in modern dairy production, and several studies have investigated the epidemiology of HL in freestall dairy herds [3, 8–14]. Similar to pressure ulcers in bedridden human patients, these lesions may develop

*Correspondence: lisa.ekman@sva.se
[1] Department of Animal Health and Antimicrobial Strategies, National Veterinary Institute, 75189 Uppsala, Sweden

due to prolonged pressure on soft tissues between bony prominences and the underlying surface, causing reduced blood flow, lack of oxygen, and tissue necrosis in the affected area [15]. Hock lesions may also result from direct trauma to the hock, caused by abrasive lying surfaces or other physical conflicts between the cow and her surroundings [3, 9]. Presence of HL can be painful for affected animals and is also associated with lameness [9, 16] and high culling rates [6, 17]. Moreover, HL might have a negative impact on udder health [6, 18].

As there is no widely adapted definition of HL the scoring of lesions differs between studies, which makes comparisons of results difficult [11]. The most common, and mildest, form of HL is localized hair loss on the lateral aspect of the hock [8, 19] while more severe lesions with swelling of the hock region or skin ulceration are seen less often. Different symptoms of HL (e.g. hair loss, swelling, and ulceration) may occur separately or in combination with each other, and the underlying cause may differ depending on the type of lesion [8, 16]. Despite the variation in scoring systems, the prevalence of HL in freestalls is high in several studies, ranging from 50 to 87% [3, 8–10]. There is a lack of large-scale Swedish studies on HL epidemiology, especially in freestalls, although one study investigated HL prevalence and risk factors in 55 Swedish dairy herds (that included 18 freestall herds) [20]. The observed prevalence was 30%, with a higher risk for cows housed in freestalls than tie-stalls [21].

The complex relationships between individual cow factors, housing- and management factors, and HL are not fully understood. Moreover, risk factors may differ depending on the type of HL [16]. This indicates that mild and severe HL should be modelled separately.

Previous studies from other countries have found risk factors for HL, including higher parity [3, 17], increased milk yield [16], and Holstein breed [16]. Other factors that affect the occurrence of HL include housing- and management-related factors such as the production system (organic or conventional) [3, 17]; bedding material [17, 22]; and cubicle size [3, 16, 23]. However, results from previous studies are not uniform and even contradictory for some risk factors (e.g., herd size [16, 17], and cow hygiene [16, 22]).

As dairy production conditions differ between regions and countries, e.g. depending on legislation, traditions and climate, risk factors for HL might differ even though similar production systems are used. This warrants investigating risk factors for different types of HL in Swedish dairy production conditions, as there are very few such studies performed. In addition, HL is important to study because it has been associated with high bulk-tank somatic cell count (SCC) [6] and clinical mastitis [18], which might lead to impaired animal welfare as well as production losses for the farmer.

Our aims were to investigate the prevalence of HL of different severity in Swedish freestall dairy herds, and to identify cow- and herd-related risk factors. Identification of HL risk factors is necessary to improve recommendations on how to prevent such lesions. The associations between HL and mastitis and culling were also investigated.

Methods

Herd selection and data collection

Herd selection and data collection were performed as described in Ekman et al. [24]. Briefly, 100 randomly selected Swedish dairy herds with freestall housing, herd size of 50–210 cows, and affiliation with the Swedish Official Milk Recording Scheme (SOMRS) were enrolled in a cross-sectional study. Each herd was visited during one milking in the winter housing season, i.e., February–April 2014 (39 herds) or December–March 2014–2015 (61 herds). All visits and registrations were performed by the first author. Additional cow and herd data were obtained from the SOMRS.

Cow data

A detailed list of cow-related variables (n = 16) and how they were obtained is given in Additional file 1. At the herd visit, a random number of cows (every second to third cow to enter the milking parlor depending on the speed of the milking process) was examined for HL and assigned a hygiene score. For practical reasons, the presence of HL was assessed on the lateral side of the hock visible from the operating area of the milking parlor, thus, one hock per cow was examined. A HL was registered as mild when there was loss of hair (regardless of the size of the hairless area) and as severe when there was evident swelling and/or ulceration in the hock area, with or without hair loss, according to the Hock Assessment Chart for Cattle [25]. Cow hygiene scores were based on the cleanliness of the udder and the hind limb above the hock visible from the operating area. Scores ranged from 1 to 4, where 1 was completely clean; 2 indicated manure stains on hind limb and/or udder; 3 was one to two areas of manure patches of at least 10 cm in diameter; and 4 was more than two areas of manure patches as described for score 3 (modified from Cook [26]).

Information on breed, parity and days in milk (DIM) for individual cows at the time of the visit was obtained from the SOMRS, as was information on individual milk yield [kg energy corrected milk (ECM)/day], cow composite milk somatic cell count (SCC), and milk urea levels from test milkings within 34 days before or after the visit. Registrations of veterinary-treated diseases and results from hoof trimmings (when available within 90 days before or after the visit) were collected from the SOMRS, as well as registrations on culling within 90 days post-visit. The 90 day limit was set to avoid investigating events too distant in time from the registered HL.

Herd data

The list of collected herd-related variables and how they were obtained is given in Additional file 2. Table 1 presents an overview of these herd-related variables, grouped into general herd factors, housing-related factors, management-related factors, and herd health-related factors. Milking routines, housing-related factors, and other management-related factors were registered while at the farms, through observations or interviews with the farm owner or staff. Additional herd data were obtained from the SOMRS, including herd performance indicators, for the 12 months preceding the herd visit. These herd performance indicators, designed by Växa Sverige (a Swedish organization for dairy farmers, Stockholm, Sweden), include calf, young stock and cow mortality; incidence of culling and veterinary-treated diseases; and percentage of cows with abnormal milk urea levels and fertility traits.

Data editing and statistical analyses

Cow and herd data registered in handwritten protocols were transferred to Excel sheets. The data were imported and analyzed with Stata (release 13.1; StataCorp LP, College Station, TX, USA) after verification by an additional person that the transfer of data from the protocols was correct. The prevalence of mild, severe, and all HL was calculated for all examined cows, and within each herd.

Risk factors for mild and severe HL

Associations between the presence of mild or severe HL and the explanatory variables were analysed with univariable mixed-effect logistic regression or mixed-effect linear regression models. The analyses were done at cow-level (both for cow and herd related risk factors), with herd as a random factor using an identity covariance structure (equal variances for random effects; all covariances are zero). Continuous variables were assessed if they were linearly related to the outcome. Where they were not, they were categorized using percentiles as cut-offs, or transformed using the natural logarithm. Cows with severe HL were excluded from the analyses with mild HL as dependent variable and vice versa. In total, 15 cow-related factors and 66 herd-related ones were analyzed for their association with mild and severe HL. All variables with a *P*-value of 0.20 or less were kept for further analyses in multivariable mixed-effect logistic regression models with herd as random factor.

Due to the large number of independent variables, four separate multivariable mixed-effect logistic regression sub-models were constructed for each of the outcomes (mild or severe HL). Sub-model 1 included cow-related factors (Additional file 1) and sub-model 2–4 included herd-related factors divided into three categories: general herd and housing, management, and herd health (Additional file 2). Spearman rank correlations were used to test collinearity between variables in all multivariable models. If two variables showed collinearity ($r \geq 0.7$), the one with the lowest *P*-value was kept in the model. Models were then built using a manual, stepwise backward variable-selection procedure where the initial model included all independent variables as main effects. Variables with a significant association ($P \leq 0.05$) with the dependent variable were kept in the models. Visit period (February–April 2014 or December–March 2014–2015) was included in all multivariable models as a potential confounder. Cows with missing data for a specific independent variable were omitted when that variable was in the model. Two herds left the SOMRS shortly before or after the visit and were therefore excluded in the multivariable analyses due to missing data. If less than 5% of cows belonged to a specific category within a variable, that category was removed from the multivariable analyses. In addition, variables with many missing values

Table 1 Herd-related variables analyzed for associations with hock lesions (HL) in 99 Swedish dairy herds

Group of variables	Number of variables	Examples of variables
General herd factors	4	Herd size (cows/year), production system, milk production, slaughter weights
Housing-related factors	17	Cubicle dimensions, year of cubicle installation, cubicle base, bedding material, stocking ratio (cows/cubicle)
Management -related factors	18	Pasture period, cubicle and alley cleaning, hoof trimming, milking, and feeding routines
Herd health-related factors	27	Presence of ectoparasites and digital dermatitis, calf and cow mortality[a], incidence rate of cullings and veterinary-treated diseases[a], fertility traits[a]

[a] Based on "Welfare signals"—herd performance indicators from the Swedish Official Milk Recording Scheme (Växa Sverige, Stockholm) based on the 12 months preceding the herd visit

(> 30% missing data) were not used in the multivariable analyses.

A final, multivariable mixed-effect model for each outcome (mild or severe HL) was then built using a manual, stepwise backward variable-selection procedure, including the variables that were significant ($P \leq 0.05$) as main effects in the sub-models. Variables associated ($P \leq 0.05$) with the dependent variable were kept in the final models. All variables with $P \leq 0.20$ for mild or severe HL in the univariable analyses were then re-tested one at a time in their respective final model, and kept in the model if they were significantly associated with the dependent variable. All plausible two-way interactions between the significant main effects were tested in the final models. Model fit was assessed by visual examination of residual plots [27, 28].

Associations between HL and mastitis and culling

We also investigated possible associations between HL and mastitis incidence and culling with univariable mixed-effect logistic regression or mixed-effect linear regression analyses. Mild or severe HL was used as independent variable and the three dependent variables were: (1) milk SCC from test milking within 34 days before or after the visit; (2) veterinary-treated clinical mastitis (VTCM) within 90 days before or after the visit; and (3) culling of the cow within 90 days post-visit. Herd was included as random factor in all models. Parity, breed, DIM, milk yield, and visit period were added to the model if there was an association ($P \leq 0.05$) between the dependent and the independent variable. This was to investigate them as confounding effects in the multivariable mixed-effect logistic model. Collinearity between variables was tested for all multivariable models, by calculations of Spearman rank correlations. Model fit for all models was assessed by visual examination of residual plots [27, 28].

Results

Herd and cow characteristics

In total, 3755 cows were examined (mean 38 cows/herd (SD 12.2); range 17–68 cows/herd), including 1901 Swedish Holstein (SH), 1300 Swedish Red (SR), 289 crossbreeds (SH × SR) and 265 cows of other breeds (mainly Jersey cows). There were few cows of other breeds in the herds, except for one herd with only Jersey cows; for this reason, cows of other breeds (n = 265) were excluded from the statistical analyses, including the Jersey herd. In addition, 273 cows were excluded because their hocks were too dirty for assessment of HL status. Thus, 3217 cows from 99 herds were included in the prevalence calculations and available for the statistical analyses. The mean annual herd size was 106 cows (SD 41.6; range 49–223 cows) and the mean annual milk production 9914 kg ECM/cow-year (SD 1236 kg; range–13,225 kg). Mean annual herd SCC was 247,000 cells/ml (SD 78,000; range 103,000–523,000 cells/ml).

Prevalence of mild and severe HL

The overall cow prevalence of HL was 74% (2388 of 3217 cows; CI 73–76%), divided in 68% (2182 of 3217 cows; CI 66–69%) for mild HL and 6% (206 of 3217 cows; CI 6–7%) for severe HL. The within-herd prevalence of HL (Fig. 1) varied among the herds between 23 and 100% (mean 73%, SD 16%). For mild HL, the within-herd prevalence varied between 23 and 100% (mean 67%, SD 15%), and for severe HL, it varied between 0 and 32% (mean 6%, SD 6%). The herd prevalence for mild lesions was 100% (99/99 herds) and for severe lesions 76% (75/99 herds).

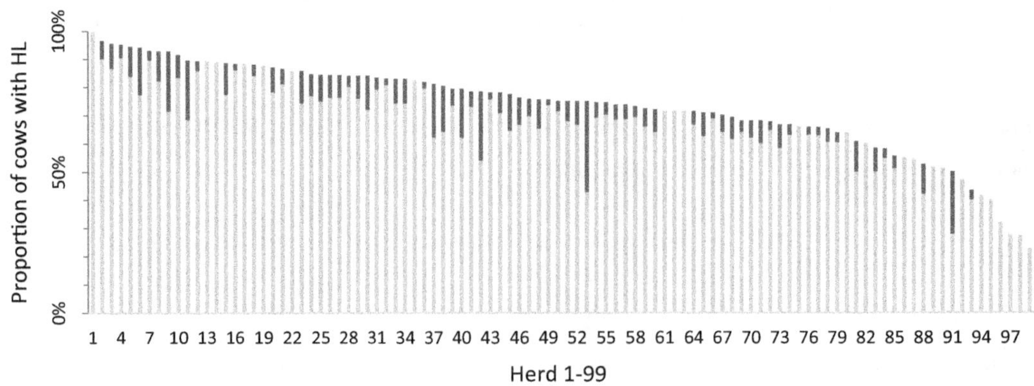

Fig. 1 Prevalence (%) of mild (light grey) and severe (dark grey) hock lesions (HL) in 99 Swedish dairy herds sorted from highest to lowest HL prevalence (n = 3217 cows)

Risk factors associated with mild HL

In total, 3009 cows from 99 herds were included in the univariable analyses, excluding cows with severe lesions. Of the 81 tested variables, 35 had $P \leq 0.20$ in the univariable analysis. Thirty-two of these 35 variables were investigated in the 4 multivariable sub-models (6 in the cow-related, 11 in the general herd- and housing-related, 7 in the management-related and 8 in the herd health-related; Additional files 1 and 2). Three variables were excluded because of too many missing values (stocking ratio and farmer-reported presence of digital dermatitis in the herd), or too few cows in a specific category (reproduction disease within 90 days of visit). Independent variables associated with mild HL in the different sub-models ($P \leq 0.05$, Table 2) were then offered to the final model for mild HL. There were initially 8 variables in this final model of which 6 remained significant. After re-testing variables with $P \leq 0.20$ in the univariable analyses, bedding material was significant and included in the model. However, the association with production system (organic or conventional) was no longer significant ($P = 0.076$) and therefore removed. The total number of cows in the final model was 2447 from 79 herds.

The final multivariable mixed-effect logistic regression model is presented in Table 3. Breed and DIM were significant cow-related risk factors. The risk for

Table 2 Cow- and herd-related variables associated with mild hock lesions (HL) in four multivariable mixed-effect logistic regression sub-models

Sub-model/variable	β	SE	OR	CI	*P*-value
Sub-model 1: cow-related factors (n = 2685)					
Breed					
Swedish Holstein (SH)	Ref				
Swedish Red (SR)	−0.34	0.12	0.71	0.56–0.90	0.005
SH × SR	−0.28	0.19	0.75	0.52–1.09	0.136
DIM (days)					
0–90	Ref				
91–180	0.27	0.12	1.31	1.04–1.65	0.022
180–305	0.62	0.12	1.87	1.46–2.38	< 0.001
> 305	0.24	0.16	1.28	0.93–1.74	0.127
Sub-model 2: general herd and housing-related factors (n = 2545 cows)					
Cubicle base					
Rubber mats	Ref				
Mattress	−0.43	0.15	0.65	0.48–0.87	0.004
Production system					
Conventional	Ref				
Organic	−0.47	0.19	0.62	0.43–0.91	0.014
Sub-model 3: management-related factors (n = 2685 cows)					
Cow diet include maize silage					
No	Ref				
Yes	0.40	0.20	1.50	1.01–2.21	0.042
Type of feeding system					
Automatic feeding stations for individual concentrate rations	Ref				
Total mixed rations (TMR)	−0.54	0.23	0.58	0.37–0.90	0.016
Combination of TMR and individual concentration rations	−0.11	0.17	0.90	0.64–1.26	0.535
Type of milking parlor					
Herringbone	Ref				
Tandem	−0.47	0.15	0.62	0.46–0.84	0.002
Sub-model 4: herd health-related factors (n = 2587 cows)					
Heifers > 17 months not inseminated (%)[a]					
0–16	Ref				
≥ 17	−0.45	0.14	0.64	0.48–0.85	0.002

β regression coefficients, *OR* odds ratio, *CI* 95% confidence interval, *Ref* reference level

[a] Based on data from the Swedish Official Milk Recording Scheme for the 12 months preceding the herd visit

mild HL was lower in SR than in SH cows (OR 0.74; CI 0.59–0.94), whereas SH × SR cows had no difference in risk compared to either SH or SR cows. The risk for mild HL increased with higher DIM up to 305 DIM compared to 0–90 DIM (OR 1.35 and 2.06 for 91–180 days and 181–305 days respectively). This risk was higher for cows within 181–305 DIM than for cows in all other categories. Cows with more than 305 DIM did not differ significantly from cows within 0–90 or 91–180 DIM. Cows housed with mattresses as cubicle base had lower risk for mild HL than cows housed on rubber mats (OR 0.66). There was also a higher risk for cows housed on other bedding material categories compared to peat [sawdust (OR 2.39; CI 1.38–4.12), straw (OR 1.88; CI 1.04–3.4), or combinations of different bedding materials (OR 2.6; CI 1.25–5.39)]. The other categories of bedding material did not differ between each other. In addition, cows in herds with tandem milking parlors had a lower risk of mild HL than those in herringbone milking parlors (OR 0.75). Cows in herds with a high proportion of not yet inseminated heifers older than 17 months had a lower risk of mild HL than the herds with a low proportion (OR 0.61). There were no significant two-way interactions in this model.

Table 3 Cow- and herd-related factors associated with mild hock lesions (HL) in the final multivariable mixed-effect logistic regression model including 2447 cows in 79 Swedish dairy herds

Variables and categories	β	SE	OR	CI	P-value
Intercept	−0.18	0.33			0.579
Breed					
Swedish Holstein (SH)	Ref				
Swedish Red (SR)	−0.29	0.12	0.74	0.59–0.94	0.012
SH × SR	−0.24	0.20	0.78	0.53–1.15	0.215
Days in milk (DIM)					
0–90	Ref				
91–180	0.30	0.12	1.35	1.05–1.72	0.017
181–305	0.72	0.13	2.06	1.59–2.66	<0.001
>305	0.30	0.17	1.35	0.97–1.88	0.074
Bedding material					
Peat	Ref				
Sawdust	0.87	0.28	2.39	1.38–4.12	0.002
Straw	0.63	0.30	1.88	1.04–3.40	0.035
Combination	0.95	0.37	2.60	1.25–5.39	0.011
Cubicle base					
Rubber mat	Ref				
Mattress	−0.42	0.13	0.66	0.51–0.84	0.001
Heifers > 17 months not inseminated (%)[a]					
0–16	Ref				
≥17	−0.49	0.13	0.61	0.48–0.79	<0.001
Type of milking parlor					
Herringbone	Ref				
Tandem	−0.28	0.13	0.75	0.59–0.97	0.027

β regression coefficients, *OR* odds ratio, *CI* 95% confidence interval, *Ref* reference level

[a] Based on data from herd performance indicators from the Swedish Official Milk Recording Scheme

Risk factors associated with severe HL

The evaluation of risk factors for severe HL included 1035 cows from 98 herds in the univariable analyses. Cows with mild lesions were excluded, including one herd with a prevalence of 100% mild HL. Of 81 analyzed variables, 22 had a $P \leq 0.20$ and were kept for further analyses in one of the four multivariable sub-models (6 in the sub-model for cow-related, 6 in the herd and housing-related, 3 in the management-related, and 5 in the herd health-related factors sub-model; Additional files 1 and 2). Two risk factors were excluded (stocking ratio and farmer-reported presence of digital dermatitis in the herd) because of too many missing values. All variables significantly associated ($P \leq 0.05$) with severe HL in the sub-models are presented in Table 4. These were then entered as main effects into the final model that initially contained 10 independent variables of which 6 remained significant. Variables with $P \leq 0.20$ in the univariable analyses were re-tested and kept in the final model if they had $P \leq 0.05$. Breed, cow hygiene, and use of teat disinfectant or other spray/dip applied after milking were variables that became significant at re-testing. Registered hoof disorder within 90 days was not significant ($P = 0.057$) and therefore removed from the final model. The random effect of cows within herd was not significant ($P = 0.12$), hence, a multivariable logistic regression model was used for the analysis instead of the mixed-effect model, this had a small effect (< 5% change) on the coefficients of the included variables.

The final model for factors associated with severe HL included 919 cows from 88 herds (Table 5). Cow-related risk factors for severe lesions included breed and DIM. There was a lower risk for SR than SH cows (OR 0.6; CI 0.41–0.87). The risk increased with higher DIM (OR 1.59; CI 1.01–2.51) and OR 2.47 (CI 1.57–3.91) for 91–180 days and 181–305 days respectively when compared to 0–90 days), except for cows with >305 DIM; for these cows there was no difference in risk compared to cows with 0–90 DIM. In addition, cows with hygiene score 4 (i.e., dirtier cows) had a lower risk of severe HL than cows with hygiene score 1–2 (OR 0.42; CI 0.23–0.79), and third or higher parity were associated with a higher risk of severe HL compared to first parity (OR 2.16; CI 1.45–3.23). Risk for severe HL was lower in cows milked in tandem milking parlors than in cows milked in herringbone ones (OR 0.47; CI 0.31–0.69). Furthermore,

Table 4 Cow- and herd-related variables associated with severe hock lesions (HL) in four multivariable mixed-effect logistic regression sub-models

Sub-model/variable	β	SE	OR	CI	*P*-value
Sub-model 1: cow-level factors (n = 936)					
Breed					
Swedish Holstein (SH)	Ref				
Swedish Red (SR)	− 0.76	0.24	0.47	0.29–0.75	0.002
SH × SR	− 0.49	0.34	0.61	0.31–1.19	0.149
DIM (days)					
0–90	Ref				
91–180	0.53	0.25	1.31	1.05–2.76	0.031
180–305	0.88	0.24	1.87	1.49–3.88	< 0.001
> 305	0.11	0.34	1.11	0.58–2.15	0.745
Parity					
First parity	Ref				
Second parity	− 0.24	0.25	0.79	0.49–1.28	0.34
Third or higher parity	0.68	0.22	1.96	1.29–3.0	0.002
Registered hoof disorder of any type (registered at hoof trimmings within 90 days from herd visit)					
No	Ref				
Yes	0.75	0.29	2.11	1.19–3.74	0.011
Hoof trimming records not available	0.24	0.29	1.28	0.72–2.27	0.408
Sub-model 2: general herd and housing-related factors (n = 880 cows)					
Average milk production (kg ECM/cow and year)[a]					
< 9800	Ref				
≥ 9800	0.51	0.24	1.66	1.04–2.65	0.032
Cubicle width					
Below recommendation	Ref				
As recommended	− 0.80	0.24	0.45	0.28–0.73	0.001
Production system					
Conventional	Ref				
Organic	− 1.07	0.33	0.34	0.18–0.66	0.001
Sub-model 3: management-related factors (n = 936 cows)					
Type of milking parlor					
Herringbone	Ref				
Tandem	− 0.84	0.27	0.43	0.25–0.74	0.002
Sub-model 4: herd health-related factors (n = 897 cows)					
Heifers > 17 months not inseminated (%)[a]					
0–16	Ref				
≥ 17	− 0.59	0.25	0.55	0.34–0.91	0.02
Presence of ectoparasites in cows during the last year according to farm owner/staff					
No	Ref				
Yes	0.73	0.25	2.01	1.26–3.43	0.004

β regression coefficients, *OR* odds ratio, *CI* 95% confidence interval, *Ref* reference level

[a] Based on data from the Swedish Official Milk Recording Scheme for the 12 months preceding the herd visit

cows in herds with recommended cubicle widths had lower risk (OR 0.36; CI 0.24–0.52) than cows in smaller cubicles. The risk was also lower for cows in herds that used teat dip (OR 0.47; CI 0.26–0.85) or no treatment (OR 0.32; CI 0.12–0.87) after milking than those that used teat spray. Finally, the variable with the largest effect size was that cows in organic herds had a lower risk (OR 0.21; CI 0.13–0.36) than those in conventional herds. There were no significant two-way interactions in this model. The model explained about 15% of the variation in the data ($R^2 = 0.145$).

Associations between hock lesions and mastitis and culling

The analyses of associations between mild HL and VTCM within 90 days before or after herd visit, or culling within 90 days post-visit, included 2911 cows from 97 herds. The analyses of associations between mild HL and milk SCC included 2884 cows from 97 herds. In the univariable mixed-effect linear regression analysis, mild HL showed no significant association with any of the outcomes ($P > 0.05$).

For severe HL, 996 cows from 96 herds were included in the analyses of association with VTCM within 90 days before or after herd visit, and culling within 90 days post-visit. The analysis of associations between severe HL and milk SCC included 988 cows from 96 herds. An association between severe HL and culling was seen in the univariable analysis ($P = 0.009$), but the association was no longer significant ($P = 0.11$) when parity, milk yield and DIM were included. There were no significant associations between severe HL and VTCM or milk SCC.

Discussion

This study is the first large-scale investigation on the prevalence of, and risk factors for HL in Swedish freestall dairy herds, and it contributes to better understanding of HL epidemiology in Sweden.

Hock lesions are a common problem in Swedish freestalls, affecting 74% of the cows in our study. Moreover, the true prevalence could be even higher as only the outside of one hock per cow was examined. However, a previous large-scale study on HL found that most HL were bilateral, and that medial lesions rarely occurred if the cow had no lateral lesion on the same leg [8]. Similarly, the risk for HL did not differ depending on which hock (right or left) that was examined in the present study (data not shown). Logically, if a cow spends an equal amount of time lying down on her left and right side, bilateral lesions are likely, as the external and internal conditions for both hocks are similar, at least for a

Table 5 Cow- and herd-related factors associated with severe hock lesions (HL) in the final multivariable logistic regression model including 919 cows from 88 Swedish dairy herds

Variables and categories	β	SE	OR	CI	P-value
Intercept	−0.96	0.37			0.011
Breed					
Swedish Holstein (SH)	Ref				
Swedish Red (SR)	−0.52	0.19	0.60	0.41–0.87	0.008
SH × SR	−0.16	0.31	0.78	0.46–1.55	0.596
Days in milk					
0–90	Ref				
91–180	0.46	0.23	1.59	1.01–2.51	0.047
181–305	0.91	0.23	2.47	1.57–3.91	<0.001
>305	0.11	0.31	1.12	0.60–2.07	0.723
Hygiene score[a]					
1–2	Ref				
3	−0.17	0.21	0.84	0.56–1.26	0.404
4	−0.86	0.32	0.42	0.23–0.79	0.007
Parity					
First parity	Ref				
Second parity	−0.11	0.23	0.90	0.57–1.42	0.638
Third or higher parity	0.77	0.21	2.16	1.45–3.23	<0.001
Cubicle width					
Below recommendation	Ref				
As recommended	−1.03	0.19	0.36	0.24–0.52	<0.001
Production system					
Conventional	Ref				
Organic	−1.54	0.27	0.21	0.13–0.36	<0.001
Teat disinfectant or other spray/dip applied after milking					
Spray	Ref				
Dip	−0.75	0.30	0.47	0.26–0.85	0.012
None	−1.15	0.52	0.32	0.12–0.87	0.026
Type of milking parlor					
Herringbone	Ref				
Tandem	−0.76	0.20	0.47	0.31–0.69	<0.001

β regression coefficients, *OR* odds ratio, *CI* 95% confidence interval, *Ref* reference level

[a] Hygiene score 1–4: (1) completely clean, (2) manure stains on hind limb and/or udder (1 and 2 merged due to few observations in category 1), (3) one to two areas of manure patches of at least 10 cm in diameter, and (4) more than 2 areas of manure patches as described for score 3

non-lame cow. Our reported prevalence of HL is considerably higher than that in a previous Swedish study [20]. However, that study used a different definition of HL, and the majority of included herds had tie-stalls. Our observed prevalence (68%) of mild HL (hair loss) is in line with results from studies in freestalls in other countries (ranging from 50% [3, 6] to 82% [8, 12]). We found an overall prevalence of 6% for severe HL (ulceration and/or evident swelling). Similar results have been reported from Norway [3] and northeastern USA [12], whereas other studies have reported higher prevalence of severe manifestations of HL (up to 36%) [8, 9]. Differences between scoring systems and observer subjectivity make comparisons between studies difficult. The problems associated with the lack of a common scoring system have been highlighted in several studies [8, 29, 30]. The hock assessment chart for cattle [25] in our study is easy to use in field studies and allows fast and accurate scoring of HL. However, registration of hair loss, swellings and ulcerations as separate, rather than combined, events would probably yield more information on the etiology of such lesions. In line with this, Potterton et al. [16] found that risk factors differ depending on the HL manifestation. As there are pros and cons with the current scoring systems, care must be taken in selection of the method, interpretation of the results and comparison with other studies. It is also important that the methods used are reported accurately to enable comparisons and reproducibility of studies.

Even though many herds had a high HL prevalence, the between-herd variation was large, especially for severe HL (0–32%). This variation, also seen by others [3, 8, 14], indicates that herd and management factors affect the HL occurrence. Our study identified several risk factors, especially cow-related ones, that were common to both mild and severe HL; however other risk factors were specific to the type of HL. The discussion below on risk factors for HL is based on the design of the sub-models and divided into cow-, general herd and housing-, management and herd health-related risk factors.

Cow-related risk factors

Breed and DIM were associated with both mild and severe HL in a similar way. The SH cows had a greater risk for HL than the SR cows. A higher risk for Holstein has also been seen in other studies compared to Jerseys and local breeds (e.g., Danish Red) [16, 31]. Generally, SH cows are larger and have a lower body condition score (BCS) than SR cows [32, 33]. Large cows (measured by hip width) [34] and low BCS [3] have an increased risk for HL, which could partly explain the difference in risk between SH and other breeds.

An increased risk for HL with increasing DIM is in line with other studies on all HL [3], severe HL [10], and swelling at the hock [16]. It is likely that a lesion that develops in early lactation persists throughout the lactation period. An interesting, previously unreported, observation was that cows with more than 305 DIM (i.e. a longer than average lactation period) had a lower risk of HL than cows within 91–180 and 181–305 DIM. This might be because there were fewer cows in this category, but it might also indicate that HL improve with time, perhaps due to repaired body condition. The association between HL and DIM needs further investigation.

Higher parity and lower hygiene scores (i.e., cleaner cows) were significant risk factors for severe HL, but not for mild HL. Other studies have shown the same association between parity and mild [16] or all HL [3, 17]. In our study, however, mild HL was very common in all parities. Higher parity is associated with a higher risk for other conditions, including most types of hoof lesions [35], lameness [36] and mastitis [37], which may indicate a reduced ability of older cows to cope with injuries and diseases. As indications of a causal relationship between lameness and HL was found by Lim et al. [30], the increased risk for lameness in older cows might also increase the risk of severe HL. In addition, older cows may be less physically agile, and therefore contract more injuries when rising and lying [17]. The lower risk for severe HL in the cows that were most dirty on the hind leg above the hock and on the side of the udder is in line with Potterton et al. [16]. It could be speculated that a layer of dirt may protect the skin integrity, or that certain management or housing factors, such as amount of bedding material in cubicles, affect both cow hygiene and severe HL. It may also be harder to detect HL on a dirty hock, but this should not be a major bias in our study because we excluded the cows that were too dirty for assessment of hock status.

Several studies have found associations between HL and lameness [3, 16, 17, 31]. In our study, we saw a significant association between registration of at least one hoof disorder within 90 days before or after HL registration and increased risk of severe HL. This association was seen in the univariable analysis and in the cow-related multivariable sub-model, but not in the final model. Hoof trimming records were, however, only available for 46 of the herds, which could have affected the results of the final model.

General herd and housing-related risk factors

We found no common housing-related risk factors for mild and severe HL, which is in line with Potterton et al. [16]. Cubicle base and bedding material were associated with mild HL. Mattress and peat were associated with a lower risk than rubber mats and other types of bedding material, respectively. Mattresses are usually thicker and softer than rubber mats which leads to less pressure on the hock when the cow is lying down, and thus, less risk of impaired circulation and subsequent tissue damage. This finding is supported by previous studies investigating different cubicle bases and their softness [3, 9, 23]. However, compared to deep straw or sand bedding, mattresses and rubber mats have been associated with a higher risk of HL [6, 13, 38]. The effect of bedding material on HL has also been investigated in several studies, and sand is usually associated with a lower risk for HL than traditional bedding materials such as sawdust and straw [16, 22]. However, the combination of cubicle base, and type and depth of bedding material, probably has a large effect on the risk for HL, as these all affect the conditions of the lying surface [13, 22]. In our study, there were too few (5) herds with deep straw or sand bedding to evaluate their effects on HL prevalence. Changing bedding from straw to peat reduced the severity of HL in a Swedish study [39], but we found no studies from other countries where peat was compared with other bedding materials in relation to HL.

Cows in herds with organic production had a notably lower risk for severe HL than cows in conventional herds. The trend was similar for mild HL, but not statistically significant in the final model. This finding is in line with other studies [3, 17]. Swedish regulations for dairy cow housing and management are similar in conventional and organic production, but the regulations for e.g., feed concentrate intake and access to pasture, are stricter in organic herds [40]. Cows in organic herds generally spend more time on pasture as they are required to have access to pasture for a longer time each day (12 h compared to 6 h) during the legislated pasture period (2–4 months/year depending on geographical location), and to have more of their nutritional needs fulfilled via pasture than cows in conventional herds [40, 41]. The organic herds also have part-time outdoor access for two additional months/year [40]. More time on pasture (both total length and hours/day) has been associated with reduced prevalence of HL and lameness [17, 31, 42]. In the present study, we investigated the length (days on pasture) and extent (if cows were outside for at least 12 h/day or not) of the most recent pasture period, but found no significant associations with HL. However, cows in organic herds may have other benefits from the pasture period that reduces their risk for severe HL compared to conventional herds. There may also be other, unidentified, management factors that differ between organic and conventional herds that affect the occurrence of severe HL.

The only housing-related factor associated with severe HL was cubicle width. Wider cubicles (i.e., of recommended dimensions compared to those under the recommendations) reduced the risk for severe HL, which is likely due to more space for the cow to lie down or stand up. To our knowledge, this association has not been reported previously, but several other cubicle dimensions have been associated with increased risk for HL. These include cubicle length [3, 9, 16], total standing area per cow [17], neck rail distance from curb [10, 16], height of neck rail [16] and height of lowest horizontal rail of cubicle partition [9, 16]. We had expected more cubicle dimensions to be associated with HL also in the present study, but individual housing risk factors can be difficult to identify due to complex interactions between cubicle design and type of bedding, cow factors, and management routines. In addition, most herds were in the "under recommendation"-category for some measurements (e.g. neck rail height and distance from rear curb), which makes possible effects of having correctly dimensioned cubicles hard to evaluate.

Management-related risk factors

Cows milked in tandem parlors had a lower risk of both mild and severe HL than cows milked in herringbone ones. To our knowledge this association has not been previously investigated. We speculate that the risk for traumatic skin injuries (due to crowding and physical conflicts with housing elements) may be greater in the herringbone milking parlors. In these parlors, several cows (generally 6–12 under Swedish conditions) move in and out at the same time, whereas they move one at a time in the tandem parlors. However, unidentified herd or management factors may also differ between herds in the two types of milking parlors. The reasons for the finding that use of teat spray after milking was associated with a higher risk of severe HL than use of teat dip or no dip/spray are not known. The association may reflect other management or herd factors not analyzed in this study or it could be a spurious finding due to the large number of independent variables that were analyzed.

Herd health-related risk factors

The only significant association between HL and herd health-related factors in the final models was an increased risk for mild HL in herds with a low proportion of not yet inseminated heifers >17 months. The same association was seen for severe HL in the herd health-related submodel, but not in the final analysis. Similar results were obtained by Rutherford et al. [17], who discussed that their results could have been related to organic farming rather than not yet insemination per se, as organic herds mated heifers later than conventional herds. Among our included herds, 43% of the conventional herds compared to 70% of the organic herds had a high proportion of not yet inseminated heifers (data not shown), indicating that this might be true also in our study and that these associations require further investigations.

Associations between HL and udder health and culling

We found no significant associations between mild or severe HL and udder health. Overall, there were few cows with registered VTCM in the SOMRS within 90 days before or after the herd visit. However, diseases are underreported to the SOMRS database [43], which could have affected our results. Hock lesions have been associated with increased risk of clinical mastitis [18] and high herd-level SCC in freestalls [6], but our results showed no such associations. Results from a previous Swedish study indicate a role of HL in transmission of the common udder pathogen *Staphylococcus aureus* in dairy herds [44]. Thus, associations between HL and udder health should be further investigated in longitudinal studies.

The univariable analysis showed that cows with severe HL had an increased risk for culling within 90 days post-visit, but when the combined effects of parity, milk yield and DIM were included in the model, this association was not significant. However, culling decisions are often based on a combination of factors, and severe HL could contribute to such a decision for affected cows.

Additional comments

The present cross-sectional study was designed to investigate several potential cow- and herd-related risk factors in a large number of Swedish dairy herds. However, a cross-sectional study only yields a snapshot of the conditions in the herds. Moreover, the large number of investigated independent variables increases the risk of type I errors (i.e. identification of risk factors that are not true risk factors). As we use a mixed effect model, that takes into account the random effect of herd, the point estimates and their intervals move toward each other. This makes the comparisons more conservative and reduces the risk for such errors. Still, some of the findings are probably due to chance and this kind of study need to be repeated to confirm true risk factors. Moreover, when the number of observations is large, small differences in the estimates might become significant although the biological effect is not of importance on population level. There is also a risk for selection bias in this type of study, as herds with HL problems might be more inclined to participate. However, the herd characteristics and inclusion process did not indicate that this was the case for our study, as most contacted herds were willing to participate, and the study also investigated udder cleft dermatitis lesions.

As previously stated, the complexity of dairy production makes it difficult to identify individual variables affecting the prevalence of HL. In line with this, most significant variables found in our study had relatively low effect size. Moreover, the final model for severe HL only explained 15% of the variation in the dataset. Thus, there might be other factors of importance that we did not register in the present study. In our study we combined cow- and herd-related factors in the statistical analyses, which could make it difficult to find significant herd-related factors as the cow-related factors seem to be more closely associated with HL. Moreover, farmers' attitudes and awareness of HL may influence management routines and HL occurrence. Benchmarking of cow comfort in dairy herds in Canada and the USA reduced HL prevalence in 14 dairy herds, because the farmers became more aware of the lesions and addressed the issue, mainly by improving cubicle bedding [45]. Mild HL is such a common finding in dairy herds that farmers might not notice them or consider them a problem [8]. However, mild HL have been associated with lameness [16] and may also contain udder pathogens [44], and should not be overlooked as a welfare problem in dairy herds.

Conclusions

HL is a common finding in Swedish freestall dairy herds. Hair loss (i.e., mild HL) was observed on cows in all herds, with more than 50% of cows affected in 88 of the 99 herds. The overall prevalence of severe lesions was 6%, but markedly higher within-herd prevalence was seen in some herds (up to 32%). Several cow- and herd-related risk factors were identified. Some were common to both mild and severe lesions, such as breed, DIM and type of milking parlor. Other risk factors were associated only with mild lesions, (e.g., cubicle base and bedding material), or severe lesions, (e.g., production system and cubicle width). Our results, combined with those of previous studies on HL, indicate that there are ways to reduce HL prevalence in Swedish dairy herds. Preventive measures may include providing a soft lying area for the cows, such as mattresses or deep bedding. Using peat as bedding material and providing cubicles with appropriate width could also reduce the risk of HL. Longitudinal studies of HL are warranted to further increase the understanding of the etiology and pathogenesis of these lesions.

Additional files

Additional file 1. Results of univariable analyses of cow-related risk factors analyzed in mixed-effect logistic regression models for their association with mild and severe hock lesions (HL), based on observations of 3217 cows in 99 Swedish dairy herds, including how the information was obtained and the number of cows in each category.

Additional file 2. Results of univariable analyses of 3 sub-groups of herd-related risk factors (general herd and housing-related, management-related and health-related factors) analyzed in mixed-effect logistic regression models for their association with mild and severe hock lesions (HL) based on observations of 3479 cows in 99 Swedish dairy herds. The table also contains information on how the information was obtained and the number of cows in each category.

Authors' contributions

LE performed all herd visits. LE and AN performed the statistical analyses. LE wrote the main part of the manuscript with major contribution from KPW. All authors were part of planning the study and commented on the manuscript. All authors read and approved the final manuscript.

Author details

[1] Department of Animal Health and Antimicrobial Strategies, National Veterinary Institute, 75189 Uppsala, Sweden. [2] Department of Clinical Sciences, Swedish University of Agricultural Sciences, 75007 Uppsala, Sweden. [3] Växa Sverige, 10425 Stockholm, Sweden.

Acknowledgements

We are grateful to the herd owners for their helpful participation. We would also like to thank Ulf Magnusson, Swedish University of Agricultural Sciences, Uppsala, Sweden, for helpful input on the study design and manuscript and Maria "Maja" Persson, National Veterinary Institute, Uppsala, Sweden, for excellent technical assistance.

Competing interests

The authors declare that they have no competing interests.

Funding

This study was financially supported by The Swedish Research Council Formas (Grant No: 221-2013-269) and The Swedish Farmers Foundation for Agricultural Research (Grant No: V1430006).

References

1. Bergsten C, Carlsson J, Jansson Mork M. Influence of grazing management on claw disorders in Swedish freestall dairies with mandatory grazing. J Dairy Sci. 2015;98:6151–62.
2. Oltenacu PA, Broom DM. The impact of genetic selection for increased milk yield on the welfare of dairy cows. Anim Welfare. 2010;19:39–49.
3. Kielland C, Ruud LE, Zanella AJ, Osteras O. Prevalence and risk factors for skin lesions on legs of dairy cattle housed in freestalls in Norway. J Dairy Sci. 2009;92:5487–96.
4. Swedish Board of Agriculture: Statens jordbruksverks föreskrifter och allmänna råd om djurhållning inom lantbruket m.m. SJVFS. 2010:15. https://www.jordbruksverket.se/download/18.6b0af7e81284865248a800024 67/2010-015.pdf. Accessed 7 Aug 2018.
5. Sogstad AM, Fjeldaas T, Osteras O. Lameness and claw lesions of the Norwegian red dairy cattle housed in free stalls in relation to environment, parity and stage of lactation. Acta Vet Scand. 2005;46:203–17.
6. Fulwider WK, Grandin T, Garrick DJ, Engle TE, Lamm WD, Dalsted NL, et al. Influence of free-stall base on tarsal joint lesions and hygiene in dairy cows. J Dairy Sci. 2007;90:3559–66.
7. de Vries M, Bokkers EA, van Reenen CG, Engel B, van Schaik G, Dijkstra T, et al. Housing and management factors associated with indicators of dairy cattle welfare. Prev Vet Med. 2015;118:80–92.
8. Potterton SL, Green MJ, Millar KM, Brignell CJ, Harris J, Whay HR, et al. Prevalence and characterisation of, and producers' attitudes towards, hock lesions in UK dairy cattle. Vet Rec. 2011;169:634.
9. Brenninkmeyer C, Dippel S, Brinkmann J, March S, Winckler C, Knierim U. Hock lesion epidemiology in cubicle housed dairy cows across two breeds, farming systems and countries. Prev Vet Med. 2013;109:236–45.
10. Heyerhoff JCZ, LeBlanc SJ, DeVries TJ, Nash CGR, Gibbons J, Orsel K, et al. Prevalence of and factors associated with hock, knee, and neck injuries on dairy cows in freestall housing in Canada. J Dairy Sci. 2014;97:173–84.
11. Kester E, Holzhauer M, Frankena K. A descriptive review of the prevalence and risk factors of hock lesions in dairy cows. Vet J. 2014;202:222–8.

12. Barrientos AK, Chapinal N, Weary DM, Galo E, von Keyserlingk MA. Herd-level risk factors for hock injuries in freestall-housed dairy cows in the northeastern United States and California. J Dairy Sci. 2013;96:3758–65.
13. Lombard JE, Tucker CB, von Keyserlingk MAG, Kopral CA, Weary DM. Associations between cow hygiene, hock injuries, and free stall usage on US dairy farms. J Dairy Sci. 2010;93:4668–76.
14. von Keyserlingk MAG, Barrientos A, Ito K, Galo E, Weary DM. Benchmarking cow comfort on North American freestall dairies: lameness, leg injuries, lying time, facility design, and management for high-producing Holstein dairy cows. J Dairy Sci. 2012;95:7399–408.
15. Defloor T. The risk of pressure sores: a conceptual scheme. J Clin Nurs. 1999;8:206–16.
16. Potterton SL, Green MJ, Harris J, Millar KM, Whay HR, Huxley JN. Risk factors associated with hair loss, ulceration, and swelling at the hock in freestall-housed UK dairy herds. J Dairy Sci. 2011;94:2952–63.
17. Rutherford KM, Langford FM, Jack MC, Sherwood L, Lawrence AB, Haskell MJ. Hock injury prevalence and associated risk factors on organic and nonorganic dairy farms in the United Kingdom. J Dairy Sci. 2008;91:2265–74.
18. Sogstad AM, Osteras O, Fjeldaas T. Bovine claw and limb disorders related to reproductive performance and production diseases. J Dairy Sci. 2006;89:2519–28.
19. Laven R, Livesey C. Getting to grips with hock lesions in cattle. Vet Rec. 2011;169:632–3.
20. Rytterlund E. Hasskador hos mjölkkor-riskfaktorer och juverhälsa [master thesis on the internet]. Uppsala: Swedish University of Agricultural Sciences; 2009. https://stud.epsilon.slu.se/745/. Accessed 5 May 2018.
21. Sandgren CH, Lindberg A, Keeling LJ. Using a national dairy database to identify herds with poor welfare. Anim Welfare. 2009;18:523–32.
22. Norring M, Manninen E, de Passille AM, Rushen J, Munksgaard L, Saloniemi H. Effects of sand and straw bedding on the lying behavior, cleanliness, and hoof and hock injuries of dairy cows. J Dairy Sci. 2008;91:570–6.
23. Livesey CT, Marsh C, Metcalf JA, Laven RA. Hock injuries in cattle kept in straw yards or cubicles with rubber mats or mattresses. Vet Rec. 2002;150:677–9.
24. Ekman L, Nyman AK, Landin H, Magnusson U, Waller KP. Mild and severe udder cleft dermatitis-Prevalence and risk factors in Swedish dairy herds. J Dairy Sci. 2018;101:556–71.
25. Cornell University: Hock Assessment Chart for Cattle. https://ahdc.vet.cornell.edu/programs/NYSCHAP/docs/HockScoringChart-NYSCHAP-4-04.pdf. Accessed 7 Aug 2018.
26. Cook NB, Reinemann DJ. A tool box for assessing cow, udder and teat hygiene. University of Wisconsin-Madison. 2007. https://milkquality.wisc.edu/wp-content/uploads/sites/212/2011/09/toolbox-for-assessing-cow-udder-and-teat-hygiene.pdf. Accessed 7 Aug 2018.
27. Hosmer DW, Lemeshow S. Applied logistic regression. 2nd ed. New York: Wiley; 2000.
28. Dohoo I, Martin W, Stryhn H. Veterinary epidemiologic research. 2nd ed. Charlottestown: VER Inc.; 2010.
29. Laven RA. Systematically tackling hock lesions. Vet J. 2015;203:2–3.
30. Lim PY, Huxley JN, Green MJ, Othman AR, Potterton SL, Brignell CJ, et al. Area of hock hair loss in dairy cows: risk factors and correlation with a categorical scale. Vet J. 2015;203:205–10.
31. Burow E, Thomsen PT, Rousing T, Sorensen JT. Daily grazing time as a risk factor for alterations at the hock joint integument in dairy cows. Animal. 2013;7:160–6.
32. Växa Sverige: Avelsvärdering Version VIII. 2008. http://www.sweebv.info/Dokument/Avelsv%C3%A4rdering%20versionVIII.pdf. Accessed 7 Aug 2018.
33. O'Hara LA, Bage R, Holtenius K. The impact of body condition after calving on metabolism and milk progesterone profiles in two breeds of dairy cows. Acta Vet Scand. 2016;58:68.
34. Haskell MJ, Rennie LJ, Bowell VA, Bell MJ, Lawrence AB. Housing system, milk production, and zero-grazing effects on lameness and leg injury in dairy cows. J Dairy Sci. 2006;89:4259–66.
35. Solano L, Barkema HW, Mason S, Pajor EA, LeBlanc SJ, Orsel K. Prevalence and distribution of foot lesions in dairy cattle in Alberta, Canada. J Dairy Sci. 2016;99:6828–41.
36. Solano L, Barkema HW, Pajor EA, Mason S, LeBlanc SJ, Zaffino Heyerhoff JC, et al. Prevalence of lameness and associated risk factors in Canadian Holstein-Friesian cows housed in freestall barns. J Dairy Sci. 2015;98:6978–91.
37. Växa Sverige: Redogörelse för husdjursorganisationens Djurhälsovård 2015/2016. 2017. https://www.vxa.se/globalassets/dokument/statistik/redogorelse-for-husdjursorganisationernas-djurhalsovard-2015-2016.pdf.pdf. Accessed 7 Aug 2018.
38. Weary DM, Taszkun I. Hock lesions and free-stall design. J Dairy Sci. 2000;83:697–702.
39. Andersson K: Peat Litter to Swedish Dairy Cows [master thesis on the internet]. Uppsala: Swedish University of Agricultural Sciences; 2007. https://stud.epsilon.slu.se/12027/1/andersson_k_171113.pdf. Accessed 7 Aug 2018.
40. KRAV: KRAV Regler 2017. http://www.krav.se/kravdrupal/sites/default/files/kravs_regler_2017.pdf. Accessed 7 Aug 2018.
41. Alvåsen K. Ekonomiska konsekvenser av krav på bete för mjölkkor. Uppsala: Swedish University of Agricultural Sciences. 2015 http://pub.epsilon.slu.se/13055/1/alvasen_k_160317.pdf. Accessed 7 Aug 2017.
42. Hernandez-Mendo O, von Keyserlingk MA, Veira DM, Weary DM. Effects of pasture on lameness in dairy cows. J Dairy Sci. 2007;90:1209–14.
43. Wolff C, Espetvedt M, Lind AK, Rintakoski S, Egenvall A, Lindberg A, et al. Completeness of the disease recording systems for dairy cows in Denmark, Finland, Norway and Sweden with special reference to clinical mastitis. BMC Vet Res. 2012;8:131.
44. Capurro A, Aspan A, Ericsson Unnerstad H, Persson Waller K, Artursson K. Identification of potential sources of Staphylococcus aureus in herds with mastitis problems. J Dairy Sci. 2010;93:180–91.
45. Chapinal N, Weary DM, Collings L, von Keyserlingk MA. Lameness and hock injuries improve on farms participating in an assessment program. Vet J. 2014;202:646–8.

Identification of matrix metalloproteinase-2 and -9 activities within the intestinal mucosa of dogs with chronic enteropathies

Mohsen Hanifeh[1,2*], Minna Marjaana Rajamäki[1], Pernilla Syrjä[3], Laura Mäkitalo[4], Susanne Kilpinen[1] and Thomas Spillmann[1]

Abstract

Background: Matrix metalloproteinases (MMPs) 2 and 9 are zinc- and calcium-dependent endopeptidases involved in the breakdown and reconstitution of extracellular matrix under both physiological and pathological conditions. Mucosal MMP-2 and -9 activities have been reported to be upregulated in the intestine of humans with inflammatory bowel disease (IBD), and in animal models of IBD. However, their involvement in the pathogenesis of canine chronic enteropathies (CE) is unknown. This study investigated mucosal pro- and active MMP-2 and -9 activities in dogs with CE and healthy dogs using gelatin zymography, and also to determine the association of their activities in dogs with CE with the canine IBD activity index (CIBDAI), histopathologic findings, the clinical outcome, and hypoalbuminemia. Intestinal mucosal samples from duodenum, ileum, colon, and cecum were collected from 40 dogs with CE and 18 healthy Beagle dogs.

Results: In dogs with CE, the number of samples positive for mucosal pro- and active MMP-2 was significantly higher in the duodenum ($P < 0.0001$ and $P = 0.011$, respectively), ileum ($P = 0.002$ and $P = 0.018$, respectively), and colon ($P < 0.0001$ and $P = 0.002$, respectively), compared with healthy controls. Mucosal pro-MMP-9-positive samples in the duodenum and colon were significantly more frequent in dogs with CE than in healthy dogs ($P = 0.0004$ and $P = 0.001$, respectively). Despite the presence of mucosal samples positive for active MMP-9 in the intestinal segments of dogs with CE, the difference compared to healthy controls did not reach statistical significance. None of the intestinal mucosal samples in healthy dogs showed gelatinolytic activity corresponding to the control bands of active MMP-2 and -9. Mucosal active MMP-9 activities displayed a significant positive association with the severity of neutrophil infiltration in the duodenum ($P = 00.040$), eosinophils in the cecum ($P = 00.037$), and the CIBDAI score for ileum samples ($P = 0.023$). There was no significant association of pro- and active MMP-2 and -9 levels with the clinical outcome or hypoalbuminemia.

Conclusions: This study is the first to demonstrate upregulation of mucosal pro- and active MMP-2 and pro-MMP-9 in the intestine of dogs with CE compared to healthy dogs. The results provide supporting evidence for the possible involvement of MMP-2 and -9 in the pathogenesis of canine CE.

Keywords: Chronic enteropathies, Dog, Matrix metalloproteinase 2, Matrix metalloproteinase 9, Zymography

*Correspondence: Mohsen.Hanifeh@helsinki.fi
[1] Department of Equine and Small Animal Medicine, Faculty of Veterinary Medicine, University of Helsinki, P.O. Box 57, (Viikintie 49), 00014 Helsinki, Finland
Full list of author information is available at the end of the article

Background

Chronic enteropathy (CE) is a term used to describe a group of inflammatory conditions of the intestinal tract of unknown cause in dogs [1]. Canine CE causes chronic gastrointestinal signs such as vomiting, diarrhea, tenesmus, hematochezia, and decreased appetite and leads to weight loss [1, 2]. There are different clinical types of CE in dogs, which are determined by their response to treatment and defined as food-responsive diarrhea or enteropathy (FRD or FRE), antibiotic-responsive diarrhea or enteropathy (ARD or ARE), steroid-responsive diarrhea or enteropathy (SRD or SRE), or steroid-non-responsive diarrhea or enteropathy (SNRD or SNRE) [3, 4]. Synonymous for CE, the term inflammatory bowel disease (IBD) has also been used in dogs, for example in a review determining canine IBD/CE according to the response to treatment [3]. While the etiology and pathophysiology of canine CE are not fully understood, interactions between the mucosal immune system, the host genetic susceptibility, and the environment such as microbial antigens and dietary antigens, have been identified as potential causative factors in the development of chronic gastrointestinal inflammation [3, 5–8]. The occurrence of an aberrant immune response to antigens derived from endogenous microbiota is likely to play an important role in CE pathogenesis; however, the specific pathways leading to tissue injury and intestinal inflammation are not fully understood [3, 8, 9].

Matrix metalloproteinases (MMPs) are a group of zinc- and calcium-dependent endopeptidases that are important in the turnover of extracellular matrix (ECM) and cell migration [10, 11]. In addition, MMPs proteolytically activate or degrade a variety of non-matrix substrates, including chemokines, cytokines, growth factors, and junctional proteins. Therefore, they play important roles in inflammatory responses [10]. MMPs have been divided according to their domain structure and substrate specificity into gelatinases, collagenases, stromelysins, elastases, and membrane-type MMPs [12]. Gelatinases are composed of two members: MMP-2 (gelatinase A) and MMP-9 (gelatinase B), which degrade similar substrates, such as gelatin, collagen types IV and V, elastin, laminin, fibronectin, and proteoglycans [12–14]. Both MMP-2 and -9 have pro and active forms with different molecular weights. MMP-2 is primarily produced by stromal cells, including fibroblasts, myofibroblasts, and endothelial cells [15, 16]. MMP-9 is mainly produced by neutrophils and to a lesser extent by eosinophils, monocytes, macrophages, lymphocytes, and epithelial cells [14, 15, 17–19]. Intestinal mucosal MMP-2 and -9 activities have been reported to be upregulated in humans with IBD (in both Crohn's disease [CD] and ulcerative colitis [UC]), and also in animal models of human IBD [13–15, 20, 21]. In a mouse model of colitis, MMP-2 was observed to play a protective role against tissue damage, possibly through the regulation of epithelial barrier function [10, 13, 14]. However, in humans with IBD, it contributes to ECM remodeling and the degradation of basal membrane type IV collagen, leading to intestinal ulceration, epithelial damage, and/or fistula formation [12, 15, 22–24]. In both humans with IBD and animal models of human IBD, MMP-9 plays a crucial role in both the induction of intestinal inflammation and wound healing. It promotes neutrophil migration, increases paracellular permeability, and reduces the adhesion complex integrity of the epithelium. In addition, MMP-9 interferes with re-epithelialization, resulting in impaired wound healing in cornea, skin, endothelial cells, and also in cultured intestinal epithelial cells [10, 13–15, 25].

In healthy dogs, we determined mucosal MMP-2 and -9 activities in different intestinal segments of Beagles in a previous study [26]. Only inactive pro-forms of MMP-2 and -9 were detected in the intestinal mucosa. Thus far, it has been unknown whether MMP-2 and -9 are also involved in the pathogenesis of canine CE. However, in dogs with CE, gene expression of MMP-1, -3, and -13 has been reported to be upregulated in the intestinal mucosa [27].

Therefore, the hypothesis of this study was that dogs with CE have higher MMP-2 and -9 activities in their intestinal mucosa than healthy dogs. The study also aimed at evaluating the association of intestinal mucosal MMP-2 and -9 activities with histological changes, the canine inflammatory bowel disease activity index (CIBDAI), the clinical outcome, and hypoalbuminemia in dogs with CE.

Methods

Animals

In this study, 52 dogs were included when undergoing routine gastroduodenoscopy and/or colonoscopy at the Veterinary Teaching Hospital, Faculty of Veterinary Medicine, University of Helsinki, Finland, due to chronic gastrointestinal (GI) signs such as vomiting, diarrhea, tenesmus, hematochezia, and/or weight loss. The study was prospectively planned and ethically approved by the Finnish National Animal Experiment Board (study license numbers: ESAVI/6973/04.10.03/2011 and ESAVI/10384/04.10.07/2014). Informed owner consent was obtained at the time the dogs were enrolled for performing gastroduodenoscopy and/or colonoscopy.

As a control group, we used stored intestinal tissue samples taken from 18 healthy laboratory Beagle dogs that underwent post-mortem examinations when finishing other unrelated studies. These studies were approved by the Finnish National Animal Experiment Board (study license numbers: ESLH-2007-09833/Ym-23, ESAVI 2010-04178/Ym-23 and ESAVI/7290/04.10.03/2012). The dogs were housed according to European Union guidelines in groups in indoor pens with access to outdoor runs. The indoor environmental temperature was maintained between 15 and 24 °C. The dogs were exposed to both natural and artificial light (from 7:00 to 16:00). They were fed a standard commercial diet and were evaluated as healthy based on history, physical examination, a complete blood count, serum biochemistry, and fecal examination. Intestinal mucosal samples were collected from the duodenum, ileum, and colon (n = 18, each, and cecum (n = 6), snap-frozen in liquid nitrogen, and stored at − 80 °C for MMP-2 and -9 determination.

For canine patients, the inclusion criteria were chronic gastrointestinal signs such as vomiting, diarrhea, tenesmus, hematochezia, and/or weight loss lasting longer than 3 weeks. Diagnostic tests were performed on each dog to exclude underlying infectious or extraintestinal disorders, which included a complete blood count, serum biochemical analysis, fecal examination for parasites, abdominal ultrasound, and gastroduodenoscopy/colonoscopy with biopsy. The diagnosis of chronic enteropathy (CE) was based on clinical, laboratory, endoscopic, and histopathologic criteria [28, 29].

Clinical examinations of dogs with CE

The clinical severity of disease in dogs with CE was determined by the CIBDAI score at the time of entering the study and after treatment [30]. In brief, the CIBDAI score was evaluated using six prominent GI related signs (attitude and activity, appetite, vomiting, stool consistency, stool frequency, and weight loss). These were scored based on their severity from 0 to 3. The total CIBDAI score represents the summation of all individual scores and was classified as insignificant (score 0–3), mild (score 4–5), moderate (score 6–8), or severe (score ≥ 9). The clinical outcome of dogs with CE was determined based on their response to treatment and since not all included dogs developed diarrhea as a clinical sign, the type of CE was defined as FRE, ARE, SRE, and SNRE [3, 4].

Serum albumin concentration in dogs with CE

The concentration of serum albumin was measured in each dog with CE and an albumin level of < 20 g/L was considered to indicate hypoalbuminemia. The severity of hypoalbuminemia was classified with a score of 1 (15–19.9 g/L), 2 (12–14.9 g/L), or 3 (< 12 g/L) [1].

Histological examinations

For histologic examination of canine patients and controls, mucosal tissue samples collected from the intestine by endoscopy or necropsy were fixed in 4% formaldehyde solution in phosphate buffered saline, embedded in paraffin, sectioned (3–5 μm), and stained with hematoxylin and eosin (HE). The intestinal tissue samples were evaluated and scored by a single pathologist (PS) using the guidelines of the World Small Animal Veterinary Association (WSAVA) Gastrointestinal Standardization Group [28, 29]. The pathologist was blinded to the results of clinical and laboratory examinations, as well as the mucosal MMP-2 and -9 activities of each case. The severity of histological changes in different segments of the intestine was evaluated and scored as 0 = normal, 1 = mild, 2 = moderate, or 3 = severe according to the WSAVA standardization guidelines. The total histological change score, representing the sum of morphologic and inflammatory scores, was classified as insignificant (score 0–4), mild (score 5–9), moderate (score 10–14), severe (score 15–19), or very severe (score ≥ 20). Ileal and cecal biopsies were scored using the guidelines provided for the interpretation of duodenal and colonic biopsies due to the lack of specific templates for these intestinal parts in the guidelines of the WSAVA Gastrointestinal Standardization Group.

Gelatin zymography

In control dogs, the intestinal mucosa was separated from the underlying muscularis layer in the snap-frozen intestinal tissue samples and stored in − 80 °C for further analysis. Snap-frozen intestinal mucosal samples from healthy dogs and dogs with CE were homogenized using Precellys 24 ceramic beads (Bertin Technologies, Paris, France) in ice-cold extraction buffer at an extraction buffer to tissue ratio of 20:1, as previously described [26]. Samples were then centrifuged and the supernatants were collected and stored at − 80 °C for MMP-2 and -9 determination. Protein concentrations of the supernatants were measured with bicinchoninic acid protein assay reagents (Pierce, Rockford, IL, USA). MMP-2 and MMP-9 activities in supernatant were measured by gelatin zymography in mini-gels as previously described in detail [26]. Briefly, supernatants were separated by electrophoresis in an 11% polyacrylamide gel impregnated with 0.7 mg/mL of gelatin as a substrate. Each lane of the gel was loaded with 20 μL of supernatant containing 10 μg of total protein mixed with a 10 μL aliquot of loading buffer. After electrophoresis, the gels were first soaked in renaturing buffer (2.5% Triton X-100) and then in zymogram developing buffer (50 mM Tris Base, pH 7.5, containing 200 mM NaCl, 5 mM $CaCl_2.2H_2O$, and 0.02% Brilj-35). They were then incubated for 18 h at 37 °C and were finally stained. Zymogram developing buffer contains divalent metal cations, which are required for enzymatic activation of both the pro and active enzymes. The areas of proteinase activity were visualized as clear bands by washing the gels with distilled water. As a control, each gel was loaded with diluted (1:600) recombinant human MMP-2 (9 μL) and -9 (8 μL) (R&D Systems, Minneapolis, MN, USA), respectively. The activities of pro- and active MMP-2 and -9 for each sample were expressed in arbitrary units (AU) related to the level of pro-MMP-2 of the positive-control standard loaded on each gel. Each band's activity was reported as the mean of two different measurements of the same sample due to the duplication of each sample in the gel.

Statistical analysis

Data are presented as the number (and percentage) of samples positive for MMP-2 and -9 or the median (range) of their activities, as appropriate. The differences in pro- and active MMP-2 and -9 positive samples in the duodenum, ileum, colon, and cecum between dogs with CE and healthy dogs were analyzed using Fisher's exact test. Associations of the CIBDAI score and pro- and active MMP-2 and -9 activities were evaluated using Spearman's correlation test. The same test was used to analyze the correlation between hypoalbuminemia and pro- and active MMP-2 and -9 activities in dogs with CE. The Kruskal–Wallis test was used to analyze the association between pro- and active MMP-2 and -9 activities and histological changes and the clinical outcome (FRE, ARE, SRE, and SNRE) in dogs with CE. P values < 0.05 were considered statistically significant. All statistical analyses were performed using SAS 9.3 statistical software (SAS Institute Inc., Cary, NC, USA).

Results

Demographics of dogs with CE and healthy dogs

The median age (range) of dogs with CE and healthy dogs was 5 years (1–13 years) and 10.5 (6–13), respectively. In the CE group, 15 dogs were intact males, 11 dogs were castrated males, 5 dogs were intact females, and 9 dogs were spayed females. In the healthy Beagle control group, 8 dogs were intact males and 10 dogs were intact females. The breeds of dogs with CE were mixed breed (6), Rottweiler (2), German Shepherd dog (2), Shetland Sheepdog (2), Parson Russell Terrier (2), Rough Collie (2), Standard Poodle (2), and one each of the following: Alaskan Malamute, Bichon Frise, Border Terrier, Chow Chow, Dalmatian, English Bulldog, Golden Retriever, Havanese, Irish Terrier, Jack Russell Terrier, Long-haired Dachshund, Mudi, Norwegian Lundehund, Rhodesian Ridgeback, Siberian Husky, Silky Terrier, Smooth Collie, Spanish Water Dog, Staffordshire Bull Terrier, Toy Poodle, West Highland White Terrier, and White Shepherd dog.

Of the 52 dogs with chronic GI signs, 12 dogs needed to be excluded from further analysis. Four dogs had primary esophageal disorders, and one dog was positive for *Giardia* sp. on fecal examination. Seven dogs had gastrointestinal neoplasia (3 gastric adenocarcinoma, 2 lymphoma, 1 rectal adenocarcinoma, and 1 rectal plasma cell tumor). Finally, 40 dogs with CE were included in the study analysis. Gastroduodenoscopy was performed in 25 dogs, gastroduodenoscopy and colonoscopy in 10 dogs, and only colonoscopy in five dogs. During the endoscopic examinations, a total of 68 intestinal mucosal biopsies were collected from four different parts of the intestine [duodenum (n = 35), ileum (n = 12), colon (n = 15), and cecum (n = 6)] (Fig. 1). The flow diagram in Fig. 1 shows the group distribution and inclusion/exclusion criteria of all dogs enrolled in the study.

Mucosal MMP-2 and -9 activities

The zymographic analyses revealed that gelatinolytic activities in positive samples were at the same molecular weights as the positive control bands of pro- and active MMP-2 and -9, and were therefore considered to represent canine pro- and active MMP-2 and -9 (Fig. 2). The median and range of mucosal pro- and active MMP-2

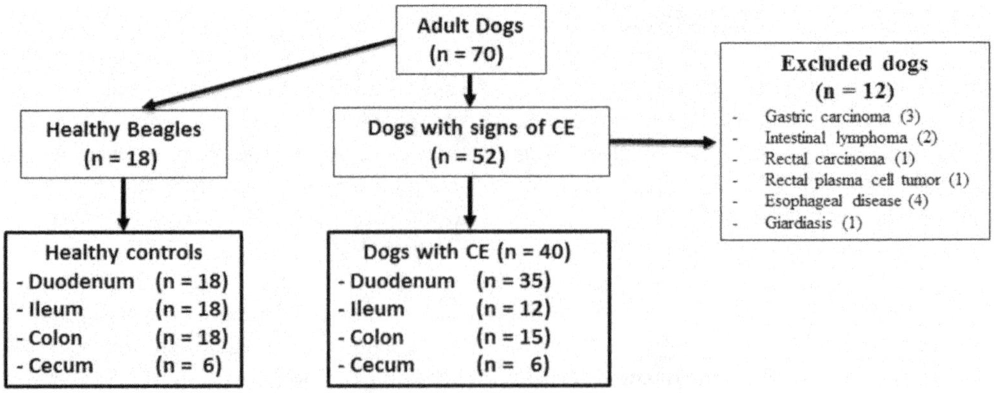

Fig. 1 Flow diagram displaying inclusion/exclusion criteria and group distribution of all dogs enrolled in the study. *CE* chronic enteropathies

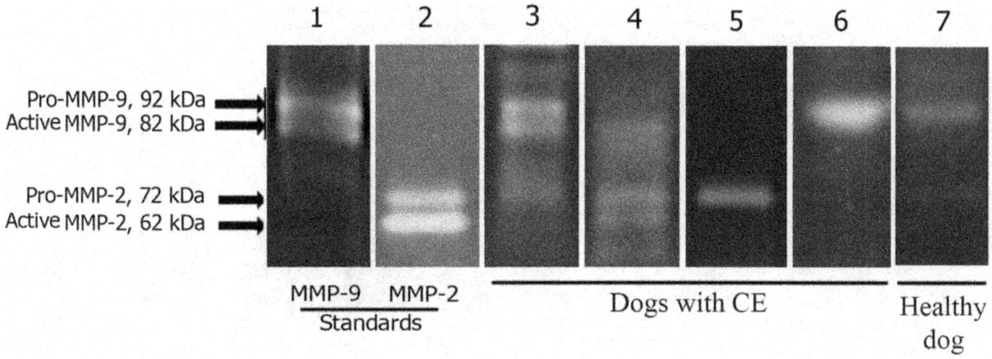

Fig. 2 Representative zymogram from intestinal mucosa samples. Recombinant human pro- and active MMP-2 (lane 2) and -9 (lane 1), pro- and active MMP-2 and -9 positive samples in dogs with CE (lanes 3–4), pro-MMP-2 and -9 positive samples in dogs with CE (lanes 5–6), and a healthy dog (lane 7)

Table 1 Mucosal pro- and active MMP-2 and -9 activities in dogs with CE and healthy dogs

Intestinal part	Group	Activity			
		Pro MMP-2 (AU) median (range)	Active MMP-2 (AU) median (range)	Pro MMP-9 (AU) median (range)	Active MMP-9 (AU) median (range)
Duodenum	Dogs with CE (n = 35)	0.01 (0–1.66)	0 (0–0.02)	0.06 (0–3.86)	0 (0–0.21)
	Healthy dogs (n = 18)	0 (0–0.64)	0 (0–0)	0.03 (0–3.32)	0 (0–0)
Ileum	Dogs with CE (n = 12)	0.02 (0–0.83)	0 (0–0.01)	0.06 (0–0.5)	0 (0–0.28)
	Healthy dogs (n = 18)	0 (0–0.52)	0 (0–0)	0.03 (0–0.45)	0 (0–0)
Colon	Dogs with CE (n = 15)	0.03 (0–0.55)	0 (0–0.05)	0.07 (0.02–0.92)	0 (0–0.04)
	Healthy dogs (n = 18)	0 (0–0.64)	0 (0–0)	0 (0–0.79)	0 (0–0)
Cecum	Dogs with CE (n = 6)	0.0 (0.01–1.48)	0 (0–0.01)	0.09 (0.02–0.59)	0.005 (0–0.05)
	Healthy dogs (n = 6)	0 (0–0.3)	0 (0–0)	0.18 (0–0.82)	0 (0–0)

Pro- and active MMP-2 and -9 activities were measured in the mucosal samples from duodenum, ileum, colon, and cecum of dogs with CE and healthy dogs

AU arbitrary units; *CE* chronic enteropathies; *Pro* pro-enzyme

and -9 activities in each intestinal segment in dogs with CE and healthy dogs are presented in Table 1.

In the duodenum, dogs with CE compared to healthy dogs had a significantly higher number (and percentage) of samples positive for mucosal pro-MMP-2 (32/35 [91.4%] vs. 3/18 [16.7%]; $P < 0.0001$), active MMP-2 (10/35 [28.6%] vs. 0/18 [0%]; $P = 0.011$), and pro MMP-9 (34/35 [97.1%] vs. 10/18 [55.6%]; $P = 0.0004$) (Fig. 3). For active MMP-9, two positive samples were recorded in dogs with CE compared to none in healthy dogs, but this difference was not significant (Fig. 3). None of the intestinal mucosal samples in healthy dogs showed gelatinolytic activity corresponding to the control bands of active MMP-2 and -9.

In the ileum, dogs with CE compared to healthy dogs had significantly higher numbers (and percentage) of samples positive for mucosal pro-MMP-2 (11/12 [91.7%] vs. 6/18 [33.3%]; $P = 0.002$) and active MMP-2 (4/12 [33.3%] vs. 0/18 [0%]; $P = 0.018$; Fig. 3). For pro- and active MMP-9, dogs with CE had more positive samples compared to healthy dogs, but the differences were not significant (Fig. 3).

In the colon, dogs with CE compared to healthy dogs had a significantly higher number (and percentage) of samples positive for mucosal pro-MMP-2 (13/15 [86.7%] vs. 3/18 [16.7%]; $P < 0.0001$), active MMP-2 (7/15 [46.7%] vs. 0/18 [0%]; $P = 0.002$), and pro-MMP-9 (15/15 [100%] vs. 8/18 [44.4%]; $P = 0.001$, Fig. 3). However, in dogs with CE, only one had active MMP-9-positive samples compared to healthy dogs with none (Fig. 3).

In the cecum, despite a higher percentage of samples positive for pro- and active MMP-2 and -9 in dogs with CE compared to healthy dogs, the differences between them did not reach statistical significance (Fig. 3).

Mucosal pro- and active MMP-2 and -9 activities and histological changes

In the ileum, pro-MMP-2 activities were significantly higher in mucosal samples with a normal epithelium ($P = 0.032$) and with no neutrophilic infiltration ($P = 0.034$).

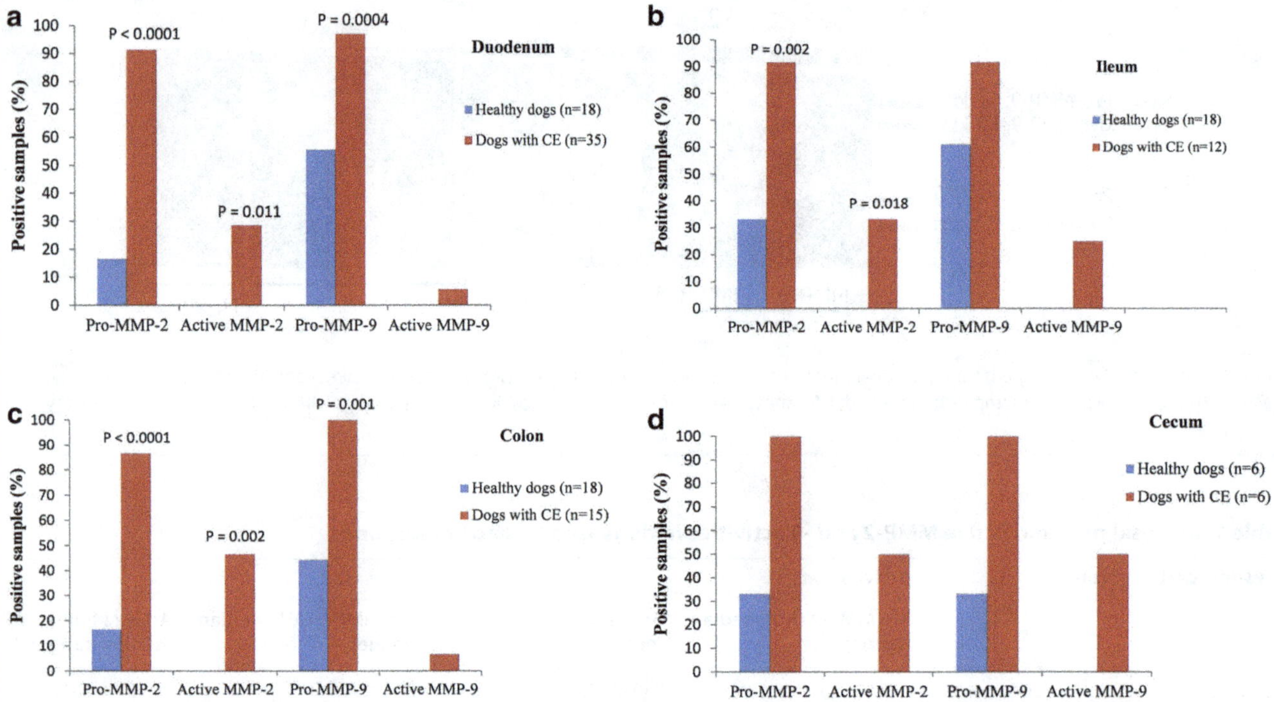

Fig. 3 Intestinal mucosal pro- and active MMP-2 and -9 activities in CE dogs and healthy dogs. This graph shows the presence of samples positive for pro- and active MMP-2 and -9 in the mucosa of duodenum (**a**), ileum (**b**), colon (**c**), and cecum (**d**) of dogs with CE and healthy dogs. P values are based on the comparison of pro- and active MMP-2 and-9 activities in the different part of the intestine of dogs with CE versus healthy dogs

There was a significant positive association between the active MMP-2 activities and the severity of eosinophilic infiltration in cecal samples (P =0.034). In addition, the association of active MMP-9 activities with the severity of neutrophilic infiltration in the duodenum (P = 0.040), and the severity of eosinophilic infiltration in the cecum (P = 0.037) were positive and significant. Active MMP-9 activities were also significantly higher in cecal samples with normal lamina propria lymphocyte/plasma cell scores (P = 0.049).

Mucosal pro- and active MMP-2 and -9 activities in relation to the CIBDAI and the clinical outcome

It was only possible to record the CIBDAI score before and after treatment in 30 out of 40 dogs with CE. The CIBDAI score before and after treatment was based on either available scores taken by the clinician in charge before and after the treatment (in 13/30 and 5/30 of dogs, respectively) or retrospectively calculated by the investigators (in 17/30 and 25/30 of dogs, respectively) from information in the clinical history (before the treatment) and from telephone interviews with the owners (after the treatment). Based on the response to treatment, the outcomes of 30 dogs with CE were classified as follows: 10 dogs with FRE, 4 dogs with ARE, 13 dogs with SRE, and 3 dogs with SNRE. For pro- and active MMP-2 and -9, only active MMP-9 activities in the ileal mucosa had a strong positive correlation with the CIBDAI score before treatment in dogs with CE (r=0.71, P=0.023). In dogs with CE, we did not find a significant association between the mucosal pro- and active MMP-2 and -9 activities and the clinical outcome in each intestinal segment.

Steroid non-responsive dogs (SNRE, n=3) either died or were euthanized due to severe clinical signs. When comparing duodenal samples, the median (range) of the CIBDAI score before treatment was higher in SNRE dogs (n=3) than in SRE dogs (n=12) (7 [4–7] vs. 4.5 [0–7]). Hypoalbuminemia (<20 g/L) was present in one SNRE and two SRE dogs. The median (range) of the total histological change score was slightly higher for SNRE dogs than SRE dogs (7 [5–7] vs. 6 [1–11]). The median (range) of the pro- and active MMP-2 and -9 activities in the duodenal mucosa of SNRE dogs compared to SRE dogs were as follows: pro-MMP-2 (0.01 [0–0.02] AU vs. 0.01 [0–1.66] AU), active MMP-2 (0 [0–0.01] AU vs. 0 [0–0.01] AU), pro-MMP-9 (0.07 [0.02–0.16] AU vs. 0.09 [0–3.86] AU), and active MMP-9 (0 [0–0.21] AU vs. 0 [0–0] AU. The number of SNRE dogs was too low for statistical analysis other than descriptive comparison.

Mucosal pro- and active MMP-2 and-9 activities in relation to hypoalbuminemia in dogs with CE

In this study, 36 dogs out of 40 (90%) had a serum albumin level of > 20 g/L, with a median (range) of 32.65 g/L (24.9–39 g/L). A total of 4 out of 40 dogs (10%) had serum albumin concentrations of < 20 g/L (median 12.2 g/L; range 11–13 g/L), with a hypoalbuminemia severity scores of 2 for two dogs and of 3 for another two [1]. Duodenal biopsy samples were taken from the four hypoalbuminemic CE dogs, and the correlations between mucosal pro- and active MMP-2 and-9 activities and hypoalbuminemia were evaluated. However, there was no significant correlation between pro-MMP-2 or active MMP-9 activities in the duodenal mucosa and hypoalbuminemia in dogs with CE. In hypoalbuminemic dogs with CE, compared to normoalbuminemic dogs with CE, the number (percentage) of positive samples in the duodenal mucosal was as follows: pro-MMP-2 (3/4 [75%] vs. 29/31 [93.5%]), active MMP-2 (1/4 [25%] vs. 9/31 [29%], pro-MMP-9 (3/4 [75%] vs. 31/31 [100%]), and active MMP-9 (1/4 [25%] vs. 1/31 [3.2%]). The median (range) of the pro- and active MMP-2 and -9 activities in the duodenal mucosa of hypoalbuminemic dogs with CE compared to normoalbuminemic dogs with CE was as follows: pro-MMP-2 (0.01 [0–0.017] AU vs. 0.01 [0–1.66] AU), active MMP-2 (0 [0–0.01] AU vs. 0 [0–0.02] AU), pro-MMP-9 (0.14 [0–0.74] AU vs. 0.05 [0.01–3.86] AU), and active MMP-9 (0 [0–0.21] AU vs. 0 [0–0.1] AU.

Discussion

This study is the first to report mucosal MMP-2 and -9 activities in the intestine of dogs with CE. The number of samples positive for pro- and active MMP-2 and pro-MMP-9 was higher in the mucosa of dogs with CE compared to healthy dogs in all intestinal segments when determined using gelatin zymography. Similar findings were also reported for active MMP-2 and pro-MMP-9 in the colonic mucosa of humans with IBD compared to healthy controls [20]. A significantly higher percentage of colonic mucosal samples in dogs with CE had pro-MMP-2 activity compared to healthy dogs (86.7% vs. 16.7%). However, the percentage of samples with colonic mucosal pro-MMP-2 activity was the same in human patients with IBD and healthy controls, and activity was detected in 80% of the samples [20]. Active MMP-2 was detected in 46.7% of the colonic samples of dogs with CE. However, no activity was found in colonic mucosal samples of healthy dogs. Similarly to our findings, Baugh et al. [20] did not detect active MMP-2 activities in the colonic mucosa of healthy humans. However, they found active MMP-2 activities in 35% of samples in humans with IBD. Under normal conditions, MMP-2 is believed to participate in the maintenance of collagen homeostasis and intestinal tissue remodeling. In human IBD, MMP-2 has been reported to contribute to ECM remodeling and the degradation of basal membrane type IV collagen, leading to intestinal ulceration, epithelial damage, and/or fistula formation [12, 15, 22–24]. It appears that intestinal tissue turnover is increased during intestinal inflammation, tissue destruction, and healing processes, and demands greater MMP-2 activities in human IBD [15]. In contrast, it has been reported that MMP-2 plays a protective role against tissue damage, possibly through the regulation of epithelial barrier function, in an MMP-2 knockout mouse model of IBD [10, 13, 14]. In our study, it appears that having higher activities of pro- and active MMP-2 in dogs with CE indicates the possible involvement of this enzyme in the pathogenesis of canine chronic enteropathies. In addition, we showed that the samples with higher pro-MMP-2 activities have an association with a normal epithelium and lamina propria without neutrophils in the ileum. Similarly to the study on an MMP-2 knockout mouse model of IBD, it is possible that MMP-2 has a protective role against tissue damage through the regulation of epithelial barrier function in dogs; however, more research is needed to clarify the role of MMP-2 in canine CE.

Mucosal pro-MMP-9 was detected in more than 90% of the samples in the intestinal segments of dogs with CE, while this form of enzyme was detected in 33–61% of the intestinal mucosal samples of healthy dogs. Therefore, pro-MMP-9 activities are elevated in dogs with CE compared to healthy dogs, which is similar to the findings of Baugh et al. [20] in humans with IBD. In our study, we did not detect the active form of MMP-9 in the mucosa of healthy dogs. Similar findings were also reported in the colonic mucosa of healthy humans [20]. In dogs with CE, the active form of MMP-9 was detected in 5.7, 25, 5.6, and 50% of duodenal, ileal, colonic, and cecal samples, respectively. In the duodenal and cecal samples, we also found a positive and significant association between active MMP-9 activities and the severity of lamina propria neutrophilic and eosinophilic infiltration, with these cells being proposed as sources of MMP-9. In comparison to human IBD, the percentage of active MMP-9-positive samples in the colon of dogs with CE was much lower (55% vs. 5.6%) [20]. This difference could be due to the different pathophysiology of canine and human chronic colitis. A higher number of infiltrated neutrophils and more ulcerative lesions in humans with chronic colitis could be the possible reasons for the higher active MMP-9 activities in humans [15]. In future studies, immunohistochemistry should also be included to assess the localization of MMP-2 and -9 in the intestinal mucosa and their correlation with intestinal pathologies in dogs.

We found a positive correlation between active MMP-9 activities in the ileal mucosa and the CIBDAI score before treatment in dogs with CE, which is similar to the relationship between mucosal MMP-9 and the disease activity index in a rat model of colitis [31], and between fecal MMP-9 and clinical activities of ulcerative colitis in humans [32]. However, due to the low number of active MMP-9-positive samples (n = 3) in the ileal samples of dogs with CE in our study, the results should not be over-interpreted.

The association between an aberrant intestinal expression of MMP-2 and -9 and human IBD is now well established [33]. MMP-2 and -9 have been investigated as biomarkers and diagnostic tool for human IBD. The level of fecal MMP-9 in UC patients correlates with disease activity and has recently been proposed as a biomarker of the disease. By measuring fecal MMP-9 levels, it was possible to distinguish UC from diarrhea predominant irritable bowel syndrome with 85% sensitivity and 100% specificity [34]. Serum level of MMP-9 have also been shown as a potential tool in the prediction of CD activity status in children [35]. In addition, MMP-2 and MMP-9 levels in urine of pediatric patients with IBD have been reported as useful novel non-invasive biomarkers to predict CD and UC independently in children [33]. Our study is the first to demonstrate an upregulation of mucosal pro- and active MMP-2 and pro-MMP-9 in the intestine of dogs with CE. This is a promising indication that MMPs play a role in canine CE with the potential of being used as biomarkers of active disease and disease severity. In the present study, however, we did not find a significant association between mucosal MMP-2 and -9 activities and the type of clinical outcome in dogs with CE which could be due to the low number of dogs with a certain clinical outcome (especially SNRE dogs, n = 3). In addition, the comparison between intestinal segments led to rather low case numbers when assessing the association between mucosal MMP-2 and -9 activities with the type of clinical outcome. Further studies with sufficient number of canine patients in each types of CE is needed to evaluate the relationship between MMP-2 and -9 activities and canine CE subtypes. MMP expression in the intestine or elsewhere in the body, e.g. serum or feces, may in the future help in properly differentiating disease subtypes and severity, and to enable tailored treatment choices for individuals.

A unique therapeutic option for human IBD is targeting MMPs which has been investigated in animal models of IBD. Inhibition of MMPs with non-selective inhibitors (e.g. Marimastat, Batimastat) has been shown to reduce mucosal damage and colitis induced by dextran sodium sulfate (DSS) in animal models [33]. However, the development of MMP inhibitors in humans has been limited by their poor selectivity [33]. To target MMPs, monoclonal antibodies against MMP-2 and MMP-9 have been developed and tested on murine models of IBD. These antibodies were significantly reducing the severity of the DSS induced colitis in mice [33, 36]. However, due to the myriad roles of MMPs in vivo and their ubiquitous expression throughout the body, using monoclonal antibodies remains a serious concern and a barrier to their current therapeutic use in human IBD [33]. Whether targeting MMPs using monoclonal antibodies in canine CE patients is beneficial for CE treatment is not known yet and needs to be studied.

It has been shown that treatment of human IBD with immunosuppressive medications could reduce the levels of MMPs in the intestinal mucosa and serum. Makitalo et al. [37] showed in people that the treatment of CD patients with anti-TNF-α therapy (infliximab or adalimumab) or with corticosteroids and other immunosuppressive drugs (methotrexate or azathioprine) decreased stromal MMP-9 and epithelial MMP-7 as assessed by immunohistochemistry methods. However, there are different reports regarding the response of MMP-9 to therapy in serum. Gao et al. [38] reported that serum levels of MMP-9 decrease in adults in response to infliximab therapy; however, Makitalo et al. [39] reported no significant changes in serum MMP-9 levels after therapy. In mice, mangiferin, a bioactive compound of the mango, attenuated DSS induced colitis through directly reducing the activity of mucosal TNF-α and MMP-9 [40]. Future studies in CE dogs should be planned as treatment follow up studies with repeated biopsies to evaluate the treatment effects of different medication especially immunosuppressive drugs such as prednisolone on the intestinal mucosal MMP-2 and -9 activities.

We did not find significant correlations between pro- and active MMP-2 and -9 activities in the duodenal mucosa and hypoalbuminemia in dogs with CE. Since only 10% (4/40) of the dogs had hypoalbuminemia (< 20 g/L), the number of samples was too low for an appropriate power of analysis and it could be the reason why we did not find significant correlations between MMP2 and 9 activities. In humans, to our knowledge, there has been so far no report studying MMP-2 and -9 activities in patients with protein losing enteropathies. In future prospective studies, the necessary number of cases of CE dogs with hypoalbuminemia should be prospectively estimated by using power analysis, for which the data of the current study are helpful. In the future, it will also be necessary to focus more on advanced cases with intestinal protein loss, a patient group that was underrepresented in this study and also looking for other MMPs. Another limitation of our study is that the cobalamin and folate concentrations were not measured in a sufficient number of dogs with CE to allow statistical analysis. Therefore, future prospective studies need to include a variety of laboratory data to assess possible associations/correlations.

Conclusions

This is the first study to demonstrate that mucosal pro- and active MMP-2 and pro-MMP-9 are upregulated in the intestine of dogs with CE compared to healthy dogs. Compared to humans with IBD, the active form of MMP-9 has been detected in a rather small number of canine patients, which could be due to the low number of granulocytes found in the intestinal mucosa of dogs with CE. The results provide supporting evidence for the possible involvement of MMP-2 and -9 in the pathogenesis of canine CE. Further research is needed to assess the localization of MMP-2 and -9 in the canine intestinal mucosa, their presence and activity level in advanced CE with intestinal protein loss, and their relationship with other inflammatory markers in canine chronic enteropathies. Furthermore, their activities in fecal samples should be determined to examine their possible usefulness as non-invasive biomarkers of intestinal inflammation.

Abbreviations

ARD: antibiotic-responsive diarrhea; ARE: antibiotic-responsive enteropathy; AU: arbitrary unit; CD: Crohn's disease; CE: chronic enteropathy; CIBDAI: canine inflammatory bowel disease activity index; cTLI: canine trypsin-like immunoreactivity; DSS: dextran sodium sulfate; ECM: extracellular matrix; FRD: food-responsive diarrhea; FRE: food-responsive enteropathy; GI: gastrointestinal; HE: hematoxylin and eosin; IBD: inflammatory bowel disease; MMPs: matrix metalloproteinases; SRD: steroid-responsive diarrhea; SRE: steroid-responsive enteropathy; SNRD: steroid non-responsive diarrhea; SNRE: steroid non-responsive enteropathy; TNF-α: tumor necrosis factor-alpha; UC: ulcerative colitis; WSAVA: World Small Animal Veterinary Association.

Authors' contributions

MH, MMR, LM, and TS conceived the study design. SK performed sample collection. MH measured MMP-2 and-9 activities. PS performed histology diagnosis. All authors read and approved the final manuscript.

Author details

[1] Department of Equine and Small Animal Medicine, Faculty of Veterinary Medicine, University of Helsinki, P.O. Box 57, (Viikintie 49), 00014 Helsinki, Finland. [2] Department of Clinical Sciences, Faculty of Veterinary Medicine, University of Tabriz, 5166616471 Tabriz, Iran. [3] Department of Veterinary Biosciences, Faculty of Veterinary Medicine, University of Helsinki, P.O. Box 66, (Agnes Sjöberginkatu 2), 00014 Helsinki, Finland. [4] Children's Hospital, Helsinki University Central Hospital, University of Helsinki, P.O. Box 63, (Haartmaninkatu 8), 00014 Helsinki, Finland.

Acknowledgements

The authors would like to thank Jouni Junnila and Tommi Pesonen, 4Pharma, Finland, for performing statistical analysis of the data and Laura Parikka for technical assistance.

Competing interests

The authors declare that they have no competing interests.

Funding

This work was supported by the Finnish Veterinary Foundation, Finland (Grant Decision Year: 2013, 2014, 2015) and the Doctoral Program in Clinical Veterinary Medicine, University of Helsinki, Helsinki, Finland (Grant Decision Year: 2013, 2014). The funders had no role in study design, data collection and analysis, decision to publish, or preparation of the manuscript.

References

1. Allenspach K, Wieland B, Grone A, Gaschen F. Chronic enteropathies in dogs: evaluation of risk factors for negative outcome. J Vet Intern Med. 2007;21:700–8.
2. Wennogle SA, Priestnall SL, Webb CB. Histopathologic characteristics of intestinal biopsy samples from dogs with chronic inflammatory enteropathy with and without hypoalbuminemia. J Vet Intern Med. 2017;31:371–6.
3. Simpson KW, Jergens AE. Pitfalls and progress in the diagnosis and management of canine inflammatory bowel disease. Vet Clin North Am Small Anim Pract. 2011;41(2):381–98.
4. Dandrieux JR. Inflammatory bowel disease versus chronic enteropathy in dogs: are they one and the same? J Small Anim Pract. 2016;57:589–99.
5. German AJ, Hall EJ, Day N. Chronic intestinal inflammation and intestinal disease in dogs. J Vet Intern Med. 2003;17:8–20.
6. Jergens AE, Simpson KW. Inflammatory bowel disease in veterinary medicine. Front Biosci (Elite Ed). 2012;4:1404–19.
7. Jergens AE, Sonea IM, O'Connor AM, Kauffman LK, Grozdanic SD, Ackermann MR, et al. Intestinal cytokine mRNA expression in canine inflammatory bowel disease: a meta-analysis with critical appraisal. Comp Med. 2009;59:153–62.
8. Cassmann E, White R, Atherly T, Wang C, Sun Y, Khoda S, et al. Alterations of the ileal and colonic mucosal microbiota in canine chronic enteropathies. PLoS ONE. 2016;11:e0147321.
9. Schmitz S, Glanemann B, Garden OA, Brooks H, Chang YM, Werling D, et al. A prospective, randomized, blinded, placebo-controlled pilot study on the effect of Enterococcus faecium on clinical activity and intestinal gene expression in canine food-responsive chronic enteropathy. J Vet Intern Med. 2015;29:533–43.
10. Ravi A, Garg P, Sitaraman SV. Matrix metalloproteinases in inflammatory bowel disease: boon or a bane? Inflamm Bowel Dis. 2007;13:97–107.
11. Naito Y, Yoshikawa T. Role of matrix metalloproteinases in inflammatory bowel disease. Mol Aspects Med. 2005;26:379–90.
12. O'Sullivan S, Gilmer JF, Medina C. Matrix metalloproteinases in inflammatory bowel disease: an update. Mediators Inflamm. 2015;2015:964131.
13. Garg P, Rojas M, Ravi A, Bockbrader K, Epstein S, Vijay-Kumar M, et al. Selective ablation of matrix metalloproteinase-2 exacerbates experimental colitis: contrasting role of gelatinases in the pathogenesis of colitis. J Immunol. 2006;177:4103–12.
14. Garg P, Vijay-Kumar M, Wang LX, Gewirtz AT, Merlin D, Sitaraman SV. Matrix metalloproteinase-9-mediated tissue injury overrides the protective effect of matrix metalloproteinase-2 during colitis. Am J Physiol Gastrointest Liver Physiol. 2009;296:G175–84.
15. Gao Q, Meijer MJW, Kubben F, Sier CFM, Kruidenier L, van Duijn W, et al. Expression of matrix metalloproteinases-2 and-9 in intestinal tissue of patients with inflammatory bowel diseases. Dig Liver Dis. 2005;37:584–92.
16. Kirkegaard T, Hansen A, Bruun E, Brynskov J. Expression and localisation of matrix metalloproteinases and their natural inhibitors in fistulae of patients with Crohn's disease. Gut. 2004;53:701–9.
17. Hogan SP. Functional role of eosinophils in gastrointestinal inflammation. Immunol Allergy Clin North Am. 2009;29:129–40.
18. Kim JH, Lee SY, Bak SM, Suh IB, Shin C, Shim JJ, et al. Effects of matrix metalloproteinase inhibitor on LPS-induced goblet cell metaplasia. Am J Physiol Lung Cell Mol Physiol. 2004;287:L127–33.
19. Lubbe WJ, Zhou ZY, Fu W, Zuzga D, Schulz S, Fridman R, et al. Tumor epithelial cell matrix metalloproteinase 9 is a target for antimetastatic therapy in colorectal cancer. Clin Cancer Res. 2006;12:1876–82.
20. Baugh MD, Perry MJ, Hollander AP, Davies DR, Cross SS, Lobo AJ, et al. Matrix metalloproteinase levels are elevated in inflammatory bowel disease. Gastroenterology. 1999;117:814–22.
21. Makitalo L, Kolho KL, Karikoski R, Anthoni H, Saarialho-Kere U. Expression profiles of matrix metalloproteinases and their inhibitors in colonic

inflammation related to pediatric inflammatory bowel disease. Scand J Gastroenterol. 2010;45:862–71.

22. Matsuno K, Adachi Y, Yamamoto H, Goto A, Arimura Y, Endo T, et al. The expression of matrix metalloproteinase matrilysin indicates the degree of inflammation in ulcerative colitis. J Gastroenterol. 2003;38:348–54.
23. McKaig BC, McWilliams D, Watson SA, Mahida YR. Expression and regulation of tissue inhibitor of metalloproteinase-1 and matrix metalloproteinases by intestinal myofibroblasts in inflammatory bowel disease. Am J Pathol. 2003;162:1355–60.
24. Stallmach A, Chan CC, Ecker KW, Feifel G, Herbst H, Schuppan D, et al. Comparable expression of matrix metalloproteinases 1 and 2 in pouchitis and ulcerative colitis. Gut. 2000;47:415–22.
25. Castaneda FE, Walia B, Vijay-Kumar M, Patel NR, Roser S, Kolachala VL, et al. Targeted deletion of metalloproteinase 9 attenuates experimental colitis in mice: central role of epithelial-derived MMP. Gastroenterology. 2005;129:1991–2008.
26. Hanifeh M, Rajamaki MM, Makitalo L, Syrja P, Sankari S, Kilpinen S, et al. Identification of matrix metalloproteinase-2 and -9 activities within intestinal mucosa of clinically healthy beagle dogs. J Vet Med Sci. 2014;76:1079–85.
27. Wilke VL, Nettleton D, Wymore MJ, Gallup JM, Demirkale CY, Ackermann MR, et al. Gene expression in intestinal mucosal biopsy specimens obtained from dogs with chronic enteropathy. Am J Vet Res. 2012;73:1219–29.
28. Day MJ, Bilzer T, Mansell J, Wilcock B, Hall EJ, Jergens A, et al. Histopathological standards for the diagnosis of gastrointestinal inflammation in endoscopic biopsy samples from the dog and cat: a report from the World Small Animal Veterinary Association Gastrointestinal Standardization Group. J Comp Pathol. 2008;138(Suppl 1):S1–43.
29. Washabau RJ, Day MJ, Willard MD, Hall EJ, Jergens AE, Mansell J, et al. Endoscopic, biopsy, and histopathologic guidelines for the evaluation of gastrointestinal inflammation in companion animals. J Vet Intern Med. 2010;24:10–26.
30. Jergens AE, Schreiner CA, Frank DE, Niyo Y, Ahrens FE, Eckersall PD, et al. A scoring index for disease activity in canine inflammatory bowel disease. J Vet Intern Med. 2003;17:291–7.
31. Oliveira LG, Cunha AL, Duarte AC, Castanon MC, Chebli JM, Aguiar JA. Positive correlation between disease activity index and matrix metalloproteinases activity in a rat model of colitis. Arq Gastroenterol. 2014;51:107–12.
32. Farkas K, Sarodi Z, Balint A, Foldesi I, Tiszlavicz L, Szucs M, et al. The diagnostic value of a new fecal marker, matrix metalloprotease-9, in different types of inflammatory bowel diseases. J Crohn's Colitis. 2015;9:231–7.
33. O'Shea NR, Smith AM. Matrix metalloproteases role in bowel inflammation and inflammatory bowel disease: an up to date review. Inflamm Bowel Dis. 2014;20:2379–93.
34. Dabritz J, Musci J, Foell D. Diagnostic utility of faecal biomarkers in patients with irritable bowel syndrome. World J Gastroenterol. 2014;20:363–75.
35. Kofla-Dlubacz A, Matusiewicz M, Krzystek-Korpacka M, Iwanczak B. Correlation of MMP-3 and MMP-9 with Crohn's disease activity in children. Dig Dis Sci. 2012;57:706–12.
36. Sela-Passwell N, Kikkeri R, Dym O, Rozenberg H, Margalit R, Arad-Yellin R, et al. Antibodies targeting the catalytic zinc complex of activated matrix metalloproteinases show therapeutic potential. Nat Med. 2011;18:143–7.
37. Makitalo L, Sipponen T, Karkkainen P, Kolho KL, Saarialho-Kere U. Changes in matrix metalloproteinase (MMP) and tissue inhibitors of metalloproteinases (TIMP) expression profile in Crohn's disease after immunosuppressive treatment correlate with histological score and calprotectin values. Int J Colorectal Dis. 2009;24:1157–67.
38. Gao Q, Meijer MJ, Schluter UG, van Hogezand RA, van der Zon JM, van den Berg M, et al. Infliximab treatment influences the serological expression of matrix metalloproteinase (MMP)-2 and -9 in Crohn's disease. Inflamm Bowel Dis. 2007;13:693–702.
39. Makitalo L, Rintamaki H, Tervahartiala T, Sorsa T, Kolho KL. Serum MMPs 7-9 and their inhibitors during glucocorticoid and anti-TNF-alpha therapy in pediatric inflammatory bowel disease. Scand J Gastroenterol. 2012;47:785–94.
40. Somani S, Zambad S, Modi K. Mangiferin attenuates DSS colitis in mice: molecular docking and in vivo approach. Chem Biol Interact. 2016;253:18–26.

23

Current biomarkers of canine mammary tumors

Ilona Kaszak[1*], Anna Ruszczak[1], Szymon Kanafa[1], Kamil Kacprzak[1], Magdalena Król[2] and Piotr Jurka[1]

Abstract

Mammary tumors are the second most common neoplasia in dogs. Due to the high similarity of canine mammary tumors (CMT) to human breast cancers (HBC), human biomarkers of HBC are also detectable in cases of CMT. The evaluation of biomarkers enables clinical diagnoses, treatment options and prognosis for bitches suffering from this disease. The aim of this article is to give a short summary of the biomarkers of CMT based on current literature. Very promising biomarkers are miRNAs, cancer stem cells, and circulating tumor cells, as well as mutations of the breast cancer 1 gene (BRCA1) and breast cancer 2 gene (BRCA2). Until now, the most studied and reliable biomarkers of CMT have remained antigen Ki-67 (Ki-67), endothelial growth factor receptor, human epidermal growth factor receptor 2 (HER-2), estrogen receptor, progesterone receptor and cyclooxygenase 1 (COX-2), which can be detected in both serum and tissue samples using different molecular methods. However, carcinoembryonic antigen and cancer antigen 15-3 (CA 15-3), while poorly studied, seem to be good biomarkers, especially for the early detection and prognosis of CMT. We will also mention the following: proliferative cell nuclear antigen, tumor protein p53 (p53), E-cadherin, vascular endothelial growth factor, microRNAs, cancer stem cells and circulating tumor cells, which can also be useful biomarkers. Although many studies have been conducted so far, the estimation of biomarkers in cases of CMT is still not a common practice, and more detailed research should be done.

Keywords: Biomarkers, Bitch, Canine mammary gland, Canine mammary tumors, Dog, Human breast cancer, Neoplasia, Veterinary oncology

Background

With the increase in life expectancy in both humans and dogs, the incidence of cancers has increased as well [1]. Mammary neoplasia is the most frequently diagnosed tumor in bitches; therefore, they represent a significant clinical problem [2–5]. Among canine mammary tumors, (CMT) approximately 50% are malignant [2, 3, 5]. The most common tumor type among them is tubular carcinoma (adenocarcinoma), followed by papillary carcinoma, solid carcinoma, complex carcinoma and carcinosarcoma (Table 1) [3, 4]. The benign mammary tumors are mostly fibroadenomas, ductal papillomas, benign mixed tumors and simple adenomas [3, 4]. It is also common to find more than one tumor type in different mammary glands of the same patient [2]. In contrast breast cancers in women are usually malignant, and the most common tumor type is invasive ductal carcinoma, followed by carcinoma in situ [6]. The grade of malignancy is based not only on tumor type but also on the presence of significant nuclear and cellular pleomorphism, mitotic index, the presence of necrotic areas, peritumoral and lymphatic invasion and regional lymph node metastasis [7]. CMT occur in elderly bitches, usually between 8 and 10 years old [2–5]. This problem is especially significant in Europe, where bitches are usually spayed at an older age [2]. The etiology of CMT is still unknown. However, some risk factors have been indicated, e.g., hormonal, nutritional and genetic factors [2, 8–10]. It has been demonstrated in several studies that certain breeds have a genetic tendency to suffer from CMT, e.g., Miniature Poodles, Dachshunds, Malteses, Yorkshire Terriers, Cocker Spaniels and German Shepherds [2, 3, 5]. However,

*Correspondence: ilonakaszak@gmail.com
[1] Department of Small Animal Diseases with Clinic, Veterinary Medicine Faculty, Warsaw University of Life Sciences, Nowoursynowska 166, 02-787 Warsaw, Poland

Table 1 Mammary gland neoplasias in bitches [7]

Malignant	Benign
1. Simple carcinoma* Tubopapillary carcinoma Tubular carcinoma adenocarcinoma* Solid carcinoma Anaplastic carcinoma 2. Carcinoma in situ 3. Complex carcinoma* 4. Special type of carcinomas Spindle cell carcinoma Squamous cell carcinoma Mucinous carcinoma Lipid-rich carcinoma Inflammatory carcinoma 5. Carcinoma arising in a mixed tumor 6. Carcinosarcoma 7. Sarcoma Fibrosarcoma Osteosarcoma Other sarcomas 8. Comedocarcinoma	1. Adenoma* Simple adenoma Intraductal papillary adenoma Complex adenoma Basaloid adenoma 2. Fibroadenoma* 3. Benign mixed tumor* 4. Ductal papilloma 5. Myopithelioma 6. Mammary hyperplasia and dysplasia Ductal hyperplasia Lobular hyperplasia Cysts Duct ectasia Focal fibrosis Gynecomastia

* The most frequent types

these predispositions may vary depending on the geographical location. However, no common mutations in dogs with CMT have been detected so far [2]. One of the main risk factors for tumor growth is sex hormones [8–10]. The risk of mammary tumors increases depending on the time of spaying. If the bitch is spayed before her first ovarian cycle, the risk is 0.5%, but when she is spayed just after or at any time later, the risk is 8% and 26%, respectively [2, 3, 5, 8]. Apart from that, false pregnancies and the use of progestins as contraception can contribute to tumor formation [2, 5]. Usually, the owners of animals notice tumors when macroscopic changes in the mammary gland are already visible [2]. The prognostic evaluation is usually based on the clinical stage, tumor size, lymph node status, radiographic evidence of distant metastases, lymphatic or vascular invasion and histopathological examination of the tumor according to the WHO guidelines after tumor removal [2, 7, 11–14]. So far, the only effective treatment is surgery, which consists of the removal of altered glands and local lymph nodes. Usually, at the same time, an ovariohysterectomy (OHE) is also performed. However, recent studies have demonstrated that not all CMT cases benefit from OHE [15]. The standard patient follow-up protocol includes clinical examination and a basic panel of blood tests, together with an X-ray check every 3 months. In most cases of malignant CMT, chemotherapy or radiotherapy is performed. Nevertheless, both chemotherapy and radiotherapy are costly, and there is limited information about their efficacy in the treatment of CMT [16]. Because of this, the early detection of CMT seems to be crucial for the patients' outcome. Unfortunately, little is known about cancer biomarkers. Determination of biomarkers in dogs could be a milestone for the early diagnosis of neoplasia and for evaluation of the progression of disease and its response to chemotherapy.

Biomarkers are usually proteins that can be measured in blood or other tissues (e.g., in tumor tissue) and can give information about the presence of a disease, results of treatment or further prognosis for the patient [17, 18]. Every cancer cell expresses specific proteins that are called tumor-associated antigens. In patients with tumors, these antigens are called biomarkers if they can be detected in other tissues, serum or urine in concentrations that are different from normal [17, 18]. Therefore, we can distinguish between serum and tissue/cellular biomarkers. In human medicine, biomarkers play a role in breast cancer diagnosis and follow-up. Human breast cancer (HBC) has similar immunohistochemical features to canine mammary tumors and expresses the same substances; therefore, the determination of the same markers may be considered [19]. Nevertheless, canine mammary cancers have a very heterogenous morphology and biology, and the choice of the most appropriate biomarker remains the biggest challenge.

In this article, we briefly describe the most reliable biomarkers of canine mammary tumors [17, 19–22] that are the most frequently determined in mammary gland tissue by immunohistochemical methods. However, we also mention possibilities to determine additional serum biomarkers by other molecular techniques.

Search strategy

This article is a literature review and is based on an examination of current veterinary and medical literature. A literature search was performed in PubMed (http://www.ncbinlm.nih.gov/pubmed) using the terms "canine mammary tumor biomarkers", "human breast cancer biomarkers", "Ki-67", "PCNA", "p53", "E-cadherin", "CEA", "CA 15-3", "VEGF" EGFR", "HER-2", "ER", "PR", "COX-2", "BRCA 1", "BRCA 2", "miRNA", "CSCs" and "CSCs". Only papers written in English and published within the last 20 years, until November 2017, were included. The articles most relevant to our review were selected.

Biomarkers of cancer cell proliferation and apoptosis

An estimation of a tumor's proliferation potential is useful for determining tumor malignancy. A high proliferation rate is related to fast tumor growth and its ability to cause local and distant metastases. Ki-67 and PCNA are biomarkers of proliferation, whereas p53 is a marker of neoplastic transformation and apoptosis.

Ki-67

Ki- 67 is the most studied biomarker of canine tumor proliferation and apoptosis and is detected in many tumor types. In mammary neoplasia, it is the most frequently used prognostic biomarker. Ki-67 is a nuclear, non-histone protein, which can only be detected in the cell nucleus during interphase, and during mitosis. Ki-67 is relocated to the surface of chromosomes. It can already be detected in the G1 phase of the cell cycle and increases in the S and G2 phases. It has the highest expression in the M phase, and its expression disappears rapidly after mitosis [23–28]. In G0 phase it is undetectable. It is a serum as well as a cellular biomarker, and different molecular techniques can be used for measuring its expression [23–30]. Determination of mitotic index (MI) in the hematoxylin and eosin stain routinely used in histology is not as precise as immunohistochemistry (IHC) Ki-67 staining, as MI shows only the number of cells undergoing mitosis, and Ki-67 in IHC staining is expressed in different phases of the cell cycle [26]. It can even be evaluated in cytological samples from a fine needle biopsy of the canine mammary gland, which creates an option for early tumor diagnosis [31].

In human medicine, high expression of Ki-67 in tumor tissues is correlated with a poor prognosis, but at the same time, it has been demonstrated that patients with a high Ki-67 responded well to chemotherapy, probably due to the high proliferative activity [23]. Although it seems to be a good prognostic marker, the American Society of Clinical Oncology does not recommend its use in clinical practice due to the lack of uniformity in laboratory techniques and analysis [32]. Immunohistochemical evaluation of Ki-67 expression, together with the assessment of estrogen receptor (ER), progesterone receptor (PR) and human epidermal growth factor receptor 2 (HER-2) levels, is used to define different subtypes of breast cancer [32].

So far, only one study has been conducted to evaluate its value as a serum biomarker, using a canine-specific ELISA kit for its determination [33]. The Ki-67 was undetectable in healthy dog serum, while serum levels in tumor bearing dogs correlated positively with tumor grade [30]. The levels of Ki-67 in IHC staining (only cells with nuclear staining were recorded as positive) were determined and are significantly lower in benign than in malignant mammary tumors, and high values correlated positively with metastasis, poor prognosis and poor survival [24, 25, 28]. Ki-67 expression is the highest in tumors with poor clinical and histopathological characteristics, such as large tumor size, inflammation and ulceration of the mammary gland, invasion into the surrounding tissues, and metastases to the lymph nodes [25, 34, 35]. Another study demonstrated that the expression level of Ki-67 measured in metastases to lymph nodes had a positive correlation with its expression in the tumor tissue [36]. However, levels of Ki-67 in older bitches tend to be lower than in younger bitches, probably due to the fact that tumor proliferation processes are slower at older ages [25].

This biomarker seems to be very promising; however, more studies on a more homogenous group should be carried out.

PCNA

PCNA is also a marker of the proliferation index (PI). PCNA is an auxiliary protein of DNA polymerase δ, which is expressed in the nuclei of cells during the DNA synthesis phase of the cell division cycle. It is involved in the DNA repair process, cell cycle control, chromatin assembly and in RNA transcription [19, 32]. It increases in the late G1 phase, reaches its peak in the S-phase and remains high in the G2 and M- phases due to its long half-life [26, 37]. It is responsible for maintaining the cell cycle continuity. PCNA has a role on both the leading and lagging strands [32].

In human medicine, PCNA is considered a good proliferation biomarker, but only when evaluated together with other HBC biomarkers, such as ER, PR, Ki-67 or HER-2. The disadvantage of PCNA as a marker is that it is not proliferation specific, but it is also involved in DNA repair [32, 37].

In veterinary medicine, the PCNA level is frequently evaluated in cases of mammary cancer [20]. PCNA expression in IHC staining (cells with nuclear staining were recorded as positive) also has a positive correlation with tumor size, tumor histological type, differentiation grade, nuclear grade, mitotic index, histological grade of malignancy, and lymph node metastasis [29]. Additionally, similar to Ki 67, its expression is greater in tumors that show more malignancy, have a large tumor size, skin ulceration, histological grade II or III, and presence of regional lymph node metastases [29]. In one study, analysis of the expression of PCNA was also confirmed in non-neoplastic, adjacent tissues, suggesting the presence of early micrometastases and higher tumor aggressiveness, which was histologically confirmed [29]. Therefore, the high expression of PCNA is associated with poor disease prognosis and decreased survival [29].

However, it is believed that PCNA expression may be stimulated by cytokines (e.g., transforming growth factor, epidermal growth factor, platelet-derived growth factor) without inducing DNA synthesis and may also be due to PCNA's association with DNA repair. Therefore, its expression may not be specific for cancer. Because of this, it is also recommended to evaluate the expression of PCNA in combination with other biomarkers, especially Ki-67, as its expression is restricted to the cell cycle [26].

Protein p53

P53 is an important biomarker of cell neoplastic transformation, cell division and apoptosis programs [19, 38–43]. This protein is responsible for the control of the cell cycle and apoptosis, and it is a suppressor of tumor development. During the neoplastic process, it accumulates in tumor tissue, and due to its gene mutation, it starts to play a role as an oncogene. Mutations of the p53 gene are thought to be the most common genetic alteration in HBC, as well as CMT [2]. Its mutation is associated with tumor progression [42]. Mutated p53 also stimulates the expression of p21, a protein that belongs to cyclin-dependent kinases. However, other factors can also induce p21 expression independent of p53 [41] Still, the relationship between the expressions of those two important proteins is unclear.

In human patients, a mutation of p53 is found in the majority of HBC, especially in more aggressive types, such as triple negative breast cancer [44, 45]. High expression of p53 correlates positively with a worse prognosis and shorter survival time [45].

In veterinary medicine, high expression of p53 is also generally associated with poor overall survival. Recent studies showed a higher p53 expression in large-breed dogs, suggesting that there may be heritable gene mutations and some breed predispositions, but further studies in this field must be conducted [41].

Both in human and veterinary patients, p53 overexpression (mainly evaluated by IHC in tumor tissues) correlates with an unfavorable prognosis. Although several mutations of p53 have been identified, its functionality is still unclear and there is no evident association between these mutations and incidence of malignant CMT [21].

Biomarkers of metastatic potential of the tumor

Another important group of biomarkers are those that indicate the metastatic potential of the tumor. The ability of the tumor to metastasize depends on the cells adhesions to each other or adjacent tissues. The strength of those connections is measured by the levels of expression of the proteins involved in these processes. There are various types of adhesion molecules, such as integrins, selectins, immunoglobulin-like particles and cadherins. Cadherins are calcium-dependent transmembrane proteins and are good indicators of tumor metastasis. Additionally, CEA and CA 15-3 are glycoproteins involved in intracellular adhesions and represent one of the most often evaluated biomarkers of HBC.

E-cadherin

Cadherins are calcium-dependent transmembrane glycoproteins and are responsible for cell–cell adhesions [46]. Their function is to maintain the normal structure of a tissue. Among cadherins, there are E-, P- and N-cadherin. P-cadherin (placental-cadherin) is expressed in myoepithelial cells, and its overexpression in high-grade tumors suggests tumor aggressiveness and a poor prognosis. However, the most frequently evaluated cadherin is E-cadherin (epithelial-cadherin), which is involved in epithelial cellular adhesion [46].

In human patients, the downregulated expression of E-cadherin is correlated with tumor histological grade, tumor size, and lymph node status, and overall, it is a predictor of a worse prognosis [47]. The loss of E-cadherin expression is a sign of epithelial-mesenchymal transition (EMT), which induces cell dissemination through an increase in cell migration and invasion [48].

In veterinary medicine, because most canine mammary tumors are of epithelial origin, a lowered expression of E-cadherin is related to increased tumor development and disease progression, tumor malignancy, aggressiveness of metastases and short overall survival [19, 30, 46]. E-cadherin binds to a group of interconnected proteins called catenins, often with β-catenin. β-catenin interacts with the cytoplasmic domain of E-cadherin and enables clustering into junctional structures. Any dysfunction of that complex reduces cell adhesion. β-catenin is a cytoplasmic protein that is degraded in the neoplastic process, which results in its accumulation in the cytoplasm and nucleus of tumor cells. Its expression is associated with tumor progression, metastases and a worse prognosis for the patient [20]. Normally, levels of β-catenin expression in blood are determined together with E-cadherin.

In both human and animal patients, low expression of E-cadherin (evaluated by IHC in tumor tissues) is correlated with a worse prognosis; however, it should be evaluated together with other biomarkers, such as Ki67. Nevertheless, it is not the most commonly evaluated biomarker of canine mammary tumors.

CEA

CEA is a glycoprotein that is involved in intracellular adhesion. It is a glycoprotein produced by gastrointestinal mucosa, localized in epithelial cell membranes in small amounts, and it is overexpressed by the cancer cells of the colon, breast and lungs.

In humans, CEA was one of the first identified tumor biomarker of breast cancer [49]. Currently, together with CA 15-3, it is the most frequently used biomarker in HBC [49]. It is usually measured in serum using various immunochemical methods, such as radioimmunological methods (RIA) or electrochemistry luminescence immunoassay (ECL) [49, 52]. There is a positive correlation between changes in CEA blood levels and response to treatment in patients with metastases of breast cancer. It is also a useful marker for early detection of recurrence and metastasis [50–53]. CEA overexpression corresponds positively with tumor clinicopathological features, such as tumor size, tumor grade and lymph node status [52]. However, several studies have confirmed that only results of the measurements of levels of both glycoproteins (CEA and CA 15-3) may be considered sensitive and specific.

In veterinary medicine, there have only been a few studies carried out that have confirmed that CEA is detectable in canine tissues as well [49, 54]. In dogs with mammary gland tumors, serum levels of CEA were elevated compared to healthy dogs [54]. In reference to human CEA serum values, in veterinary medicine, these values are approximately ten times smaller and ranged from 0.00 to 0.23 ng/ml. CEA can be measured in both serum and tissue samples using different molecular techniques. Importantly, human kits can be used to evaluate serum levels of CEA and CA 15-3 [54].

Although it is a commonly used biomarker in human medicine, its usefulness in the early detection of primary breast cancers remains doubtful due to its low sensitivity and specificity. Therefore, only CEA determination, together with Cancer Antigen 15-3 (CA 15-3), may be useful in an early cancer diagnosis in both humans and dogs [52–56]. However, CEA plays an important role in the follow-up. Several studies have agreed that elevated levels of CEA, determined alone or together with CA 15-3, as well as with other biomarkers such as HER 2, may be a factor in recurrences and metastases [51–53, 55]. To confirm its application in veterinary medicine, further studies must be done.

CA 15-3

CA 15-3 (also called Mucin 1 or MUC 1) is a large transmembrane glycoprotein, a product of the *mucin 1* gene, expressed in the apical plasma membrane [56]. However, during malignant transformation, it can be overexpressed on the membrane surface, as well as in the cytoplasm [57]. In humans, it is frequently overexpressed in many adenocarcinomas [56]. This antigen possesses two epitopes that are recognized by two monoclonal antibodies: glycoprotein DF3 *(mucin* 1 derived) and 115d8 [56]. During the malignancy process, MUC1 often acts as an anti-adhesive molecule and enables the detachment of malignant cells; therefore, it increases the metastatic and invasive potential of tumor cells [56].

The CA 15-3 is a very good biomarker for monitoring therapy outcomes and detecting recurrences and metastases in humans. It correlates positively with clinical and pathological tumor features, such as lymph node status, tumor size and disease stage [51]. However, as stated before, it is recommended to determinate CA 15-3 together with CEA. [51–53].

In veterinary medicine, it has been proven that CA 15-3 has a positive correlation with tumor grade (higher CA 15-3 serum concentrations were found in grade II and III carcinomas than in grade I carcinomas) [56]. Additionally, high levels of CA 15-3 were correlated with a poor clinical stage and bad prognosis. Apart from that, studies confirmed that tumor size, skin ulceration, necrosis, inflammation and histological type of mammary cancer have no relation to the serum levels of CA 15–3. CA 15-3 was also expressed in normal mammary tissues, as well as in benign tumor tissues [56].

Although CA 15-3 is the most widely used serum biomarker in patients with breast cancer, due to its low sensitivity, determination of CA 15-3 in the diagnosis of primary breast cancer is precluded. Therefore, it is used in follow-up monitoring, especially when other biomarkers, such as CEA, are evaluated at the same time. In veterinary medicine, published studies were made based on a small number of heterogeneous patients. Therefore, more studies need to be done before it can be considered an adequate biomarker.

Biomarkers of angiogenesis

Every neoplastic process includes the formation of new blood vessels on the base of already existing vessels. This is essential for delivering nutritional supplies for the tumor and maintaining tissues homeostasis [58]. With tumor growth, the angiogenic process is advanced. Therefore, such biomarkers may be crucial for the determination of tumor progress or the presence of metastases. It has been shown that malignant CMT have significantly more blood vessel formation than benign tumors [59]. Common biomarkers of angiogenesis are vascular endothelial growth factor (VEGF), epidermal growth factor receptor (EGFR) and von Willebrand factor VIII or CD 31 [20]. VEGF is a protein, and its expression in tumors is responsible for angiogenesis and lymphangiogenesis, whereas EGFR is a tyrosine kinase receptor and acts as a promotor of cell migration and invasion [20, 60]. Von Willebrand factor VIII is a glycoprotein that participates in platelet adhesion and is expressed in both healthy and neoplastically transformed blood vessel endothelial cells and lymphatic vessels [20]. CD31, also called platelet/endothelial cell adhesion molecule, is a protein that plays a role in inflammatory processes and is expressed in vascular endothelium of arteries, veins and capillary blood vessels [20].

VEGF

VEGF is the most frequently used biomarker in human medicine, as it controls angiogenesis. VEGFs are proteins encoded by four genes: VEGF-A, VEGF-B, VEGF-C and VEGF-D. VEGF-A and VEGF- B are responsible for angiogenesis, whereas VEGF-C and VEGF-D are responsible for lymphangiogenesis [60]. In healthy tissues, VEGF is responsible for the formation of new vessels and regulates their functions and structure. VEGF stimulates cell migration and endothelial proliferation and increases microvascular permeability, which allows cells to escape from the blood vessels and form distant metastases; it also inhibits the regression of newly formed vessels stimulates endothelial cell invasion to form new vessels and, at the same time, inhibits apoptosis [58, 60–63].

In human medicine, increased expression of VEGF (evaluated by IHC in tumor tissues as well as by ELISA in serum samples) is found in different tumors, including: lung, gastric, ovarian, endometrial, and breast. Its overexpression is related to tumor growth and metastasis, while its down-regulation results in suppression of tumor development [64, 65].

In CMT, it has been shown that increased VEGF serum levels correlate positively with a worse clinical stage, bad prognosis and lower survival rate. It is usually increased in cases of more malignant tumors with infiltrative growth. This is why it is considered a marker of tumor development and metastasis. VEGF is also increased in tumors with histologically diagnosed necrosis [61].

In both human and veterinary medicine, VEGF seems to be both a good serum and cellular biomarker. It is especially useful for the early detection of HBC [64, 65], as well as CMT. The same studies also claimed that VEGF sensitivity is increased when combined with CA 15-3 determination.

EGFR (HER 1)

EGFR is a transmembrane tyrosine kinase receptor and belongs to the family of human epidermal growth factor receptors (HER). The family consists of EGFR (HER-1/ErbB-1), HER-2/ErbB-2, HER-3/ErbB-3, and HER-4/ErbB-4, which are usually located on cell membranes. They are transmembrane receptors that contain three domains: an extracellular ligand-binding domain, a transmembrane domain, and an intracellular domain with tyrosine kinase activity [66]. EGFR in malignant tumors is thought to be a promoter of cancer cell migration and invasion [67].

The EGFR increases angiogenesis and metastasis and is associated with poor clinical outcomes in breast cancer patients [68].

Several studies have revealed a role of EGFR in malignant tumor development and progression of the disease in canine mammary tumors [68, 69]. High expression of EGFR (evaluated by IHC in tumor tissues) is associated with a large tumor size, tumor necrosis, high mitotic index, the histological grade of tumor malignancy and a poor clinical stage [68–70]. An association between EGFR expression and the dog's age was also found [69]. There is a positive correlation between EGFR and CD31 and between EGFR and COX-2 expression [68, 70]. The EGFR can regulate the synthesis and secretion of other angiogenic factors, such as VEGF. There are also studies on the use of specific EGFR tyrosine kinase inhibitors in cancer treatment for both humans and dogs [68]. EGFR inhibitors alone or together with COX-2 inhibitors seem to be a good treatment option for advanced malignant CMT.

HER-2

HER-2 is also considered an important tumor marker. HER-2 functions to regulate tumor growth, survival and differentiation. It is expressed in approximately 30% of CMT, which is the same percentage as in HBC [71–75].

In HBC patients, HER-2 overexpression is strongly related to decreased survival [76]. Approximately 30% of all HBC express HER-2 [77]. Therefore, an HER-2 targeted drug, trastuzumab, combined with chemotherapy is often used in the treatment of HBC.

In veterinary medicine, a positive correlation between HER-2 serum (determined by ELISA) and tissue (determined by IHC) expression was noticed [71]. There is also a positive correlation between HER-2 expression and tumor mitotic index, high histological grade and size [72, 74, 78]. It is considered to be a marker of poor prognosis [70, 73]. However, not all studies have confirmed this [66, 71, 72, 79], and no difference between HER-2 expression in benign and malignant tumors was seen [66, 71, 79]. Surprisingly, one study showed that dogs with malignant tumors expressing HER-2 showed a longer survival rate than HER-2-negative dogs [73]. Therefore, HER-2 may participate in tumor formation, but not necessarily in malignant transformation, or at least, it is not a good marker of malignancy.

As there is high homology between human and canine HER-2 antigens, antibody-based immunotherapy with trastuzumab or cetuximab seems to be promising in canine patients with HER-2 expression [75]. In regard to the contradictory research results in veterinary medicine, further studies should be performed [80].

Hormone receptors

Estrogen and progesterone are the most studied biomarkers of CMT [10, 39, 81–101]. Estrogen and progesterone are essential for normal mammary tissue growth and development [97]. Both estrogen and progesterone are thought also to have an influence on tumor growth. The majority of CMT (benign and malignant) express ER and/or PR [86]. Additionally, prolactin and growth hormones were found to be involved in the process of tumor growth [94, 97].

HBC can either have a low or high steroid hormone expression. HBC with low expressions of ER and PR are not sensitive to endocrine therapy and are related to a poor prognosis, whereas HBC with a high expression of these steroid hormones have slightly better clinical outcomes [84, 92]. Both receptors are only detected in epithelial tumor cells [97]. Expression of ER and PR, together with HER-2, is evaluated to estimate HBC staging and improves prognostic accuracy. ER and PR targeted therapies, such as tamoxifen treatment, improve survival in women with hormone receptor-positive breast cancer [101].

In veterinary medicine, some studies have shown that the expression of one or both receptors was more frequent in benign tumors, and in general, its expression was related to a more favorable prognosis [87, 89, 91]. Though, in other studies, increased levels of estrogen, progesterone and prolactin were found in cases of malignant neoplasms [81, 95]. In one study, both serum and tissue steroid hormone expression (both determined by competitive EIA) was increased in patients with malignant tumors and a poor prognosis [95]. A recent study revealed that estrogen-negative (ER−) and progesterone-positive (PR+) tumors were correlated with a worse clinical outcome than ER+ and PR+ tumors, but at the same time, ER- and PR- tumors had the worst prognostic factor of all [86]. Another study showed that dogs with grade 2, ER− positive tumors as well as dogs with increased serum E2 level are likely to benefit from OHE [15].

Determination of both ER and PR expression should always be considered in cases of HBC as well as CMT. Nevertheless, sex hormone targeted therapy does not seem to play an important role in CMT, as it does in HBC, probably due to the appearance of multiple estrogenic side effects, such as vulva edema, purulent vaginal discharge and pyometra [102, 103]. However, in one study, safe doses of tamoxifen in canine mammary neoplasias were recommended [103]. Still, more studies concerning the efficacy of this selective estrogen-receptor modulator in the treatment of CMT must be carried out.

Biomarkers of inflammation

Chronic inflammation is always present during neoplastic processes. Inflammatory cells secrete pro-inflammatory mediators, such as cytokines and chemokines, some of which promote angiogenesis and consequently tumor growth [104]. We only briefly describe the most commonly evaluated biomarkers of inflammation in CMT.

Cox-2

The cyclooxygenase enzyme catalyzes the prostaglandin biosynthesis from arachnoid acid. Many studies have confirmed that prostaglandins play an important role in the tumor's development. Deregulation of the enzymatic pathway of prostaglandin E2 formation is strongly related to neoplasm progression [105]. There are two isoforms: cyclooxygenase 1 (COX-1) and cyclooxygenase 2 (COX-2), but they have different biological functions. COX-1 is expressed in normal tissues and is responsible for the control of renal function, reproduction and, among other things, cytoprotection of the stomach. COX-2 is undetectable in normal tissues; it is expressed in tissue due to inflammatory reactions, growth factors, tumor promoters and oncogenes.

In human medicine, COX-2 overexpression is associated with the risk of tumor recurrence, advanced cancer stage, presence of metastases and poor overall survival in patients with HBC, as well as in ovarian, pancreatic, and gastric cancers, among others [106]. COX-2 inhibitors are used in the treatment of HBC [76].

In veterinary medicine, many studies have proven the presence of COX-2 expression in mammary tumors, as well as in some normal mammary tissues [5, 61, 104–115]. In mouse models of mammary neoplasias, COX-2 inhibitors suppress tumor growth [108]. The COX-2 expression (determined by IHC) is higher in cases of malignant CMT than in benign CMT [5, 105]. Tumors that express COX-2 may be treated with COX-2 inhibitors, such as meloxicam or piroxicam (they inhibit cell proliferation and angiogenesis) [111]. However, the mechanism of their antiproliferative effect is still unclear [111]. One study demonstrated that bitches with inflammatory mammary carcinoma treated with piroxicam had better outcomes than bitches treated with traditional chemotherapy [106].

In both human and veterinary medicine, selective COX-2 inhibitors are useful in the treatment of HBC, as well as CMT, but combination with other antitumor drugs is necessary. To obtain good treatment results with COX-2 inhibitors, the expression of COX-2 in tumors should be previously determined.

Mutations of BRCA1 and BRCA2 genes

Among multiple gene mutations, the mutations of BRCA1 and BRCA2 turned out to play very important roles in the formation of both human and canine tumors of the mammary gland. The BRCA1 gene is located on human chromosome 17q21 and is expressed in many mammalian tissues. It encodes a nuclear phosphoprotein that participates in the regulation of the cell cycle of mammary epithelial cells. The loss of BRCA1 expression results in defective DNA repair, abnormal cell cycle, increased apoptosis and tumorigenesis. It was found that BRCA 1 is a tumor suppressor gene [116].

In human medicine, many gene mutations were found in cases of HBC. Mutations in BRCA1 and BRCA2 are hereditary, and affected women have a risk of 56–84% of developing HBC [116]. Statistically, approximately 5–10% of all breast cancers in women are due to mutations in BRCA1 and BRCA2 genes [117]. BRCA1 mutations are associated with tumors of a higher grade and may also indicate ovarian cancer. Interestingly, BRCA 2 was also found in cases of male breast cancer [117].

In veterinary medicine, hereditary patterns of CMT are still under investigation, but several breeds are thought to be predisposed to CMT [117]. In one study, mutations in ten different genes associated with breast cancer were evaluated in CMT (by iPLEX genotyping of sixty-three single nucleotide polymorphisms), but only BRCA1 and BRCA2 were significantly associated with the development of this tumor [117]. BRCA1 was especially associated with malignant tumors (reduced nuclear expression), which was also confirmed in previous studies [118]. There was no difference in BRCA2 expression between benign and malignant tumors [117]. However, in another study, reduced expression of BRCA2 was found in CMT compared to normal mammary tissues [116].

Although, BRCA1 and BRCA2 have been studied for a long time, little is still known about their exact mutations and the functional mechanism that reduces their expression in mammary neoplasias in both humans and dogs. Further studies of the canine genome and its mutations should be carried out.

MiRNA

MiRNAs are small, non-coding molecules involved in the post-transcriptional negative regulation of gene expression. Numerous studies have indicated that the level of miRNA expression is altered in several types of cancer, even within the same tumor. However, different miRNA expression profiles can be observed for cancer's various stages. MiRNAs were found to participate in nearly all important cellular processes, such as the regulation of cell proliferation, differentiation, angiogenesis, migration and apoptosis [119]. There is also strong evidence that miRNAs act as oncogenes or tumor suppressor genes [119, 120]. They can act as both serum or tissue biomarkers.

In human medicine, many studies have been done on miRNA expression in HBC. Several miRNAs were found to have diagnostic potential (miR-9, miR-10b and mir-17-5p), while others had a prognostic potential (mi-R-148a and miR-335) [121, 122]. Some miRNAs were found to have multiple roles in the diagnosis, prognosis and prediction of therapeutic response in HBC.

In veterinary medicine, a few analyses of the miRNA expression levels in tissues of canine mammary tumors (CMT) have been published [119, 120, 123, 124]. In one study, nine of ten miRNAs studied (miR-15a, miR-16, miR-17-5p, miR-21, miR-29b, miR-125b, miR-145, miR-155, miR-181b, let-7f) that are involved in human breast cancer appeared to have the same expression pattern in CMTs [119]. Different miRNA expression patterns (determined by qRT_PCR) have been observed in different tumor types: miR-15a and miR-16 showed a significant down-regulation in canine ductal carcinomas, while miR-181b, miR-21, miR-29b and miRlet-7f were strongly up-regulated in canine tubular papillary carcinomas [119]. In another study, the suitability of 16 miRNAs to distinguish between different stages of CMT was analyzed [123]. It was shown that metastatic cells differed from primary tumors cells in terms of mir-29b, miR-101, miR-125a, miR-143 and miR-145 levels of expression [123]. Recent studies have also indicated that microRNA expression differs significantly between metastatic and non-metastatic tumors, making it a good metastasis biomarker [120]. Studies of miRNA expression in canine mammary cancer cell lines have also shown its altered expression [124, 125].

Evaluation of miRNA is a very novel, but promising, method of cancer diagnosis. The fact that dogs follow similar miRNA expression patterns to those of humans suggests that further studies can be carried out on canine models. Recent studies in cancer patients suggest that multiple miRNA-based profiles may be very useful in the diagnosis and prognosis of both HBC and CMT, and miRNA-based drugs seem to be a promising targeted therapy for those tumors.

Cancer stem cells

CSCs, also called tumor-initiating cells (TICs), are a small subpopulation of tumor cells that have the ability to renew themselves, as well as differentiate into different cancer cells [125]. They are thought to be responsible for drug, chemotherapy and radiotherapy resistance, tumor recurrence and metastasis [125–128]. The origin of CSCs is still unclear. It is thought that they result from the malignant transformation of normal stem cells, dedifferentiation of mature cancer cells or induction of pluripotent cancer cells [126]. Identification and isolation of these cells has become an opportunity for new therapeutic strategies [127].

In human medicine, CSCs are well-described and identified by several molecular methods. They express several cell surface antigens, such as CD44, CD24 and EPCAM, which facilitate its identification. The CD44+/CD24− phenotype of CSCs has often been evaluated and was found to be related to a poor prognosis [128, 129].

It has been demonstrated that canine mammary CSC express similar surface markers to human breast CSC, and they are resistant to chemotherapy and radiotherapy [126]. The CD44+/CD24− phenotype of CSCs has been associated with high-grade canine mammary carcinoma [128]. In another study, a significant deregulation of 33 miRNAs was found in canine CSCs isolated from different CMC cell lines [127].

Due to the similar biological behavior of canine mammary and human breast CSCs, studies on canine models may result in useful breast cancer research. Nevertheless, the lack of a universal method for CSC detections, as well as the multiple phenotypes of CSCs and their heterogenic and dynamic nature, makes their exploitation as a diagnostic tool difficult to predict and assess.

Circulating tumor cells

CTCs are tumor cells that are found in the peripheral blood, originating from either the primary tumor or its metastases. Therefore, they possess antigenic or genetic characteristics of specific tumor types [130]. Their presence is necessary for the development of distant metastases, so they may play an important role as biomarkers of a tumor's metastatic potential.

In HBC, the detection of CTC is helpful in disease monitoring. CTCs can be counted in blood samples using CTC kits on the FDA-approved CellSearch System [131]. A correlation was found between the number of detected CTCs and a shorter overall survival in women with metastatic breast cancer [131, 132]. At the same time, decreasing the number of CTC was correlated with disease regression [133].

In veterinary medicine, just a few studies have been carried out so far, though a set of potential CTCs was found [130, 134]. The CTCs were identified through the expression of six specific genes: AGR2, ATP8B1, CRYAB, F3 IRX3 and SLC1A1 using DNA microarrays [134]. CRYAB was found to have the highest specificity and moderate sensitivity for CTC detection [130].

To understand the usefulness of these promising markers, further studies are required. However, CRYAB appears to be a good marker for detection of CTCs in dogs with metastasis of CMT.

Conclusions

Over the past few decades, many studies concerning biomarkers of the mammary glands have been carried out in both human and veterinary patients. However, no ideal biomarker has yet been found. A perfect biomarker should be easily measured in the blood, and its concentrations should only be elevated in cases of malignant tumors. Second, it should be tumor-specific, and its measurement should give a clear prognosis. Serum biomarkers have the advantage over tissue biomarkers, as the procedure of measurement is non-invasive, and they show dynamic changes of physiological and pathological states before the clinical signs appear. Therefore, they may be used for the early detection of cancers.

Although many studies have been carried out concerning the clinical application of mammary tumor biomarkers, no productive conclusions have been drawn. Human biomarkers of HBC have proven to be detectable in CMT; therefore, this enables clinical diagnostic and treatment options for bitches suffering from this disease.

In both human and veterinary medicine, the most promising group of HBC and CMT biomarkers are miRNAs due to their high specificity and sensitivity. MiRNAs can act as oncogenes, as well as tumor suppressor genes, and different miRNA expression levels are altered in cases of both HBC and CMT. They can be measured in both blood and tissues, so they are very useful.

The evaluation of cancer stem cells as a tissue biomarker is also very novel, but due to their multiple phenotypes and lack of a universal method for their estimation, they are not a very precise biomarker. Nevertheless, in human medicine, this tissue biomarker helps to choose new therapeutic strategies, as many CSCs show resistance to radiotherapy as well as chemotherapy.

Circulating tumor cells may act as good serum biomarkers of tumor metastatic potential in humans, but in veterinary medicine, further studies must be done.

Recently, also collagen signatures turned out to be a good prognostic biomarker and potential target for treatment as its expression (collagen density, fiber width, length and straightness) inversely correlates with patient overall survival time [135].

The mutations of BRCA1 and BRCA2 in human medicine are hereditary and an indicator of a high possibility of high-grade breast cancer development. In dogs; however, similar mutations were found and seemed to be related with tumor formation have still not been proven to be hereditary. More detailed studies concerning gene mutation inheritance and the influence of BRCA1 and BRCA2 mutations on the grade of CMT should be done.

Up to now, it seems that the most studied and reliable biomarkers of CMT are Ki-67, EGFR, HER-2, ER, PR and COX-2, which can be detected in both serum and tissue samples using different molecular methods. In human medicine, those biomarkers are also evaluated; however, they are evaluated less frequently each time due to the application of newer biomarkers. Still, particularly if more than one of these biomarkers are evaluated, they can act as a reliable prognostic biomarker.

Notably, CEA and CA 15-3, which can be measured in tissues as well as in blood, while poorly studied, seem to be good biomarkers, especially for the early detection and prognosis of CMT. In human medicine, it has been proven that if those biomarkers are evaluated together, they have quite a high specificity and sensitivity, especially in the follow-up of the patients.

The evaluation of PCNA, protein p53, E-cadherin and VEGF, only if evaluated with the abovementioned biomarkers, may be useful. In summary, it is always recommended to evaluate more than one biomarker in order to obtain more reliable results.

Nevertheless, most of the studies were conducted on small groups of patients and/or very heterogeneous groups, using different molecular techniques. Therefore, the results are not truly reliable. More detailed studies should be carried out in the near future. So far, all abovementioned biomarkers seem to have certain prognostic potential in CMT. In cases of CMT, the evaluation of some biomarkers should always be considered.

Abbreviations

BRCA1: breast cancer 1 gene; BRCA2: breast cancer 2 gene; CA15-3: cancer antigen 15-3; CEA: carcinoembryonic antigen; COX-1: cyclooxygenase 1; COX-2: cyclooxygenase 2; CMT: canine mammary tumors; CSCs: cancer stem cells; CTCs: circulating tumor cells; E-cadherin: epithelial cadherin; EGFR: endothelial growth factor receptor; ER: estrogen receptor; HER2: human epidermal growth factor receptor 2; HBC: human breast cancers; Ki-67: antigen Ki-67; miRNAs: microRNAs; OHE: ovariohysterectomy; p53: tumor protein p53; P-cadherin: placental cadherin; PCNA: proliferative cell nuclear antigen; PR: progesterone receptor; N-cadherin: neural cadherin; VEGF: vascular endothelial growth factor.

Authors' contributions

IK reviewed the literature and wrote the main body of the manuscript. AR, SK, and KK helped in reviewing the literature and designing the manuscript. MK and PJ critically reviewed and substantially contributed to the final draft of the manuscript. All authors read and approved the final manuscript.

Author details

[1] Department of Small Animal Diseases with Clinic, Veterinary Medicine Faculty, Warsaw University of Life Sciences, Nowoursynowska 166, 02-787 Warsaw, Poland. [2] Department of Physiological Sciences, Veterinary Medicine Faculty, Warsaw University of Life Sciences, Nowoursynowska 166, 02-787 Warsaw, Poland.

Competing interests

The authors declare that they have no competing interests.

Funding

Publication was funded by KNOW (Leading National Research Centre) Scientific Consortium "Healthy Animal- Safe Food", decision of Ministry of Science and Higher Education No. 05-1/KNOW2/2015.

References

1. National Cancer Institute: http://www.cancer.gov. Accessed 10 Oct 2017.
2. Sorenmo K. Canine mammary gland tumors. Vet Clin Am Small Anim Pract. 2003;33:573–96.
3. Salas Y, Marquez A, Diaz D, Romero L. Epidemiological study of mammary tumors in female dogs diagnosed during the period 2002–2012. A growing animal health problem. PLoS ONE. 2015. https://doi.org/10.1371/journal.pone.0127381.
4. Reddy GBM, Kumar P, Kumar R, Pawaiya RVS, Ravindran R. Histopathological classification and incidence of canine mammary tumours. Indian J Vet Pathol. 2009;33:152–5.
5. Benavente MA, Bianchi CP, Aba MA. Canine mammary tumors: risk factors, prognosis and treatments. J Vet Adv. 2016;6:1291–300.
6. Weigelt B, Geyer FC, Reis-Filho JS. Histological types of breast cancer: how special are they? Mol Oncol. 2010;4:192–208.
7. Goldshmidt M, Pena L, Rasotto R, Zappulli V. Classification and grading of canine mammary tumors. Vet Pathol. 2011;48:117–31.
8. Beauvais W, Cardwell JM, Brodbelt DC. The effect of neutering on the risk of mammary tumours in dogs –a systematic review. J Small Anim Pract. 2012;53:314–22.
9. Sorenmo K, Shofer FS, Goldschmidt MH. Effect of spaying and timing of spaying on survival of dogs with mammary carcinoma. J Vet Intern Med. 2000;14:266–70.
10. Chang CC, Tsai MH, Liao JW. Evaluation of hormone receptor expression for use in predicting survival of female dogs with malignant mammary gland tumors. J Am Vet Med Assoc. 2009;235:391–6.
11. Santos AA, Lopes CC, Ribeiro JR. Identification of prognostic factors in canine mammary malignant tumours: a multivariable survival study. BMC Vet Res. 2013;9:1.
12. Perez Alenza MD, Pena L, Del Castillo N. Factors influencing the incidence and prognosis of canine mammary tumors. J Small Anim Pract. 2000;41:287–91.
13. Sarli G, Preziosi R, Benazzi C. Prognostic value of histologic stage and proliferative activity in canine malignant mammary tumors. J Vet Diagn Invest. 2002;14:25–34.
14. Tavasoly A, Golshahi H, Rezaie A. Classification and grading of canine malignant mammary tumors. Vet Res Forum. 2013;4:25–30.
15. Kristiansen VM, Pena L, Diez Cordova L, Illera JC, Skjerve E, Breen AM, et al. Effect of ovariohysterectomy at the time of tumor removal in dogs with mammary carcinomas: a randomized controlled trial. J Vet Intern Med. 2016;30:230–41.
16. Cassali GD, Lavalle GE, De Nardi AB, Ferreira E, Bertagnolli AC, Estrela-Lima A, et al. Consensus for the diagnosis, prognosis and treatment of canine mammary tumors. Braz J Vet Pathol. 2011;4:153–80.
17. Mobasheri A, Cassidy J. Biomarkers in veterinary medicine: towards targeted, individualised therapies for companion animals. Vet J. 2010;185:1–3.
18. Henry JC. Biomarkers in veterinary cancer screening: applications, limitations and expectations. Vet J. 2010;185:10–4.
19. Pena L, Gama A, Goldschmidt MH, Abadie J, Benazzi C, Castagnaro M, et al. Canine mammary tumors: a review and consensus of standard guidelines on epithelial and myoepithelial phenotype markers, HER2, and hormone receptor assessment using immunohistochemistry. Vet Pathol. 2014;51:127–45.

20. Kandefer-Gola M, Nowak M, Ciaputa R. Usefulness of immunohistochemical indicators for diagnosis and prognosis of poorly differentiated tumours. J Vet Res. 2016;60:323–30.
21. Klopfleisch R, von Euler H, Sarli G. Molecular carcinogenesis of canine mammary tumors: news from an old disease. Vet Pathol. 2011;48:98–116.
22. Noronha Toledo G, Del Aguila Silva P, Nascimento Borges B. Specific cellular biomarkers for canine's breast cancer: literature review. Rev Cienc Agrar. 2016;59:212–8.
23. Emi Tokuda MD, Yoshiya Horimoto MD, Atsushi Arakawa MD, Himuro T, Senuma K, Nakai K, et al. Differences in Ki67 expressions between pre- and post-neoadjuvant chemotherapy specimens might predict early recurrence of breast cancer. Hum Pathol. 2017;63:40–5.
24. Gizinski S, Boryczko Z, Katkiewicz M. Ki-67 protein as a prognostic factor in mammary gland tumors in female dogs. Med Weter. 2003;59:888–91.
25. Nowak M, Madej JA, Pula B. Expression of matrix metalloproteinase 2 (MMP-2), E-cadherin and Ki-67 in metastatic and non-metastatic canine mammary carcinomas. Ir Vet J. 2015;69:9.
26. Pena L, Nieto A, Perez-Alenza D. Immunohistochemical detection of Ki-67 and PCNA in canine mammary tumors: relationship to clinical and pathologic variables. J Vet Diagn Invest. 1998;10:237–46.
27. Zuccari DA, Santana AE, Cury PM. Immunocytochemical study of Ki-67 as a prognostic marker in canine mammary neoplasia. Vet Clin Pathol. 2004;33:23–8.
28. Queiroga FL, Raposo T, Carvalho MI. Canine mammary tumours as a model to study human breast cancer: most recent findings. Vivo. 2011;25:455–66.
29. Carvalho MI, Pires I, Prada J. Ki-67 and PCNA expression in canine mammary tumors and adjacent nonneoplastic mammary glands: prognostic impact by a multivariate survival analysis. Vet Pathol. 2016;53:1138–46.
30. Nowak M, Madej JA, Dziegiel P. Expression of E-cadherin, β-catenin and Ki-67 antigen and their reciprocal relationships in mammary adenocarcinomas in bitches. Folia Histochem Cytobiol. 2007;45:233–8.
31. Choi US, Kim DY. Immunocytochemical detection of Ki-67 in Diff-Quik-stained cytological smears of canine mammary gland tumours. Cytopathology. 2011;22:115–20.
32. Jurikovaa M, Danihelb L, Polaka S. Ki67, PCNA, and MCM proteins: markers of proliferation in the diagnosis of breast cancer. Acta Histochem. 2016;118:544–52.
33. Neumann S, Schuettler J, Frenz M. Investigation of serum Ki-67 as a biomarker in tumor-bearing dogs. Res Vet Sci. 2017;110:16–21.
34. Lohr CV, Teifke JP, Failing K. Characterization of the proliferative state in canine mammary tumors by the standardized AgNOR method with postfixation and immunohistologic detection of Ki-67 and PCNA. Vet Pathol. 1997;34:212–21.
35. Rodrigues H, Carvalho MI, Pires I. Clinicopathological significance of caspase-3 and ki-67 expression in canine mammary gland tumours. Acta Vet Hung. 2016;64:78–89.
36. Araujo MR, Campos LC, Damasceno KA. HER-2, EGFR, Cox-2 and Ki67 expression in lymph node metastasis of canine mammary carcinomas: association with clinical-pathological parameters and overall survival. Res Vet Sci. 2016;106:121–30.
37. Zacchetti A, Van Garderen E, Teske E, Nederbragt H, Dierendonck JH, Rutteman GR. Validation of the use of proliferation markers in canine neoplastic and non-neoplastic tissues: comparison of Ki-67 and proliferating cell nuclear antigen (PCNA) expression versus in vivo bromodeoxyuridine labelling by immunohistochemistry. APMIS. 2003;111:430–8.
38. Dileepkumar KM, Maiti SK, Naveen K. Expression of p-53 and Cox-2 genes as tumour markers in spontaneous canine mammary tumours. Adv Anim Vet Sci. 2016;4:294–300.
39. Dolka I, Motyl T, Malicka E. Relationship between receptors for insulin-like growth factor-I, steroid hormones and apoptosis-associated proteins in canine mammary tumors. Pol J Vet Sci. 2011;14:245–51.
40. Kumaraguruparan R, Prathiba D, Nagini S. Of humans and canines: immunohistochemical analysis of PCNA, Bcl-2, p53, cytokeratin and ER in mammary tumours. Res Vet Sci. 2006;81:218–24.
41. Klopfleisch R, Gruber AD. Differential expression of cell cycle regulators p21, p27 and p53 in metastasizing canine mammary adenocarcinomas versus normal mammary glands. Res Vet Sci. 2009;87:91–6.
42. Lee CH, Kim WH, Lim JH. Mutation and overexpression of p53 as a prognostic factor in canine mammary tumors. J Vet Sci. 2004;5:63–9.
43. Rodo A, Malicka E. Immunohistochemical expression of protein p53 in neoplasms of the mammary gland in bitches. Pol J Vet Sci. 2008;11:89–95.
44. Pala EE, Bayol U, Keskin EU, Ozguzer A, Kucuk U, Ozer O, et al. Determination of HER2 and p53 mutations by sequence analysis method and EGFR/Chromosome 7 gene status by fluorescence in situ hybridization for the predilection of targeted therapy modalities in immunohistochemically triple negative breast carcinomas in Turkish population. Pathol Oncol Res. 2015;21:1223–7.
45. Pan Y, Yuan Y, Liu G. P53 and Ki-67 as prognostic markers in triple- negative breast cancer patients. PLoS ONE. 2017. https://doi.org/10.1371/journal.pone.0172324.
46. Matos AJ, Lopes C, Carvalheira J. E-cadherin expression in canine malignant mammary tumors: relationship to other clinico-pathological variables. J Comp Pathol. 2006;134:182–9.
47. Gama A, Paredes J, Gartner F, Alves A, Schmitt F. Expression of E-cadherin, P-cadherin and β-cadherin in canine malignant mammary tumours in relation to clinicopathological parameters, proliferation and survival. Vet J. 2008;177:45–53.
48. Li Z, Yin S, Zhang L. Prognostic value of reduced E-cadherin expression in breast cancer: a meta-analysis. Oncotarget. 2017;8:16445–55.
49. Ledecky V, Valencakova Agyagosova A, Lepej J. Determination of carcinoembryonic antigen and cancer antigen values with the radioimmunoassay method in healthy females dogs. Vet Med (Praha). 2013;58:277–83.
50. Di Gioia D, Blankenburg I, Nagel D. Tumor markers in the early detection of tumor recurrence in breast cancer patients: CA 125, CYFRA 21-1, HER2 shed antigen, LDH and CRP in combination with CEA and CA 15-3. Clin Chim Acta. 2016;461:1–7.
51. Pedersen AC, Sorensen PD, Jacobsen EH. Sensitivity of CA 15-3, CEA and serum HER2 in the early detection of recurrence of breast cancer. Clin Chem Lab Med. 2013;51:1511–9.
52. Shao Y, Sun X, He Y. Elevated levels of serum tumor markers CEA and CA15-3 are prognostic parameters for different molecular subtypes of breast cancer. PLoS ONE. 2015. https://doi.org/10.1371/journal.pone.0133830.
53. Stieber P, Nagel D, Blankenburg I, Heinemann V, Untch M, Bauerfeind I, et al. Diagnostic efficacy of CA 15-3 and CEA in the early detection of metastatic breast cancer—a retrospective analysis of kinetics on 743 breast cancer patients. Clin Chim Acta. 2015;448:228–31.
54. Campos LC, Lavalle GE, Estrela-Lima A, Melgaco de Faira JC, Guimaraes JE, Dutra AP, et al. CA15.3, CEA, and LDH in dogs with malignant mammary tumors. J Vet Int Med. 2012;26:1383–8.
55. Moazzezy N, Farahany TZ, Oloomi M. Relationship between preoperative serum CA15-3 and CEA levels and clinicopathological parameters in breast cancer. Asian Pac J Cancer Prev. 2014;15:1685–8.
56. Manuali E, De Giuseppe A, Feliziani F, Forti K, Casciari C, Marchesi MC, et al. CA 15–3 cell lines and tissue expression in canine mammary cancer and the correlation between serum levels and tumour histological grade. BMC Vet Res. 2012;8:86.
57. Duffy MJ, Evoy D, McDermott EW. CA 15-3: uses and limitation as a biomarker for breast cancer. Clin Chim Acta. 2010;411:1869–74.
58. Gobbe Moschetta M, Bazela Maschio L, Victorasso Jardim-Perassi B, Gelaleti GB, Lopes JR, Leonel C, et al. Prognostic value of vascular endothelial growth factor and hypoxia-inducible factor 1α in canine malignant mammary tumors. Oncol Rep. 2015;33:2345–53.
59. Sleeckx N, Van Brantegem L, Van den Eynden G, Fransen E, Casteleyn C, Van Cruchten S, et al. Angiogenesis in canine mammary tumours: a morphometric and prognostic study. J Comp Pathol. 2014;150:175–83.
60. Milanta F, Caneschi V, Ressel L. Expression of vascular endothelial growth factor in canine inflammatory and non-inflammatory mammary carcinoma. J Comp Pathol. 2010;142:36–42.
61. Queiroga F, Pires I, Parente M. COX-2 over-expression correlates with VEGF and tumour angiogenesis in canine mammary cancer. Vet J. 2011;189:77–82.
62. Restucci B, Papparella S, Maiolino P. Expression of vascular endothelial growth factor in canine mammary tumors. Vet Pathol. 2002;39:488–93.
63. Santos AA, Oliveira JT, Lopes CC, Amorim IF, Vincente CM, Gartner FR, et al. Immunohistochemical expression of vascular endothelial growth factor in canine mammary tumours. J Comp Pathol. 2010;143:268–75.

64. Zajkowska M, Glazewska EK, Będkowska GE. Diagnostic power of vascular endothelial growth factor and macrophage colony-stimulating factor in breast cancer patients based on ROC analysis. Mediators Inflamm. 2016. https://doi.org/10.1155/2016/5962946.
65. Lawicki S, Zajkowska M, Glazewska EK. Plasma levels and diagnostic utility of VEGF, MMP-2 and TIMP-2 in the diagnostics of breast cancer patients. Onco Targets Ther. 2016;9:911–9.
66. Kim JH, Im KS, Kim NH. Expression of HER-2 and nuclear localization of HER-3 protein in canine mammary tumors: histopathological and immunohistochemical study. Vet. J. 2011;189:318–22.
67. Masuda H, Zhang D, Bartholomeusz C. Role of epidermal growth factor receptor in breast cancer. Breast Cancer Res Treat. 2012;136:331–45.
68. Carvalho MI, Guimaraes MJ, Pires I, Prada J, Silva-Carvalho R, Lopes C, et al. EGFR and microvessel density in canine malignant mammary tumours. Res Vet Sci. 2013;95:1094–9.
69. Gama A, Gartner F, Alves A. Immunohistochemical expression of epidermal growth factor receptor (EGFR) in canine mammary tissues. Res Vet Sci. 2009;87:432–7.
70. Guimaraes MJ, Carvalho MI, Pires I, Prada J, Gli AG, Lopes C, et al. Concurrent expression of cyclo-oxygenase-2 and epidermal growth factor receptor in canine malignant mammary tumours. J Comp Pathol. 2014;150:27–34.
71. Campos LC, Silva JO, Santos FS, Araujo MR, Lavalle GE, Ferreira E, et al. Prognostic significance of tissue and serum HER2 and MUC1 in canine mammary cancer. J Vet Diagn Invest. 2015;27:531–5.
72. Dutra AP, Granja NV, Schmitt FC. c-erbB-2 expression and nuclear pleomorphism in canine mammary tumors. Braz J Med Biol Res. 2004;37:1673–81.
73. Hsu WL, Huang HM, Liao JW. Increased survival in dogs with malignant mammary tumours overexpressing HER-2 protein and detection of a silent single nucleotide polymorphism in the canine HER-2 gene. Vet J. 2009;180:116–23.
74. Muhammadnejad A, Keyhani E, Mortazavi P. Overexpression of HER-2/neu in malignant mammary tumors; translation of clinicopathological features from dog to human. Asian Pac J Cancer Prev. 2012;13:6415–21.
75. Singer J, Weichselbaumer M, Stockner T, Mechtcheriakova D, Sobanov Y, Bajna E, et al. Comparative oncology: ErbB-1 and ErbB-2 homologues in canine cancer are susceptible to cetuximab and trastuzumab targeting. Mol Immunol. 2012;50:200–9.
76. De Pedro M, Baeza S, Escudero MT, Dierssen-Sotos T, Gomez-Acebo I, Pollan M, et al. Effect of COX-2 inhibitors and other non-steroidal inflammatory drugs on breast cancer risk: a meta-analysis. Breast Cancer Res Treat. 2015;149:525–36.
77. Worzfeld T, Swiercz JM, Looso M. ErbB-2 signals through Plexin-B1 to promote breast cancer metastasis. J Clin Invest. 2012;122:1296–305.
78. Silva ILD, Dias APM, Bertagnolli AC. Analysis of EGFR and HER-2 expressions in ductal carcinomas in situ in canine mammary glands. Arq Bras Med Vet Zootec. 2014;66:763–8.
79. Ressel L, Puleio R, Loria GR, Vannozzi I, Millanta F, Caracappa S, et al. HER-2 expression in canine morphologically normal, hyperplastic and neoplastic mammary tissues and its correlation with the clinical outcome. Res Vet Sci. 2013;94:299–305.
80. Burrai GP, Tanca A, De Miglio MR, Abbondio M, Pisanu S, Polinas M, et al. Investigation of HER2 expression in canine mammary tumors by antibody-based, transcriptomic and mass spectrometry analysis: is the dog a suitable animal model for human breast cancer? Tumour Biol. 2015;36:9083–91.
81. Caceres S, Peña L, Silvan G, Illera MJ, Woodward WA, Reuben JM, et al. Steroid tumor environment in male and female mice model of canine and human inflammatory breast cancer. Biomed Res Int. 2016. https://doi.org/10.1155/2016/8909878.
82. De Andres PJ, Caceres S, Clemente M. Profile of steroid receptors and increased aromatase immunoexpression in canine inflammatory mammary cancer as a potential therapeutic target. Reprod Domest Anim. 2016;51:269–75.
83. De las Mulas M, Millan Y, Dios R. A prospective analysis of immunohistochemically determined estrogen receptor and progesterone receptor expression and host and tumor factors as predictors of disease-free period in mammary tumors of the dog. Vet Pathol. 2005;42:200–12.
84. Dowsett M, Houghton J, Iden C, Salter J, Farndon J, A'Hern R, et al. Benefit from adjuvant tamoxifen therapy in primary breast cancer patients according oestrogen receptor, progesterone receptor, EGF receptor and HER2 status. Ann Oncol. 2006;17:818–26.
85. Illera JC, Perez-Alenza MD, Nieto A, Jimenez MA, Silvan G, Dunner S, et al. Steroids and receptors in canine mammary cancer. Steroids. 2006;71:541–8.
86. Kim NH, Lim KY, Im KS. Evaluation of clinicopathological characteristics and oestrogen receptor gene expression in oestrogen receptor-negative, progesterone receptor- positive canine mammary carcinomas. J Comp Pathol. 2014;151:42–50.
87. Mainenti M, Rasotto R, Carnier P. Oestrogen-α and progesterone receptor expression in subtypes of canine mammary tumours in intact and ovariectomised dogs. Vet J. 2014;202:62–8.
88. Manee-in S, Srisuwatanasagul S, Lohachit C. The number of ERa and PR in the mammary glands of bitches with and without tumor mass using immunohistochemical assay. Comp Clin Pathol. 2009;18:221–7.
89. Millanta F, Calandrella M, Bari G. Comparison of steroid receptor expression in normal, dysplastic, and neoplastic canine and feline mammary tissues. Res Vet Sci. 2005;79:225–32.
90. Mohr A, Ripolli LF, Hammer SC, Willenbrock S, Hewicker-Trautwein M, Kielbowicz Z, et al. Hormone receptor expression analyses in neoplastic and non neoplastic canine mammary tissue by a bead based multiplex branched DNA assay: a gene expression study in fresh frozen and formalin-fixed, paraffin-embedded samples. PLoS ONE. 2016. https://doi.org/10.1371/journal.pone.0163311.
91. Nieto A, Pena L, Perez-Alenza MD. Immunohistologic detection of estrogen receptor alpha in canine mammary tumors: clinical and pathologic associations and prognostic significance. Vet Pathol. 2000;37:239–47.
92. Osborne CK, Schiff R, Arpino G. Endocrine responsiveness: understanding how progesterone receptor can be used to select endocrine therapy. Breast. 2005;14:458–65.
93. Port Louis LR, Varshney KC, Nair MG. An immunohistochemical study on the expression of sex steroid receptors in canine mammary tumors. ISRN Vet Sci. 2012. https://doi.org/10.5402/2012/378607.
94. Queiroga FL, Perez-Alenza MD, Silvan G. Role of steroid hormones and prolactin in canine mammary cancer. J Steroid Biochem Mol Biol. 2005;94:181–7.
95. Queiroga F, Perez-Alenza MD, Gonzalez-Gil A. Serum and tissue steroid hormone levels in canine mammary tumours: clinical and prognostic implications. Reprod Domest Anim. 2015;50:858–65.
96. Queiroga F, Perez-Alenza D, Silvan G. Positive correlation of steroid hormones and EGF in canine mammary cancer. J Steroid Biochem Mol Biol. 2009;115:9–13.
97. Spoerri M, Guscetti F, Hartnack S, Boos A, Oei C, Balogh O, et al. Endocrine control of canine mammary neoplasms: serum reproductive hormone levels and tissue expression of steroid hormone, prolactin and growth hormone receptors. BMC Vet Res. 2015;11:235.
98. Thuroczy J, Reisvaag GJ, Perge E. Immunohistochemical detection of progesterone and cellular proliferation in canine mammary tumours. J Comp Pathol. 2007;137:122–9.
99. Toniti W, Buranasinsup S, Kongcharoen A. Immunohistochemical determination of estrogen and progesterone receptors in canine mammary tumors. Asian Pac J Cancer Prev. 2009;10:907–11.
100. Yang WY, Liu CH, Chang CJ. Proliferative activity, apoptosis and expression of oestrogen receptor and Bcl-2 oncoprotein in canine mammary gland tumours. J Comp Pathol. 2006;134:70–9.
101. Yip CH, Rhodes A. Estrogen and progesterone receptors in breast cancer. Future Oncol. 2014;10:2293–301.
102. Morris JS, Dobson JM, Bostock DE. Use of tamoxifen in the control of canine mammary neoplasia. Vet Rec. 1993;133:539–42.
103. Tavares WL, Lavelle GE, Figueiredo MS, Souza AG, Bertagnolli AC, Viana FA, et al. Evaluation of adverse effects in tamoxifen exposed healthy female dogs. Acta Vet Scand. 2010;52:67. https://doi.org/10.1186/1751-0147-52-67.
104. Carvalho MI, Silva-Carvalho R, Pires I, Prada J, Bianchini R, Jensen-Jarolim E, et al. A comparative approach of tumor-associated inflammation in mammary cancer between humans and dogs. BioMed Res Int. 2016. https://doi.org/10.1155/2016/4917387.
105. Queiroga FL, Pires I, Lobo L. The role of Cox-2 expression in the prognosis of dogs with malignant mammary tumours. Res Vet Sci. 2010;88:441–5.

106. Hugo HJ, Saunders C, Ramsay RG. New insights on COX-2 in chronic inflammation driving breast cancer growth and metastasis. J Mammary Gland Biol Neoplasia. 2015;20:109–19.
107. Clemente M, Rodriguez Sanchez-Archidona A, Sardón D, Diez L, Martin-Ruiz A, Caceres S, et al. Different role of COX-2 and angiogenesis in canine inflammatory and non-inflammatory mammary cancer. Vet J. 2013;197:427–32.
108. De M, Souza CH, Toledo-Piza E, Amorin R. Inflammatory mammary carcinoma in 12 dogs: clinical features, cyclooxygenase-2 expression, and response to piroxicam treatment. Can Vet J. 2009;50:506–10.
109. Dore M, Lanthier I, Sirois J. Cyclooxygenase-2 expression in canine mammary tumors. Vet Pathol. 2003;40:207–12.
110. Huang J, Zhang D, Xie F. The potential role of COX-2 in cancer stem cel mediated canine mammary tumor initiation: an immunohistochemical study. J Vet Sci. 2015;16:225–31.
111. Knottenbelt C, Chambers G, Gault E. The in vitro effects of piroxicam and meloxicam on canine cell lines. J Small Anim Pract. 2006;47:14–20.
112. Millanta F, Citi S, Della Santa D. COX-2 expression in canine and feline invasive mammary carcinomas: correlation with clinicopathological features and prognostic molecular markers. Breast Cancer Res Treat. 2006;98:115–20.
113. Queiroga FL, Perez-Alenza MD, Silvan G. Cox-2 levels in canine mammary tumors, including inflammatory mammary carcinoma: clinicopathological features and prognostic significance. Anticancer Res. 2005;25:4269–75.
114. Saito T, Tamura D, Asano R. Usefulness of selective COX-2 inhibitors as therapeutic agents against canine mammary tumors. Oncol Rep. 2014;31:1637–44.
115. Brunelle M, Sartin EA, Wolfe LG. Cyclooxygenase-2 expression in normal and neoplastic canine mammary cell lines. Vet Pathol. 2006;43:656–66.
116. Yoshikawa Y, Morimatsu M, Ochiai K, Ishiguro-Oonuma T, Wada S, Orino K, et al. Reduced canine BRCA2 expression levels in mammary gland tumors. BMC Vet Res. 2015;11:159.
117. Rivera P, Melin M, Biagi T, Fall T, Haggstrom J, Lindblad-Toh K, et al. Mammary tumor development in dogs is associated with BRCA1 and BRCA2. Cancer Res. 2009;69:8770–4.
118. Nieto A, Perez-Alenza MD, Del Castillo N. BRCA1 Expression in canine mammary dysplasias and tumours: relationship with prognostic variables. J Comp Pathol. 2003;128:260–8.
119. Boggs RM, Wright ZM, Stickney MJ. MicroRNA expression in canine mammary cancer. Mamm Genome. 2008;19:561–9.
120. Bulkowska M, Rybicka A, Mert Senses K, Ulewicz K, Witt K, Szymanska J, et al. MicroRNA expression patterns in canine mammary cancer show significant differences between metastatic and non-metastatic tumours. BMC Cancer. 2017;17:728.
121. Bertoli G, Cava C, Castiglioni I. MicroRNAs: new biomarkers for diagnosis, prognosis, therapy prediction and therapeutic tools for breast cancer. Theranostics. 2015;5:1122–43.
122. Zhang K, Wang YW, Wang YY, Song Y, Zhu J, Si PC, et al. Identification of microRNA biomarkers in the blood of breast cancer patients based on microRNA profiling. Gene. 2017;619:10–20.
123. Von Deetzen MC, Schmeck BT, Gruber AD. Malignancy associated microRNA expression changes in canine mammary cancer of different malignancies. ISRN Vet Sci. 2014. https://doi.org/10.1155/2014/148597.
124. Osaki T, Sunden Y, Sugiyama A, Azuma K, Murahata Y, Tsuka T, et al. Establishment of a canine mammary gland tumor cell line and characterization of its miRNA expression. J Vet Sci. 2016;17:385–90.
125. Pang LY, Argyle D. Cancer stem cells and telomerase as potential biomarkers in veterinary oncology. Vet J. 2010;185:15–22.
126. Rybicka A, Krol M. Identification and characterization of cancer stem cells in canine mammary tumors. Acta Vet Scand. 2016;58:86.
127. Rybicka A, Mucha J, Majchrzak K, Taciak B, Hellmen E, Motyl T, et al. Analysis of microRNA expression in canine mammary cancer stem-like cells indicates epigenetic regulation of transforming growth factor-Beta signaling. J Physiol Pharmacol. 2015;66:29–37.
128. Im KS, Jang JG, Shin JI, Kim NH, Lim HY, Lee SM, et al. CD44+/CD24− cancer stem cells are associated with higher grade of canine mammary carcinomas. Vet Pathol. 2015;52:1041–4.
129. Akrap N, Andersson D, Bom E, Gregersson P, Stahlberg A, Landberg G. Identification of distinct breast cancer stem cell populations based on single-cell analyses of functionally enriched stem and progenitor pools. Stem Cell Reports. 2016;6:121–36.
130. Da Costa A, Kohn B, Gruber AD. Multiple RT-PCR markers for the detection of circulating tumour cells of metastatic canine mammary tumours. Vet J. 2013;196:34–9.
131. Mu Z, Wang C, Ye Z, Austin L, Civan J, Hyslop T, et al. Prospective assessment of the prognostic value of circulating tumor cells and their clusters in patients with advanced-stage breast cancer. Breast Cancer Res Treat. 2015;154:563–71.
132. Shiomi-Mouri Y, Kousaka J, Ando T, Tetsuka R, Nakano S, Yoshida M, et al. Clinical significance of circulating tumor cells (CTCs) with respect to optimal cut-off value and tumor markers in advanced/metastatic breast cancer. Breast Cancer. 2016;23:120–7.
133. Hayes DF, Cristofanilli M, Budd GT, Ellis MJ, Stopeck A, Miller MC, et al. Circulating tumor cells at each follow-up time point during therapy of metastatic breast cancer patients predict progression-free and overall survival. Clin Cancer Res. 2006;12:4218–24.
134. Da Costa A, Lenze D, Hummel M. Identification of six potential markers for the detection of circulating canine mammary tumour cells in the peripheral blood identified by microarray analysis. J Comp Pathol. 2012;146:143–51.
135. Case A, Brisson BK, Durham AC, Rosen S, Monslow J, Buza E, et al. Identification of prognostic collagen signatures and potential therapeutic stromal targets in canine mammary gland carcinoma. PLoS ONE. 2017. https://doi.org/10.1371/journal.pone.0180448.

Permissions

All chapters in this book were first published in AVS, by BioMed Central; hereby published with permission under the Creative Commons Attribution License or equivalent. Every chapter published in this book has been scrutinized by our experts. Their significance has been extensively debated. The topics covered herein carry significant findings which will fuel the growth of the discipline. They may even be implemented as practical applications or may be referred to as a beginning point for another development.

The contributors of this book come from diverse backgrounds, making this book a truly international effort. This book will bring forth new frontiers with its revolutionizing research information and detailed analysis of the nascent developments around the world.

We would like to thank all the contributing authors for lending their expertise to make the book truly unique. They have played a crucial role in the development of this book. Without their invaluable contributions this book wouldn't have been possible. They have made vital efforts to compile up to date information on the varied aspects of this subject to make this book a valuable addition to the collection of many professionals and students.

This book was conceptualized with the vision of imparting up-to-date information and advanced data in this field. To ensure the same, a matchless editorial board was set up. Every individual on the board went through rigorous rounds of assessment to prove their worth. After which they invested a large part of their time researching and compiling the most relevant data for our readers.

The editorial board has been involved in producing this book since its inception. They have spent rigorous hours researching and exploring the diverse topics which have resulted in the successful publishing of this book. They have passed on their knowledge of decades through this book. To expedite this challenging task, the publisher supported the team at every step. A small team of assistant editors was also appointed to further simplify the editing procedure and attain best results for the readers.

Apart from the editorial board, the designing team has also invested a significant amount of their time in understanding the subject and creating the most relevant covers. They scrutinized every image to scout for the most suitable representation of the subject and create an appropriate cover for the book.

The publishing team has been an ardent support to the editorial, designing and production team. Their endless efforts to recruit the best for this project, has resulted in the accomplishment of this book. They are a veteran in the field of academics and their pool of knowledge is as vast as their experience in printing. Their expertise and guidance has proved useful at every step. Their uncompromising quality standards have made this book an exceptional effort. Their encouragement from time to time has been an inspiration for everyone.

The publisher and the editorial board hope that this book will prove to be a valuable piece of knowledge for researchers, students, practitioners and scholars across the globe.

List of Contributors

Stanislav Katina
Department of Mathematics and Statistics, Masaryk University, Kotlarska 2, Brno, Czech Republic

Jana Farbakova and Aladar Madari
University of Veterinary Medicine and Pharmacy, Komenskeho 73, Kosice, Slovak Republic

Michal Novak and Norbert Zilka
Institute of Neuroimmunology,Slovak Academy of Sciences, Dubravska cesta 9, Bratislava, Slovak Republic

Norbert Zilka
Institute of Neuroimmunology, No., Dvorakovo Nabrezie 45, Bratislava, Slovak Republic

Aage Kristian Olsen Alstrup and Ole Lajord Munk
Department of Nuclear Medicine and PET Center, Institute of Clinical Medicine, Aarhus University Hospital, Nørrebrogade 44, 10C, 8000 Aarhus, Denmark

Trine Hammer Jensen
Department of Chemistry and Bioscience, Aalborg University/Aalborg Zoo, Mølleparkvej 63, 9000 Aalborg, Denmark

Lasse Fast Jensen
Fisheries and Maritime Museum, Tarphagevej 2, 6710 Esbjerg, Denmark

Abdi Hedayat
Natural History Museum of Denmark, University of Copenhagen, Universitetsparken 15, 2100 Copenhagen, Denmark

Brian Hansen
Center of Functionally Integrative Neuroscience, Aarhus University Hospital, Nørrebrogade 44, 10G, 8000 Aarhus, Denmark

Anna Malmsten and Anne-Marie Dalin
Division of Reproduction, Department of Clinical Sciences, Swedish University of Agricultural Sciences, SE-750 07 Uppsala, Sweden

Mai Louise Grandsgaard Mikkelsen, James Edward Miles, Helle Harding Poulsen and Thomas Eriksen
Department of Veterinary Clinical Sciences, Faculty of Health and Medical Sciences, University of Copenhagen, 16 Dyrlægevej, 1870 Frederiksberg C, Denmark

Rikard Ambrus
Department of Surgical Gastroenterology C, Rigshospitalet, Faculty of Health and Medical Sciences, University of Copenhagen, 9 Blegdamsvej, 2100 Copenhagen Ø, Denmark

Rune Rasmussen
Department of Neurosurgery, The Neuroscience Centre, Rigshospitalet, Faculty of Health and Medical Sciences, University of Copenhagen, 9 Blegdamsvej, 2100 Copenhagen Ø, Denmark

Finn Borgbjerg Moltke
Department of Neuroanaesthesia, Rigshospitalet, University of Copenhagen, 9 Blegdamsvej, 2100 Copenhagen Ø, Denmark
Department of Anaesthesia, Bispebjerg and Frederiksberg Hospitals, Faculty of Health and Medical Sciences, University of Copenhagen, 23 Bispebjerg Bakke, 2400 Copenhagen NV, Denmark

Malgorzata Domino, Bartosz Pawlinski, Romuald Zabielski and Zdzislaw Gajewski
Department of Large Animal Diseases with Clinic, Faculty of Veterinary Medicine, Warsaw University of Life Sciences (WULS-SGGW), Nowoursynowska 100, 02-797 Warsaw, Poland
Veterinary Research Centre and Center for Biomedical Research, Warsaw University of Life Sciences (WULS-SGGW), Nowoursynowska 100, 02-797 Warsaw, Poland

Stine Billeschou Christiansen and Peter Sandøe
Department of Large Animal Sciences, Faculty of Health and Medical Sciences, University of Copenhagen, Grønnegårdsvej 8, 1870 Frederiksberg C, Denmark

Annemarie Thuri Kristensen
Department of Veterinary Clinical and Animal Sciences, Faculty of Health and Medical Sciences, University of Copenhagen, Dyrlægevej 16, 1870 Frederiksberg C, Denmark

Jesper Lassen and Peter Sandøe
Department of Food and Resource Economics, Faculty of Science, University of Copenhagen, Rolighedsvej 25, 1958 Frederiksberg C, Denmark

Maaike Catteeuw, Eline Wydooghe and Ann Van Soom
Department of Reproduction, Obstetrics, and Herd Health, Faculty of Veterinary Medicine, Ghent University, Salisburylaan 133, 9820 Merelbeke, Belgium

Erik Mullaart and Hiemke M. Knijn
CRV BV, Wassenaarweg 20, 6843 NW Arnhem, The Netherlands

Anna Rave Vestberg
Anicura Regional Animal Hospital, Ljusnevägen 17, 12848 Bagarmossen, Sweden

Anna Tidholm
Anicura Albano Animal Hospital, Rinkebyvägen 21a, 18236 Danderyd, Sweden

Anna Tidholm and Ingrid Ljungvall
Department of Clinical Sciences, Faculty of Veterinary Medicine and Small Animal Sciences, Swedish University of Agricultural Sciences, 75007 Uppsala, Sweden

Ann Essner, Lena Zetterberg and Karin Hellström
Department of Neuroscience, Faculty of Physiotherapy, Uppsala University, Husargatan, Biomedical Centre, 751 24 Uppsala, Sweden

Ann Essner
Evidensia Djurkliniken Gefle, Norra Gatan 1, 803 21 Gävle, Sweden

Pia Gustås
Department of Clinical Sciences, Faculty of Veterinary Medicine and Animal Husbandry, Swedish University of Agricultural Sciences, Uppsala, Sweden

Hans Högberg
Department of Health and Caring Sciences, Faculty of Health and Occupational Studies, University of Gävle, 801 76 Gävle, Sweden

Rita Sjöström
Unit of Research Education and Development, Region Jämtland Härjedalen, Östersund, Sweden
Department of Community Medicine and Rehabilitation, Faculty of Physiotherapy, Umeå University, 901 87 Umeå, Sweden

Rita Payan-Carreira, Sónia Miranda and Severiano R. Silva
Zootecnia Department, CECAV-Centro de Ciência Animal e Veterinária, Universidade de Trás-os-Montes e Alto Douro, Quinta de Prados, 5000-801 Vila Real, Portugal

Luis Martins, Sónia Miranda and Pedro Olivério
EUVG-Escola Universitária Vasco da Gama, Campus Universitário, Bloco B, Lordemão, 3020-210 Coimbra, Portugal

Sónia Miranda
HVBV-Hospital Veterinário do Baixo Vouga, Segadães, 3750-742 Águeda, Portugal

Marte Ekeland Fergestad and Ellen Skancke
Department of Companion Animal Clinical Sciences, Faculty of Veterinary
Medicine and Biosciences, Norwegian University of Life Sciences, Dep, 0033 Oslo, Norway.

Tuva Holt Jahr
Department of Companion Animal Clinical Sciences, Faculty of Veterinary Medicine and Biosciences, Norwegian University of Life Sciences, Dep, 0033 Oslo, Norway

Randi I. Krontveit
Department for Pharmacoeconomics, Norwegian Medicines Agency, Kalbakken 0901 Oslo, Norway
Department of Food Safety and Infection Biology, Faculty of Veterinary Medicine and Biosciences, Norwegian University of Life Sciences, Dep, 0033 Oslo, Norway

Julie Melsted Birch, Jens Frederik Agger, Christina Dahlin, Anne Sofie Hammer and Henrik Elvang Jensen
Department of Veterinary and Animal Sciences, Faculty of Health and Medical Sciences, University of Copenhagen, Ridebanevej 3, 1870 Frederiksberg C, Denmark

Vibeke Frøkjær Jensen
National Veterinary Institute, Technical University of Denmark, Kemitorvet, 2800 Kongens Lyngby, Denmark

Tina Struve
Kopenhagen Diagnostics, Kopenhagen Fur, Langagervej 60, 2600 Glostrup, Denmark

Sarah Stadig
Department of Clinical Sciences, Faculty of Veterinary Medicine and Animal Husbandry, Swedish University of Agricultural Sciences,, S532 23 Skara, Sweden

B. Duncan X. Lascelles
Comparative Pain Research, Department of Clinical Sciences, College of Veterinary Medicine, North Carolina State University, Raleigh, NC 27606, USA
Center for Pain Research and Innovation, School of Dentistry, University of North Carolina, Chapel Hill, NC, USA

Anna Bergh
Department of Anatomy, Physiology and Biochemistry, Faculty of Veterinary Medicine and Animal Husbandry, Swedish University of Agricultural Sciences, S750 07 Uppsala, Sweden

Elżbieta Gabriela Giza, Marta Płonek, Józef Marian Nicpoń and Marcin Adam Wrzosek
Department of Internal Medicine and Clinic of Horses, Dogs and Cats, Faculty of Veterinary Medicine, Wroclaw University of Environmental and Life Sciences, pl. Grunwaldzki 47, 50-366 Wroclaw, Poland

Johanna Vakkamäki, Suvi Taponen and Satu Pyörälä
Department of Production Animal Medicine, Faculty of Veterinary Medicine, University of Helsinki, Paroninkuja 20, 04920 Saarentaus, Finland

Anna-Maija Heikkilä
Natural Resources Institute Finland (Luke), Koetilantie 5, 00790 Helsinki, Finland

Jan Hultgren
Department of Animal Environment and Health, Swedish University of Agricultural Sciences, 53223 Skara, Sweden

Bo Algers
Department of Animal Environment and Health, Swedish University of Agricultural Sciences, 53223 Skara, Sweden

Sophie Atkinson
Department of Animal Environment and Health, Swedish University of Agricultural Sciences, 75007 Uppsala, Sweden

Kristian Ellingsen and Cecilie Marie Mejdell
Veterinary Public Health, Norwegian Veterinary Institute, Sentrum, 0106 Oslo, Norway

Sofia Eriksson
Vallnäsvägen 3, 70358 Örebro, Sweden

Kjartan Hreinsson
Icelandic Food and Veterinary Authority, Austurvegur 64, 800 Selfoss, Iceland

Lotta Nordensten
Swedish Board of Agriculture, 551 82 Jönköping, Sweden

Heidi Valtari
Brahea Centre for Training and Development, University of Turku, 20014 Turku, Finland

Mohamed Ibrahim Shaalan, Mansour El-Matbouli and Mona Saleh
Clinical Division of Fish Medicine, University of Veterinary Medicine, Veterinärplatz 1, 1210 Vienna, Austria

Mohamed Ibrahim Shaalan and Magdy Mohamed El-Mahdy
Department of Pathology, Faculty of Veterinary Medicine, Cairo University, Giza 12211, Egypt

Sarah Theiner
Institute of Analytical Chemistry, University of Vienna, Währinger Straße 38, 1090 Vienna, Austria

Ronja Mathiesen and Peter Mikael Helweg Heegaard
Innate Immunology Group, National Veterinary Institute, Technical University of Denmark, Kemitorvet, Building 204, 2800 Kgs. Lyngby, Denmark

Innate Immunology Group, Department of Biotechnology and Biomedicine, Technical University of Denmark, Kemitorvet, Building 204, 2800 Kgs. Lyngby, Denmark

Julie Melsted Birch, Henrik Elvang Jensen and Jens Frederik Agger
Department of Veterinary and Animals Sciences, Faculty of Health and Medical Sciences, University of Copenhagen, Ridebanevej 3, 1870 Frederiksberg C, Denmark

Mariann Chriél
Diagnostics & Scientific Advice, National Veterinary Institute, Technical University of Denmark, Kemitorvet, Building 204, 2800 Kgs. Lyngby, Denmark

Tina Struve
Kopenhagen Fur, Langagervej 60, 2600 Glostrup, Denmark

Marcus Vinicius Candido, Susanne Kilpinen and Thomas Spillmann
Department of Equine and Small Animal Medicine, Faculty of Veterinary Medicine, University of Helsinki, Helsinki, Finland

Pernilla Syrjä
Department of Veterinary Biosciences, Faculty of Veterinary Medicine, University of Helsinki, Helsinki, Finland

Lisa Ekman and Karin Persson Waller
Department of Animal Health and Antimicrobial Strategies, National Veterinary Institute, 75189 Uppsala, Sweden

Department of Clinical Sciences, Swedish University of Agricultural Sciences, 75007 Uppsala, Sweden

Ann-Kristin Nyman and Håkan Landin
Växa Sverige, 10425 Stockholm, Sweden

Mohsen Hanifeh, Minna Marjaana Rajamäki, Susanne Kilpinen and Thomas Spillmann
Department of Equine and Small Animal Medicine, Faculty of Veterinary Medicine, University of Helsinki, (Viikintie 49), 00014 Helsinki, Finland

Mohsen Hanifeh
Department of Clinical Sciences, Faculty of Veterinary Medicine, University of Tabriz, 5166616471 Tabriz, Iran

Pernilla Syrjä
Department of Veterinary Biosciences, Faculty of Veterinary Medicine, University of Helsinki, (Agnes Sjöberginkatu 2), 00014 Helsinki, Finland

Laura Mäkitalo
Children's Hospital, Helsinki University Central Hospital, University of Helsinki, (Haartmaninkatu 8), 00014 Helsinki, Finland

Ilona Kaszak, Anna Ruszczak, Szymon Kanafa, Kamil Kacprzak and Piotr Jurka
Department of Small Animal Diseases with Clinic, Veterinary Medicine Faculty, Warsaw University of Life Sciences, Nowoursynowska 166, 02-787 Warsaw, Poland

Magdalena Król
Department of Physiological Sciences, Veterinary Medicine Faculty, Warsaw University of Life Sciences, Nowoursynowska 166, 02-787 Warsaw, Poland

Index

CPSIA information can be obtained
at www.ICGtesting.com
Printed in the USA
LVHW062321230820
663958LV00008B/393

9 781632 428684